BSAVA Guide to Pain Management in Small Animal Practice

Editor:

Ian Self
BSc BVSc PGCertVetEd FHEA CertVA DipECVAA MRCVS

School of Veterinary Medicine and Science, University of Nottingham,
College Road, Sutton Bonington, Loughborough,
Leicestershire, LE12 5RD, UK

Published by:

British Small Animal Veterinary Association
Woodrow House, 1 Telford Way,
Waterwells Business Park, Quedgeley,
Gloucester GL2 2AB

A Company Limited by Guarantee in England
Registered Company No. 2837793
Registered as a Charity

Copyright © 2010 BSAVA

All rights reserved. No part of this publication may be reproduced, stored in a retrieval system, or transmitted, in form or by any means, electronic, mechanical, photocopying, recording or otherwise without prior written permission of the copyright holder.

Figures 6.14, 7.13, 7.14, 7.15 and those in Appendix 2 were drawn by
S.J. Elmhurst BA Hons (www.livingart.org.uk) and are printed with her permission.

A catalogue record for this book is available from the British Library.

ISBN 978 1 910443 00 2

The publishers, editors and contributors cannot take responsibility for information provided on dosages and methods of application of drugs mentioned or referred to in this publication. Details of this kind must be verified in each case by individual users from up to date literature published by the manufacturers or suppliers of those drugs. Veterinary surgeons are reminded that in each case they must follow all appropriate national legislation and regulations (for example, in the United Kingdom, the prescribing cascade) from time to time in force.

Printed in India by Parksons Graphics
Printed on ECF paper made from sustainable forests

4756PUBS18

Contents

Contributors

Briony Alderson BVSc CertVA DipECVAA MRCVS
Small Animal Teaching Hospital, Institute of
Veterinary Science, University of Liverpool,
Leahurst Campus, Chester High Road,
Neston CH64 7TE, UK

Dominic Barfield BSc BVSc MVetMed DipACVECC
DipECVECC FHEA MRCVS
Queen Mother Hospital for Animals, The Royal
Veterinary College, Hawkshead Lane, North
Mymms, Hatfield, Hertfordshire AL9 7TA, UK

Carl Bradbrook BVSc CertVA DipECVAA MRCVS
Anderson Moores Veterinary Specialists, The
Granary, Bunstead Barns, Poles Lane, Hursley,
Winchester, Hampshire, SO21 2LL

Federico Corletto PhD CertVA DipECVAA MRCVS
Dick White Referrals, Station Farm, London Road,
Six Mile Bottom, Cambridgeshire CB8 0UH, UK

Kevin Eatwell BVSc CertZooMed DZooMed(Reptilian)
DipECZM MRCVS
Royal (Dick) School of Veterinary Medicine,
The University of Edinburgh, Easter Bush,
Midlothian EH25 9RG, UK

Cecilia Gorrel BSc MA VetMB DDS HonFAVD DipEVDC
MRCVS
Veterinary Dentistry and Oral Surgery Referrals,
Veterinary Oral Health Consultancy,
Southampton, UK

Tamara Grubb BS MS DVM PhD DipACVAA IVAPM
Board of Directors
Washington State University, Department of
Veterinary Clinical Sciences, Pullman, WA,
99164-6610, USA

Joanna Hedley BVM&S DZooMed(Reptilian)
DipECZM(Herpetology) MRCVS
Beaumont Sainsbury Animal Hospital,
Royal Veterinary College, Royal College Street,
London NW1 0TU, UK

Jenny Helm BVMS CertSAM DipECVIM-CA FHEA
MRCVS
School of Veterinary Medicine, College of Medical,
Veterinary & Life Sciences, University of Glasgow,
Bearsden Road, Glasgow G61 1QH, UK

James Hunt BVetMed MSc CertVA
DipECAWBM(AWSEL) MRCVS
Cave Veterinary Specialists, George's Farm,
West Buckland, Somerset TA21 9LE, UK

Colette Jolliffe BVetMed CertVA DipECVAA MRCVS
Animal Health Trust, Lanwades Park, Kentford,
Newmarket, Suffolk CB8 7UU, UK

Caroline Kisielewicz MVB CertSAM DipECVIM-CA
MRCVS
Pride Veterinary Centre, Riverside Road,
Derby DE24 8HX, UK

Samantha Lindley BVSc MRCVS
Hon Associate, Glasgow University Veterinary School, UK
Longview Veterinary Services, Glasgow, UK

Ana Marques DVM MACVSc CertSAS DipECVS MRCVS
Royal (Dick) School of Veterinary Medicine,
The University of Edinburgh, Easter Bush,
Midlothian EH25 9RG, UK

Jo Murrell BVSc PhD DipECVAA MRCVS
Highcroft Veterinary Referrals, 615 Wells Road,
Whitchurch, Bristol BS14 9BE, UK

Fiona Scarlett RVN BSc(Hons) (AnSci) VTS(anesthesia/
analgesia) GPCert(Western Veterinary Acupuncture &
Chronic Pain Management)
University of Glasgow, School of Veterinary
Medicine, 464 Bearsden Road, Bearsden,
Glasgow G61 1QH, UK

Ian Self BSc BVSc PGCertVetEd FHEA CertVA DipECVAA
MRCVS
School of Veterinary Medicine and Science,
University of Nottingham, College Road,
Sutton Bonington, Loughborough,
Leicestershire LE12 5RD, UK

Kinley Smith MA VetMB CertSAS DipECVS PhD MRCVS
Willows Veterinary Centre and Referral Service,
Highlands Road, Shirley, Solihull,
West Midlands B90 4NH, UK

Steve Smith BVetMed CertZooMed DipECZM(Avian)
MRCVS
Tiggywinkles Wildlife Hospital, Aston Road,
Haddenham, Buckinghamshire HP17 8AF, UK

Annette Wessman DrMedVet DipECVN PGCertAcPrac
FHEA MRCVS
Pride Veterinary Centre, Riverside Road,
Derby DE24 8HX, UK

Kate White MA VetMB DVA DipECVAA MRCVS
School of Veterinary Medicine and Science,
University of Nottingham, College Road,
Sutton Bonington, Loughborough,
Leicestershire LE12 5RD, UK

Foreword

Our understanding of pain in small animals has increased exponentially over the past 20 years or so. For wild animals, showing signs of pain or injury will often result in being killed by predators or dominant members of their own species – a good reason for evolving to hide signs of pain very effectively. We now have a much better understanding of behavioural changes associated with pain in animals and are better equipped to anticipate and treat pain in an effective manner. For instance, techniques have been developed to reduce surgical pain such as in my own field of minimally invasive surgery; however, this does not eliminate the need for effective pain control both in the surgical patient and those with disease. This book provides a comprehensive and detailed overview of pain management in small animals and will provide an extremely useful and concise resource for the busy practitioner on a day-to-day basis.

This guide includes extensive coverage of types and causes of pain and how to prevent or minimise, as well as treat, pain in a variety of situations and species. There is a liberal use of bullet points, tables and photographs, together with case studies and examples that make this a really useful manual for getting information quickly in a practice setting.

This new guide provides a wealth of information and practical advice that will benefit both the general practitioner and the veterinary nurse, and more importantly, their patients. It is a really valuable addition to the BSAVA range of titles.

Philip Lhermette
FRCVS
BSAVA President 2018–2019

Chapter 1

Introduction

Ian Self

The recognition and treatment of pain has always been a vital aspect of small animal practice. Good pain management improves patient care and owner satisfaction, as well as contributing to greater professional satisfaction for veterinary personnel involved in treating patients. Over the last 10 years, management of small animal pain has progressed rapidly. This is in no small part due to the introduction of a number of validated pain scales, which have vastly improved our ability to detect pain and, more importantly, to assess the effectiveness of analgesic interventions and decide if further treatment is necessary.

Despite these advances in the basic understanding of pain, veterinary surgeons (veterinarians) and nurses are faced with a larger variety of cases of increasing complexity as the knowledge and ability to treat previously untreatable conditions increases. This inevitably presents us with new challenges when dealing with pain in unfamiliar clinical situations where there may be multiple co-morbidities to consider. In addition to new clinical techniques and recognized conditions, there are increasing numbers of licensed analgesic agents being introduced into the veterinary market. Whilst offering greater scope for pain treatment, this can also lead to confusion over suitability of a particular drug for a particular presentation.

This BSAVA Guide has been produced with the busy practitioner in mind. Although there are many excellent pain and analgesia textbooks available, this Guide has been designed to be a 'bedside' companion for pain and analgesia practitioners. It is divided into sections examining acute and chronic pain, together with the physiological basis of pain and the pharmaceutical options available for treatment. The Guide then discusses common clinical conditions by systems/diseases to allow easy identification of where to seek help when faced with a patient in pain. It also examines pain in exotic pet species, as well as having important sections on physical therapies and the role of nursing in the alleviation of suffering.

The contributors who have written the individual chapters are all specialists in their respective fields and are currently working in first-opinion or referral practice. They all share first-hand knowledge of the effects of pain on their patients and are uniquely placed to be able to advise on the most useful analgesia techniques in particular clinical situations. With this in mind, whilst all the chapters are based on published evidence, a unique feature of this

Guide is the 'Author's perspective'. This allows the reader to see how a specialist in the field would or has treated similar cases in the past, with information on the pros and cons of each treatment mentioned. We hope that this will allow the reader to see that there are many suitable methods to approach a situation ensuring patient welfare. Indeed, this Guide is not to be seen as an instruction manual, rather a helping hand. For each case discussed and analgesic approach explained, there are multiple valid alternative approaches that would ensure the same outcome. Nevertheless, when seeking inspiration or information when faced with a patient in pain, we hope that the information presented here will assist in reaching a satisfactory clinical response.

The motto on the Royal College of Anaesthetists' crest reads, 'Divinum sedare dolorem' which translates as 'It is divine (or praiseworthy) to alleviate pain'. We hope this Guide will contribute to this goal.

Chapter 2

Physiology of pain

Ian Self and Tamara Grubb

Introduction

What is pain?

Pain has been defined by the International Association for the Study of Pain (IASP) as 'an unpleasant sensory or emotional experience associated with actual or potential tissue damage, or described in terms of such damage' (IASP, 1994). This immediately raises problems for veterinary professionals attempting to treat pain as we are extremely limited in terms of examining whether our patients experience the sensory or emotional aspects of true pain. Indeed, the emotional and sensory components of pain are difficult to understand even in human pain medicine, where different people with the same condition describe their pain as different in terms of quality, intensity, and how it makes them feel. Nevertheless, there is little doubt amongst most veterinary surgeons (veterinarians) that the behaviours seen in painful animals are the expression of such 'emotions'. A more recent addition to the IASP's definition has attempted to encompass the non-verbal situation encountered by veterinary pain professionals: 'The inability to communicate in no way negates the possibility that an individual is experiencing pain and is in need of appropriate pain-relieving treatment'. This shifts the onus on to veterinary professionals as carers to realize that a patient who may be expected to be painful (e.g. following major surgery) but is not yet demonstrating classical signs of pain should nevertheless be regarded as probably requiring analgesic intervention.

An alternative definition for pain in animals is 'an aversive sensory and emotional experience which elicits protective motor actions, results in learned avoidance and may modify species-specific traits of behaviour including social behaviour' (Morton et al., 2005). This is arguably a better working definition as it takes into account the altered behaviour commonly seen in animals experiencing pain, although the sensory and emotional components are still difficult to evaluate.

Why is pain detrimental and why should it be treated aggressively?

Veterinary professionals have both a professional and moral duty of care to animals. On entering the profession, UK veterinary surgeons take an oath to 'ensure the welfare of animals committed to my care', as per the Royal College of Veterinary Surgeons (RCVS). In addition, most small animals are companion animals, and rely on us to protect their welfare, including their day-to-day requirements and freedom from pain. It has been argued that animal pain is 'worse' than human pain. Animals are thought to live in the 'now' and, unlike a human being in pain, are not aware that the pain is only temporary and will be relieved given time or treatment (Robertson, 2002).

In addition to the ethical arguments, there are a number of well recognized physiological consequences of untreated pain. These include:

- Release of catecholamines and pituitary hormones and, therefore, a catabolic state leading to weight loss and potential wound breakdown
- Hyperglycaemia and insulin resistance
- Leucocytosis (neutrophilia)
- Cytokine production
- Poor immune function
- Poor appetite
- Impaired respiratory function
- Increased blood pressure.

It is also likely that failure to manage pain may lead an animal to self-traumatize, potentially leading to the development of chronic (pathological) pain.

In general, these physiological changes are likely to lead to an increase in postoperative complications in surgical patients with poorly controlled pain, as well as client dissatisfaction with the veterinary practice. Indeed, the economic and time losses alone could be significant as complications are generally treated by the practice at a reduced rate.

The physiological basis of pain: neural pathways and where they can be interrupted

The major physiological pathways involved in mammalian pain, although well characterized, are subject to a high degree of plasticity and alteration depending on the disease status of the animal. However, it is useful to appreciate the major steps in the transmission of pain to the central nervous system (CNS), as this allows the judicious application of multimodal analgesia (MMA). MMA refers to the concept of using multiple analgesic agents acting at different sites in the pain pathway. In this way, the dose of any one agent, and hence the potential side effects, is kept to a minimum, yet the analgesic effect is often enhanced leading to better clinical pain control. An example of MMA in small animal practice is the use of a centrally acting opioid given as part of a premedication protocol for a dog admitted for dental extractions followed by a suitable dental block using local anaesthetic. In this case the block is designed to stop transmission of the pain sensation from the periphery, whereas the opioid works centrally to decrease the projection and appreciation of any pain within the CNS.

The physiology of pain can be divided into four processes: transduction, transmission (and projection), modulation and perception.

Transduction is the process by which afferent nerve endings participate in translating noxious stimuli (e.g. a pinprick) into nociceptive impulses (Figure 2.1). Signal transduction can only be initiated by a mechanical, thermal or chemical stimulus. These stimuli can be converted into an electrical signal at a nociceptor via a stimulus-gated ion channel. Nociceptors are present on specific nerve endings spread throughout the body and respond to potentially painful inputs, thus allowing pain perception and localization. Different afferent nerve fibres (see below) have differing nociceptors. Aδ fibres possess thermal and mechanical nociceptors with higher activation thresholds than Aβ (touch) receptors. C fibre nociceptors are polymodal receptors with even higher activation thresholds than Aδ fibre receptors and respond to all three stimulus types. An example of such a nociceptor is the transient receptor potential vanilloid-1 receptor (TRPV-1), which responds to capsaicin in chilli peppers to give a burning sensation.

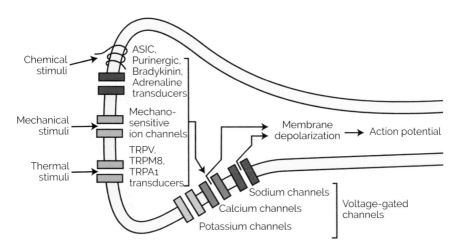

2.1 Diagram of a nociceptor terminal illustrating various transducers sensitive to noxious stimuli and ion channels. Influx of calcium and sodium ions in sufficient concentration will cause an action potential along the nerve axon. Potassium ions are usually inhibitory. ASIC = acid-sending ion channels; TRPA1 = transient receptor potential ankyrin 1; TRPM8 = transient receptor potential cation channel subfamily M member 8; TRPV = transient receptor potential channel subfamily V.
(© Juliane Deubner, University of Saskatchewan, Canada)

Nociception is a term frequently used and can be considered to be 'physiological pain', which is not necessarily perceived as pain. For example, anaesthetized patients with inadequate analgesia will often show marked increases in heart rate and respiratory rate during surgery, yet be unaware of the surgery because they are anaesthetized. This represents activation of the pain pathways without conscious perception of the pain and steps should be taken to provide analgesia to avoid pain perception in recovery.

Transmission is the process by which impulses are sent via primary afferent nerves to the dorsal horn of the spinal cord (Figure 2.2), and then along the sensory tracts to the brain. The transmission from the dorsal horn to the brain is sometimes termed **projection**. As previously mentioned, there are two major fibres transmitting to the spinal cord. Aδ fibres are smaller diameter, thinly myelinated (fast transmitting) fibres carrying thermal/mechanical information responsible for the

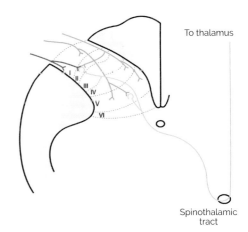

2.2 Diagram of a transverse section of the spinal cord, illustrating the central terminals of the first-order Aβ (green), Aδ (orange) and C (red) neurons within the dorsal horn of the grey matter. The numerals represent the position of the terminals in Rexed's laminae of the spinal cord.
(© Juliane Deubner, University of Saskatchewan, Canada)

initial sharp pain sensations. C fibres are small, unmyelinated (slow transmitting) nerves, which selectively carry nociceptive stimuli from the high activation, polymodal nociceptors. They are responsible for carrying dull/burning pain sensations.

The dorsal horn of the spinal cord has been classified into physiological zones or 'laminae', with lamina I being the most superficial. Aδ and C fibres terminate predominantly in laminae I–II but a few terminate deeper, with C fibres tending to communicate to deeper laminae via interneurons. Interestingly, most touch afferents also project to deeper laminae and this is thought to be the site of pain 'gating' – the phenomenon whereby rubbing a painful area can alleviate some of the acute pain after an injury. This is thought to occur by activation of inhibitory interneurons arising from the touch receptors.

One of three things may happen to the afferent signals. First, a spinal/segmental reflex (e.g. withdrawal) may occur. Secondly, the impulse may be passed on to the brain via spinoreticular and spinothalamic tracts. Thirdly, the impulse may be processed (modulated, e.g. gate theory).

The primary afferents synapse on to a variety of differing postsynaptic cell types. These include nociceptor-specific (NS) cells (Aδ and C fibres only) that fire in response to painful stimuli, proprioceptor-specific cells that respond to Aβ fibres (touch), and wide dynamic range (WDR) cells which respond to all three fibres – touch to pain. Located deep in lamina V, WDR neurons fire in a graded fashion depending on stimulus intensity and exhibit 'wind-up' (synaptic plasticity).

There are two major postsynaptic receptors involved in spinal cord pain transmission. AMPA (α-amino-3-hydroxy 5-methyl-4-isoxazeloproprionic acid) receptors are fast activation receptors that set the 'baseline' dorsal horn response to noxious and tactile stimuli. The second receptor is the NMDA (N-methyl-D-aspartate) receptor. Activated by prolonged and repetitive C fibre stimulation, this receptor allows calcium ion influx into the postsynaptic cell and is responsible for wind-up and potentially central sensitization. The NMDA receptor is therefore a good target for analgesic drugs such as ketamine, which are thought to minimize the development of chronic pain if used at the time of initial insult.

Modulation is the process of dampening or amplifying nociceptive signals. Modulation takes place primarily in the dorsal horn of the spinal cord, but also elsewhere, with input from ascending and descending pathways. It is a complex process, and the relationship between stimulus intensity and response to pain is not consistent. The output from the dorsal horn is also altered by the interaction of various neurotransmitters, all of which are subject to plasticity and alterations. It is a very labile phenomenon with several distinct components: peripheral sensitization, dorsal horn (gating), central sensitization/wind-up, descending inhibitory pathways and descending facilitatory pathways. Peripheral sensitization is a form of modulation involving local production of pro-inflammatory mediators contributing to hyperalgesia (exaggerated response to a stimulus that would be expected to be painful) around damaged tissue. This is in contrast to allodynia, which is a non-painful stimulus eliciting pain, and more likely due to central sensitization. Non-steroidal anti-inflammatory drugs (NSAIDs) are the analgesic agents of choice for treatment of peripheral sensitization. As previously mentioned, NMDA activation may lead to long-term potentiation of the pain response via elevated activity of dorsal horn neurons. This receptor is a target for analgesic drugs such as ketamine.

Descending modulatory pathways have four 'tiers' but are poorly understood. Inhibition may arise from the cortex and thalamus, the periaqueductal gray matter (PAG) in the mid-brain (which has a high opioid receptor concentration and is thought to be important in opioid-mediated analgesia), the nucleus raphe magnus (NRM) in the pons and rostral ventral medulla (RVM) and finally the medulla oblongata and spinal cord. Although descending inhibition is thought to work on many levels of the CNS, it is considered most important at the spinal level and can be very potent, for example, being able to run from a life-threatening situation with a fractured femur, which is termed 'stress-induced analgesia'.

Many descending transmitters are involved in modulating dorsal horn responsiveness but of particular interest are serotonin (pronociceptive and a component of central sensitization) and norepinephrine, which is the major transmitter involved in descending inhibition of pain transmission at the spinal level. Norepinephrine is released from brainstem nuclei (especially the NRM) and acts predominantly at α2-adrenoceptor spinal cord receptors, inhibiting transmitter release from primary afferent neurons and suppressing firing of projection neurons.

Perception, motivational, affective and behavioural aspects of pain must also be considered. Perception refers to the subjective experience of pain that results from the interaction of transduction, transmission, modulation, and the psychological aspects of the individual. Although well studied in human medicine, this is an area that is difficult to elucidate in veterinary patients due to their non-verbal status. General anaesthesia, whilst not analgesic per se, acts on perception by decreasing overall awareness, thereby eliminating the sensory component of pain.

It is recognized that fear and anxiety increase pain perception and that pain can cause fear and anxiety There are many (plastic) connections between pain pathways and neuro-endocrine, limbic (pain, pleasure, autonomic components) and withdrawal reflexes. In addition, the cortex responds to pain, giving rise to the behavioural component that can be assessed by validated small animal pain scales (see below).

Although the degree is not as completely elucidated in animals as in humans, there is no question that pain has an affective component. Affective behaviours are generally easily observed by pet owners and can be assessed/quantified using quality of life (QoL) scales in dogs, cats and other mammals. This is not a surprise, in that pain is a multidimensional experience that is not purely physiological. The affective components are likely mediated at a variety of nociceptive centres in the brain. Higher cortical centres, including the anterior cingulate, insular and prefrontal cortices, as well as the amygdala, hippocampus and parts of the limbic system, all play a role in the affective component of pain in humans (Figure 2.3) and all are present in dogs, cats and other mammals.

Location or structure	Function or role
Anterior cingulate cortex	Role in anxiety, anticipation of pain, attention to pain, and motor responses
Insular cortex	Potential role in the sensory discriminative and affective aspects of pain that contribute to the negative emotional responses and behaviours associated with painful stimuli
Prefrontal cortex	Role in sensory integration, decision making, memory retrieval, and attention processing in relation to pain
Amygdala, hippocampus, and other parts of the limbic system	Role in the formation and storage of memories associated with emotional events, which affect arousal and attention to pain and learning. The limbic system may also be partially responsible for the fear that accompanies pain

2.3 The role of higher cortical centres in the affective component of pain (Cohen and Mao, 2014).

Additional features of pain physiology

Visceral pain differs from somatic pain as pain from viscera is poorly localized. This is because viscera are innervated by very few nociceptors (C fibres) but with large overlapping receptive fields and a graded response to stimulation, although there are many mechanoreceptors present that respond to distension. Referred pain is common – visceral afferents synapse on spinal cord segments, which also receive inputs from specific somatic areas, a typical human example being arm pain in angina. This is termed somato-visceral convergence and is due to visceral afferents synapsing on spinal cord neurones that receive information from somatic nociceptors.

Pathological (chronic) pain is pain that is still present after the originating painful stimulus has disappeared. Chronic pain is mostly as a result of C fibre activity. It is not stimulus-specific or protective and inevitably leads to morbidity. Both wind-up and central sensitization are involved in the development of chronic pain states.

Phantom pain refers to perception of pain from a part of the body that has been removed. It is due to depolarization in nerve endings that originally carried sensation from the amputated limb.

Pain and quality of life assessment methods in dogs and cats

For many years pain treatment has been based on the principle of 'if it hurts us it will hurt them', which is a good starting point but is very much a generalization; this approach is almost a preconception of how likely a procedure is to be painful but takes little account of the patient's response. It could be said that this approach is a pre-emptive pain scoring system based on the science of the preservation of the pain pathway across mammalian species, with the addition of anthropomorphism and the projection of human emotions and feelings on to animals. Arguably the biggest breakthrough in small animal pain medicine has been the introduction of pain scoring systems, which have allowed us to attempt to quantify pain in patients and therefore adjust analgesia accordingly. Although incredibly helpful as a guide to pain treatment, pain scoring systems should be used to guide analgesic therapy but pain scoring should never override clinical examination and decision making. In particular, companion animals that are expected to be painful but score low on pain scales should always be given the 'benefit of doubt' and analgesia should not be withheld. Even with the utilization of pain scoring systems, the most accurate way

to determine whether or not a patient is in pain is to administer a dose of an analgesic drug and utilize pain scores to monitor the patient's response.

Acute pain scales and pain ethics

The provision of effective pain relief in small animals and its importance in relation to patient care and welfare is becoming more widely accepted by the veterinary profession (Lascelles *et al.*, 1995; Paul-Murphy *et al.*, 2004; Mathews *et al.*, 2014). Nevertheless, studies suggest that there is no agreed 'gold standard' provision of perioperative analgesia to small animal patients (Dohoo and Dohoo, 1996; Williams *et al.*, 2005). In several studies, the clinician's difficulty in recognizing and assessing pain is often raised as a reason for not administering analgesia, together with the fear of side effects. Because of this there have been major efforts to produce reliable, validated pain scoring systems taking into account the painful conditions regularly encountered in small animal practice to allow targeted analgesic therapy clinically and to support research and development of new analgesic drugs (Sharkey, 2013).

It is accepted that the recognition and assessment of pain in animals is problematic. In people, self-reporting of pain is recognized as the gold standard tool for measuring pain levels (Mathew and Mathew, 2003). In veterinary medicine the recognition of pain relies on the subjective interpretation of the patient's physiology and behaviour by an observer. Thus, unlike in human medicine where 'pain is what the patient says it is', pain in veterinary patients is better defined as 'what the observer says it is'. This leaves an unacceptable burden of proof of the existence of pain on the skill and bias of the observer unless standardized pain assessment tools are utilized. Thus, pain scales or scoring systems, with the ideal properties of validity, reliability and sensitivity to change (Mathews *et al.*, 2014), are needed for veterinary patients.

Attempts to validate and accurately assess pain in animals initially began in the 1980s by, for example, Taylor and Houlton (1984). Initial findings led to the development of scales such as numerical rating scales, simple word descriptive scales and visual analogue scales. These scales were adapted for the veterinary setting from human pain scales such as the McGill pain questionnaire (Melzack, 1975). Unfortunately, these scales tend to be unreliable in the treatment of acute pain in a hospital setting, mainly due to wide operator variability, the subjective nature of the scales and the inherent need for, and capacity of, animal patients to hide pain. This is evidenced in a study in which behavioural assessments, but not a numerical scoring system, identified dogs given analgesics *versus* those given placebo drugs (Hardie *et al.*, 1997). In addition, these scales are simple one-dimensional measurement tools that may indicate the presence, and perhaps even intensity, of pain but do not include affective and behavioural components that describe the impact of that pain on the patient. Since pain is a complex multidimensional stimulus, assessment of pain should be done with multidimensional tools.

This realization led to more advanced scales being developed that encompass physiological data such as heart rate, respiratory rate and cortisol levels, as well as behavioural scales which focused on the ethnology of animals experiencing pain (e.g. Murrell and Johnson, 2006). Currently, the most advanced veterinary pain scales available are composite-based scales such as those produced by Morton and Griffiths (1985), Hellyor and Gaynor (1998), Firth and Haldane (1999), Reid *et al.* (2007), and Brondani *et al.* (2013). The important feature of the multidimensional scales is that they take into account not only the pain intensity, but also the sensory and affective components of pain – i.e. not just how bad the pain is, but how it affects the patient.

Since sensory and affective components of pain impact patient behaviour, it is recognized that **change in behaviour** is the most predictive indicator that the patient may be in pain (Mathews *et al.*, 2014). Of course, change in behaviour is predictive for many maladies so the change must be equated to a painful incident and the patient must be examined for

other medical concerns. Gentle, respectful palpation of (or around) presumed painful areas is also very useful in detecting the presence of pain, and validated pain scales such as the Glasgow Composite Measure Pain Scale (see below) specify palpation 5 cm away from the wound as direct wound manipulation is undesirable. Other potential signs of pain, such as vocalization and changes in physiological parameters, may contribute to the prediction of pain but cannot be used in isolation. In fact, in a study in cats undergoing onychectomy, physiological parameters did not differentiate between cats that had surgery and those that were simply anaesthetized and bandaged without any painful procedure (Cambridge *et al.*, 2000). Furthermore, stress to collect physiological data may cause changes in these parameters, confounding results. Thus, many of the most useful pain scoring systems used to assess acute pain in conscious patients do not include physiological parameter changes as a component of the score. Physiological changes are more useful in anaesthetized patients where unconsciousness alleviates the impact of stress on the parameters.

Change in behaviour from before the painful incident (i.e. pre-surgery or pre-trauma) to after it is ideal for identifying pain but the patient's behaviour pre-pain may be unknown to the veterinary staff. The owner may be able to provide insight on normal behaviour for their pet but this is often more useful for chronic pain where the pet is at home and the behaviour has changed. Hospitalization itself can change behaviour, which confounds the identification of pain *versus* stress. The presence or absence of behaviours associated with pain can also be useful and are the premise for most of the multidimensional composite pain scales described in this chapter. The observer is not asked to decide whether the behaviour is normal/abnormal for the pet, but to state whether it exists or not. This simplifies the pain evaluation and makes it more robust, at least for the general population. As stated, however, individual patients should still be treated if they exhibit what the clinician presumes to be pain, even if they score outside the treatment cut-off using the scale. Pain is a very individual sensation and there is no 'one protocol fits all' answer for its assessment or its treatment.

Although scoring systems are not perfect at identifying pain in all patients and scores between assessors may vary, validated scoring systems, and training with the scoring systems, greatly decrease variability. For example, in cats, using a validated scoring system by reviewers who received 2 hours of video training on the system resulted in only a 6.1% difference between the observers regarding which cats should receive rescue analgesia (Benito *et al.*, 2017). In addition, multidimensional composite scales include both observation of the patient from a distance and hands-on interaction with the patient, which forces the observer to open the cage and put hands on the patient and not merely assume that patients that are 'sitting quietly' are pain-free. In actuality, immobility is often a sign of severe pain and failure to treat a patient with that degree of pain is unacceptable. Thus, the interactive portion of pain scales is a critical part of the most effective pain scoring systems.

Using pain scales

For all pain scales, training will improve the probability and consistency of pain identification. All team members involved in patient care should understand the importance of pain scoring and all patients that have undergone painful procedures should be assessed for pain. The scales are designed to decrease the subjectivity of pain scores and, to best support that goal, the assessment protocol outlined in the instructions that accompany the scale must be followed. It is best if the same person scores the patient at each assessment time but this is not always possible. Using validated scales promotes consistent assessment. The assessments should be repeated at scheduled times, and extra assessments added at 'important' times, such as after treatment. The interval between assessments should not be automatically set at a pre-determined interval for all patients but should be based on the nature of the pain (i.e. acute or chronic), the intensity of the pain, and the patient's response to analgesic therapy (Mathews *et al.*, 2014).

Authors' perspective

Using pain scales and scoring systems

A patient's pain score is a composite of multidimensional factors such as behaviours, body postures, facial grimaces and (for some scales) physiological parameters that might indicate pain.

- **Change** in behaviour between pre- and post-painful stimulus is the most consistent indicator of the presence of pain.
- When in doubt as to whether or not a patient is in pain, the default is administer analgesia and reassess their comfort level.

Best practice for using pain scoring systems or scales:

1. Scores are most consistent if the same person scores the patient before and after painful events. The use of validated scoring systems improves consistency of scores if different people need to score the patient.
2. A time schedule should be set for scoring so that the patient has consistent care. However, this is only a guideline and the actual schedule should be patient-based and adapted to the situation. For instance, scoring should be more frequent than the scheduled interval if the patient's analgesic protocol needs to be altered for the likelihood of breakthrough pain. If analgesic drugs are administered, patients should be reassessed within 30 minutes of the administration to ensure pain relief.
   - Never treat a patient and assume that treatment was effective. Pain – and response to analgesic drugs – are specific to each individual so assess each patient. ▶

Authors' perspective *continued*

3. The scales include observation of patients from a distance so that behaviour can be assessed in the absence of a human. This allows the patient to act 'normally' without feeling the need to hide pain. Watch the patient care fully for:
    - Abnormal body posture (e.g. hunched back, tucked abdomen)
    - Grimaced facial expressions (e.g. position of ears, 'openness' of eyes)
    - Location in the cage (e.g. at cage door or hiding or facing the back of the cage)
    - Mobility (e.g. 'frozen' stillness, excessive movement like pacing or circling)
    - Interest in surroundings (are they watching activity or just 'staring'?)
    - Abnormal behaviours (e.g. excessive grooming or licking)
    - Vocalization (e.g. howling, growling, purring)
    - Abnormal physiological parameters that can be assessed without interaction (e.g. respiratory rate, pupil size).
4. The scales include interaction with the patient so open the cage door and touch the patient. Get the patient out of the cage (if appropriate). Measure heart rate and other physiological parameters at this step. Pay close attention to response to:
    - Approach of the observer (e.g. wanting to be petted *versus* withdrawing or attacking)
    - Normal handling, such as petting
    - Gentle palpation around the painful area
    - Ability to/interest in ambulating, if appropriate (get the animal out of the cage)
    - Food, if appropriate (offer appetizing food).
5. **Ask the patient.**
    - If unsure, always 'ask' the patient, pharmacologically, if it is in pain. Administer a dose of analgesic drugs
    - Opioids and alpha-2 agonists are commonly used for this query. They are rapidly acting and their effects are reversible if the patient is not in pain and adverse effects from the drugs occur. This is actually unlikely: if you think the patient is in pain, it likely is.
6. **Reassess.**
    - If the patient is comfortable, resume the normal schedule for assessment
    - If the patient is not comfortable, add another analgesic drug to the protocol or increase the dose of the previously administered drug and reassess in 30 minutes.

Specific pain scales

Glasgow Composite Pain Scoring Scale

Of the composite multidimensional scales developed, the Glasgow Composite Pain Scoring Scale (GCPSS; see Appendix 1) or Glasgow Composite Measure Pain Scale (GCMPS) is the original scale designed using psychometric principles that are well established in human medicine to measure complex variables. The components of the scales are based on specific behaviours that have been identified to indicate pain and weighted as to their importance in pain behaviour in the dog and the cat. The composite GCMPS for dogs has a long form and short form. The long form is more robust in its guidance for the evaluator with definitions of terms used to describe the specific pain-related behaviours. The scale does take some time to complete and does not have a numeric scoring system.

The GCMPS-SF (for 'short form') is a condensation of the most important composite information in a clinically useful form (i.e. simple and quick to apply) with a numeric scoring system. Included in the GCMPS-SF is the patient's overall behaviour, including behaviour in the cage, on a leash and during palpation around the surgical site. The scale has a cut-off score above which it is suggested analgesia should be administered. The maximum score for all categories is 24, or 20 if mobility is omitted (e.g. in patients that can not ambulate). The recommended analgesic intervention level is ≥6/24 (total score) or ≥5/20 (no mobility score). This is currently the only validated dog acute pain scale available for use in veterinary practice (Reid *et al.*, 2007). It has been widely used both clinically and in research and is translated into several languages. The SF of the scale, along with the information on validation of the scale and instructions on how to use the scale, can be downloaded at: http://www.newmetrica.com/wp-content/uploads/2016/09/Reid-et-al-2007.pdf. See also Appendix 1.

The GCMPS-Feline is only available as the SF. The easy-to-use scale includes vocalization, body posture/tension/location in the cage, attention to painful area, response to palpation of the painful area, response to stroking, and a feline grimace scale with caricature diagrams of ear and whisker position (Holden *et al.*, 2014). The cut-off score for analgesic administration is ≥5 points out of 20 points total. This scale has been recently validated (Calvo *et al.*, 2014; Reid *et al.*, 2017) and its use is rapidly increasing in clinics and in research studies. The scale, along with the information on validation of the scale and instructions on how to use the scale, can be downloaded at: http://www.newmetrica.com/wp-content/uploads/2016/09/Calvo-et-al-2014.pdf. See also Appendix 1.

UNESP-Botucatu multidimensional composite pain scale

The UNESP-Botucatu scale (see Appendix 1) is also a multidimensional composite scale validated to identify acute pain in cats. The scale also focuses on the presence or absence of specific behaviours. The scale was originally validated in Brazilian Portuguese (Brondani *et al.*, 2011) but is now validated in English (Brondani *et al.*, 2013), French (Steagall *et al.*, 2017) and Italian (Della Rocca *et al.*, 2018). The English scale includes 10 items: posture,

comfort, activity, attitude, miscellaneous behaviours, reaction to palpation of the surgical wound, reaction to palpation of the abdomen/flank, arterial blood pressure, appetite and vocalization. The score indicating the need for analgesia is ≥7 points out of the 30 total points. The scale has been used both clinically and in research. The scale, along with the information on its validation, instructions on its use and videos of cats in pain for practice scoring, can be downloaded at: http://www.animalpain.com.br/en-us/avaliacao-da-dor-em-gatos.php. See also Appendix 1.

Other pain scales

Other scales to consider include the Colorado State Scale (see Appendix 1) and the Melbourne Pain Scale, both of which are multidimensional composite scales. The Colorado State Scale is available for dogs, cats and horses. The scale uses psychological and behavioural signs of pain, caricatures of facial expressions and body posture and palpation responses to create a numerical score. Although not yet validated, validation studies are in progress for the cat scale (Shipley *et al.*, 2018). The feline scale can be downloaded at: http://csu-cvmbs.colostate.edu/Documents/anesthesia-pain-management-pain-score-feline.pdf and the canine scale at: http://csu-cvmbs.colostate.edu/Documents/anesthesia-pain-management-pain-score-canine.pdf. See also Appendix 1. The Melbourne scale for dogs uses physiological (heart and respiratory rates) and behavioural responses (response to palpation, activity, mental status, posture, and vocalization) and has been validated (Firth and Haldane, 1999).

Chronic pain scales and quality of life assessments

It should be noted that the pain scales mentioned here are designed for recognition of acute pain and are likely inaccurate for recognition of chronic pain, which may be manifest by the patient in a very different way than it would manifest acute pain. However, chronic pain scales do exist and these scales are covered in the chapter on chronic pain.

Many of the scales are quality of life scales rather than true pain scales. A validated QoL scale, available at http:www.newmetrica.com/vetmetrica-hrql, has recently been introduced. Quality of life assessments are important because the bottom line for the patient is not necessarily the presence of pain, but the impact of pain on quality of life.

References and further reading

Benito J, Monteiro BP, Beauchamp G, Lascelles BDX and Steagall PV (2017) Evaluation of interobserver agreement for postoperative pain and sedation assessment in cats. *Journal of the American Veterinary Medical Association* **251**, 544–551

Brondani JT, Luna SP and Padovani CR (2011) Refinement and initial validation of a multidimensional composite scale for use in assessing acute postoperative pain in cats. *American Journal of Veterinary Research* **72**, 174–183

Brondani JT, Mama KR, Luna SP *et al.* (2013) Validation of the English version of the UNESP-Botucatu multidimensional composite pain scale for assessing postoperative pain in cats. *BMC Veterinary Research* **9**, 143

Calvo G, Holden E, Reid J *et al.* (2014) Development of a behaviour-based measurement tool with defined intervention level for assessing acute pain in cats. *Journal of Small Animal Practice* **55**, 622–629

Cambridge AJ, Tobias KM, Newberry RC and Sarkar DK (2000) Subjective and objective measurements of postoperative pain in cats. *Journal of the American Veterinary Medical Association* **217**, 685–690

Cohen SP and Mao J (2014) Neuropathic pain: mechanisms and their clinical implications. *British Medical Journal* **348**, f7656

Della Rocca G, Catanzaro A, Conti MB *et al.* (2018) Validation of the Italian version of the UNESP-Botucatu multidimensional composite pain scale for the assessment of postoperative pain in cats. *Veterinaria Italiana* **54**, 49–61

Dohoo S and Dohoo I (1996) Postoperative use of analgesics in dogs and cats by Canadian veterinarians. *Canadian Veterinary Journal* **37**, 540–551

Firth AF and Haldane SL (1999) Development of a scale to evaluate postoperative pain in dogs. *Journal of the American Veterinary Medical Association* **214**, 651–659

Hardie EM, Hansen BD and Carroll GS (1997) Behavior after ovariohysterectomy in the dog: what's normal? *Applied Animal Behaviour Science* **5**, 111–128

Hellyer PW and Gaynor JS (1998) Acute post-surgical pain in dogs and cats. *The Compendium of Continuing Education (Small Animal)* **20**, 140–153

Holden E, Calvo G, Collins M *et al.* (2014) Evaluation of facial expression in acute pain in cats. *Journal of Small Animal Practice* **55**, 615–621

IASP (1994) Pain terms, a current list with definitions and notes on usage. In: *Classification of Chronic Pain, 2nd edn*, ed. H Merskey and N Bogduk. IASP Press, Seattle

Lascelles B, Capner C and Waterman AE (1995) Survey of perioperative analgesic use in small animals. *Veterinary Record* **137**, 23–30

Mathew P and Mathew J (2003) Assessment and management of pain in infants. *Postgraduate Medical Journal* **79**, 438–443

Mathews K, Kronen PW, Lascelles D *et al.* (2014) Guidelines for recognition, assessment and treatment of pain: WSAVA Global Pain Council. *Journal of Small Animal Practice* **55**, E10–68

Melzack R (1975) The McGill pain questionnaire: major properties and scoring methods. *Journal of Pain* **1**, 277–299

Morton CM, Reid J, Scott J, Holton LL and Nolan AM (2005) Application of a scaling model to establish and validate an interval level pain scale for assessment of acute pain in dogs. *American Journal of Veterinary Research* **66**, 2154–2166

Morton DB and Griffiths PH (1985) Guidelines on the recognition of pain, distress and discomfort in experimental animals and a hypothesis of assessment. *Veterinary Record* **116**, 431–436

Murrell JC and Johnson CB (2006) Neurophysical techniques to assess pain in animals. *Journal of Veterinary Pharmacology and Therapeutics* **29**, 325–335

Paul-Murphy J, Ludders J, Robertson S *et al.* (2004) The need for a cross species approach to the study of pain in animals. *Journal of the American Veterinary Medical Association* **224**, 692–697

Reid J, Nolan AM, Hughes JML *et al.* (2007) Development of the short form Glasgow Composite Measure Pain Scale (CMPS-SF) and derivation of an analgesic intervention score. *Animal Welfare* **16**, 97–104

Reid J, Scott EM, Calvo G and Nolan AM (2017) Definitive Glasgow acute pain scale for cats: validation and intervention level. *Veterinary Record* **180**, 449

Robertson SA (2002) What is pain? *Journal of the American Veterinary Medical Association* **221**, 202–204

Sharkey M (2013) The challenges of assessing osteoarthritis and postoperative pain in dogs. *Journal of the American Association of Pharmaceutical Scientists* **15**, 598–607

Shipley H, Guedes A, Graham L, Goudie-DeAngelis E and Wendt-Hornickle E (2018) Preliminary appraisal of the reliability and validity of the Colorado State University Feline Acute Pain Scale. *Journal of Feline Medicine and Surgery*, doi: 10.1177/1098612X18777506

Steagall PV, Monteiro BP, Lavoie AM *et al.* (2017) Validation de la version francophone d'une échelle composite multidimensionnelle pour l'évaluation de la douleur postopératoire chez les chats. *Canadian Veterinary Journal* **58**, 56–64

Taylor PM and Houlton JF (1984) Postoperative analgesia in the dog: A comparison of morphine, buprenorphine and pentazocine. *Journal of Small Animal Practice* **25**, 437–451

Williams V, Lascelles B and Robson M (2005) Current attitudes to, and use of, peri-operative analgesia in dogs and cats by veterinarians in New Zealand. *New Zealand Veterinary Journal* **53**, 193–203

Useful websites

Newmetrica:
http://www.newmetrica.com/vetmetrica-hrql/
RCVS:
https://www.rcvs.org.uk/home/

Chapter 3

Acute and perioperative pain

Jo Murrell and Briony Alderson

Over the last 20 years in veterinary medicine there has been increasing recognition that surgery causes pain and, therefore, animals undergoing surgery require analgesia. This is evidenced by UK surveys investigating attitudes to perioperative analgesia in cats and dogs. A survey carried out in 1996/1997 by Capner and colleagues reported a relatively low level of analgesic administration to cats and dogs undergoing routine neutering, with only 26% of cats receiving analgesics for neutering procedures (Capner *et al.*, 1999; Lascelles *et al.*, 1999); however, when the UK survey was repeated in 2013, almost ubiquitous use of analgesia for neutering was reported, with 98% of respondents administering a non-steroidal anti-inflammatory drug (NSAID) to dogs and cats undergoing neutering (Hunt *et al.*, 2015a). Although surveys can be criticized for being biased, in that veterinary surgeons that are more likely to administer analgesia may be more likely to respond to a survey about perioperative analgesic use, it is reasonable to assume that the 2013 survey reflects a trend towards increased perioperative analgesic use in cats and dogs in the UK, which is beneficial for patient welfare. The underlying reasons for this trend are unknown, but it probably reflects increased scientific knowledge about pain following surgery in cats and dogs (Berry, 2016), changes to veterinary undergraduate and postgraduate teaching, and the greater number of licensed analgesic drugs that are now available for administration to cats and dogs in the perioperative period compared with previous years. The 2013 survey also highlighted areas for improvement in perioperative analgesic management: a low number of respondents used pain scoring tools in dogs and cats, and local anaesthesia techniques were only used by a minority of respondents. Recognition and quantification of pain is the cornerstone of effective pain management in animals; therefore, use of pain scoring tools is pivotal. Local anaesthetic techniques can reduce the requirement for systemic analgesic drugs, thereby minimizing side effects associated with drug administration; therefore, their use is to be encouraged in acute analgesia regimens for cats and dogs.

The aims of this chapter are to describe the general approach to the administration of analgesic agents to surgical patients, and to discuss clinically appropriate analgesia protocols for routine surgical procedures.

BSAVA Guide to Pain Management in Small Animal Practice. Edited by Ian Self. ©BSAVA 2019

Pre-emptive and preventive analgesia protocols

Pre-emptive analgesia can be defined as the administration of analgesic drugs before the onset of nociceptive stimulation (Kissin, 2000) and was the focus of gold standard analgesic administration for many years. Nociception refers to the sensory nervous system's response to certain harmful or potentially harmful stimuli. It was hoped that the pre-emptive administration of analgesic drugs would reduce the requirement for analgesia postoperatively and decrease pain after surgery. Despite many studies being carried out in human medicine to assess the impact of pre-emptive analgesia on postoperative pain scores, the evidence that pre-emptive analgesia strategies reduce the requirement for postoperative analgesia and reduce perioperative pain is mixed, with many clinical studies showing no benefit in administering pre-emptive analgesia compared with protocols in which analgesic drugs were administered after surgery (McQuay, 1995; Kelly et al., 2001; Moiniche et al., 2002; Grape and Tramèr, 2007). However, some experimental studies carried out in laboratory animals using induced pain models show a good evidence of efficacy of pre-emptive protocols (e.g. Nakamura and Takasaki, 2001), which may reflect differences between the complexity of clinical pain states compared with induced pain models. In veterinary medicine, a few studies have compared pre-emptive or preoperative administration of analgesics with postoperative analgesic administration and demonstrated beneficial effects of the pre-emptive strategies (Lascelles et al., 1998; Slingsby and Waterman-Pearson, 2000).

More recently the concept of pre-emptive analgesia, where it is the timing of analgesic administration that is the focus, has been replaced with an approach termed 'preventive analgesia' (Katz et al., 2011). The focus of preventive analgesia is not on the relative timing of analgesic treatments but on attenuating peripheral and central sensitization, which increase postoperative pain intensity and analgesic requirements. Generally, it is deemed that preventive analgesia has been demonstrated when postoperative pain and analgesic use are reduced beyond the duration of action of the target drug, which can be defined as 5.5 half-lives of the target drug. This definition ensures that the observed analgesic effect is not only due to a direct analgesic effect of the target drug, but also that analgesia has been sustained beyond the expected time course of the analgesic agent. However, there are few studies in people that have investigated the efficacy of preventive analgesia approaches compared with more traditional analgesia regimens. No studies of preventive analgesia regimens have been conducted in cats and dogs. Nonetheless, the types of analgesic approaches described in this chapter adopt the principles of preventive analgesia, whereby analgesics are administered as early as possible before surgery and are continued during and after surgery until the likelihood of peripheral and central sensitization as a result of tissue trauma associated with surgery has waned.

Role of premedication in preventive analgesia strategies

The addition of analgesic agents to premedication protocols is pivotal to the application of preventive analgesic strategies in cats and dogs. In animals undergoing elective surgery and not in pain, this ensures that analgesics are administered before the onset of nociceptive stimulation, which, dependent on the analgesic drug administered, may serve to reduce the likelihood of peripheral and central sensitization. In animals that are already in pain at the time of surgery, the early administration of analgesics will help limit the magnitude of changes in central and peripheral sensory processing as a result of pain. As well as contributing to preventive analgesia strategies, administration of analgesics as part of premedication protocols has a number of other advantages:

1. Provision of intraoperative analgesia. Although a patient that is adequately anaesthetized cannot by definition experience pain, nociception during surgery will still occur. Therefore, provision of intraoperative analgesia is imperative to prevent upregulation of the pain pathways during surgery.

2. The administration of opioid analgesics will increase the sedative effects of many sedative premedicant drugs including acepromazine, alpha-2 agonists, and benzodiazepines. Synergistic sedation between opioids and sedatives may allow a lower dose of the sedative premedicant to be used, while still maintaining good sedation, which may have cardiovascular and respiratory system benefits.

3. By virtue of the synergistic sedation between opioids and sedative premedicants, the administration of analgesics as part of premedication protocols should allow a lower dose of hypnotic agent to be required for induction of anaesthesia, which may reduce cardiovascular and respiratory system depression.

4. Opioids have a minimal alveolar concentration (MAC) sparing effect and reduce the concentration of inhalant agent required to maintain anaesthesia in dogs and cats (e.g. Credie et al., 2010). This is likely to lessen depression of the cardiorespiratory systems during anaesthesia.

Approach to the administration of analgesic agents to surgical patients

There are a number of principles to consider when designing effective perioperative analgesic protocols for surgical patients. The first, preventive analgesia, has been described above, and is imperative to try and prevent or limit the magnitude of central and peripheral sensitization.

The second is the principle of multimodal analgesia, the practice of using different classes of analgesic drug in combination to provide more effective pain relief while limiting side effects from the individual agents. Multimodal analgesia is widely accepted to be best practice in human anaesthesia and analgesia (Jakobsson, 2014). It is more effective than unimodal analgesia techniques utilizing one class of analgesic drug because the pain pathway is complex and comprises multiple neurotransmitters and receptors. Therefore, analgesia provision using one class of analgesic drug that acts at one receptor or only one component of the pain pathway is unlikely to provide comprehensive pain relief. Combining different classes of analgesic drug often allows lower doses of individual agents to be used, reducing the likelihood of side effects. For example, using a local anaesthetic technique will usually allow lower doses of systemic opioid drugs to be administered after surgery, thereby reducing concurrent sedation associated with opioid administration. Combining different classes of analgesic drug may also provide better temporal pain relief. For example, NSAIDs have a long duration of action, typically 24 hours, but have a relatively slow onset of action. In contrast, many parenteral opioids are short acting but have a quick onset of action, typically in the order of minutes after intravenous injection. Combining an opioid with an NSAID thereby allows a rapid onset and long duration of analgesia to be achieved. There is some evidence in veterinary medicine that multimodal analgesia techniques provide superior analgesia compared with unimodal techniques (e.g. Brondani et al., 2009; Zanuzzo et al., 2015). It is important to make a distinction between multimodal analgesia and polypharmacy. Multimodal analgesia is the strategic use of different classes of analgesic agents to combat different underlying pain mechanisms. Therefore, the combinations of drugs utilized should complement each other in terms of differing mechanisms of action to target different parts of the pain pathway. It is also important to note, for example, that combining two different opioid drugs does not constitute multimodal analgesia because the drugs are from the same class.

The third essential element to effective pain management is the coupling of analgesic drug administration to the recognition and quantification of pain. The use of pain scoring tools can be extremely helpful for improving the quantification of pain in animals. Glasgow University has recently developed two tools for the quantification of pain in dogs and cats; the Glasgow Composite Pain Scale Canine and Glasgow Composite Pain Scale Feline. Both scales can be freely downloaded from the internet, follow a similar framework to each other, and are simple to use. They comprise a series of questions about the animal, starting with the appearance of the animal from outside of the cage, their response to interaction, how the animal reacts to application of gentle pressure around the surgical wound, and finally questions about the general impression of the demeanour of the animal. The maximum possible score for the canine scale is either 20, in patients that are non-ambulatory, or 24 in ambulatory patients. In cats, the maximum possible score is 20. Importantly, the critical score above which rescue analgesia is required has been defined for both cats and dogs. In dogs, scores of ≥5/20 or ≥6/24 indicate that additional analgesia is needed, whereas in cats a score of ≥5/20 has been set as the intervention level.

Two different approaches have been advocated to combine pain scoring with drug administration. The first approach is to delay drug administration until the animal shows signs of pain and reaches the criteria for rescue analgesic administration. The disadvantage of this approach is that it requires the animal to become painful before analgesia is administered, driving upregulation of sensory processing. To ensure good patient welfare it also requires that pain assessment is very frequent, for example every 2 hours, which may be difficult to achieve in a busy practice setting. An alternative approach, favoured by the authors, is to prescribe analgesia after surgery, irrespective of the pain score, but tailor the dose according to pain assessment. The timing of analgesic administration is determined by the expected duration of action of the analgesic drugs, for example methadone may be prescribed every 4–5 hours. An inherent risk with this approach is that animals are over analgesed, resulting in an increased incidence of side effects such as sedation or dysphoria arising from opioid administration. However, this approach is more likely to prevent upregulation of the pain pathways, which is advantageous in terms of facilitating longer term pain relief and potentially reducing the likelihood of chronic pain.

Authors' perspectives on cases

A number of different drug classes are commonly used for the provision of perioperative analgesia. Opioids remain the backbone of perioperative analgesia, not least because of their important role as part of premedication protocols. However, there is widespread evidence for the analgesic efficacy of different opioid drugs in cats and dogs, supporting their use in the perioperative period. Similarly, NSAIDs also form a valuable component of analgesia regimens for acute pain because there is good evidence of efficacy for acute pain states and there are a variety of drugs licensed for perioperative administration to cats and dogs. Other classes of drug that are used include local anaesthetics, ketamine and alpha-2 agonists. When the authors consider multimodal analgesia the acronym NOLAN is useful; where N = NSAID, O = opioids, L = local anaesthetics, A = alpha-2 agonists and N = N-methyl-D-aspartate (NMDA) antagonists (e.g. ketamine). P for paracetamol can be added for dogs. Logical approaches to drug selection within each class of drug are given below.

General considerations for analgesia in all surgical cases

The selection of drugs for perioperative analgesia will depend on the surgery to be performed, the individual animal and the availability of drugs.

NSAIDs

There is very good evidence for the efficacy of NSAIDs as a component of analgesia regimens for acute pain in dogs and cats (Kamata *et al.*, 2012; Gruet *et al.*, 2013), and as such they are widely used for this purpose. The optimal timing of perioperative analgesic administration of NSAIDs remains contentious. Preoperative administration is recommended in animals that are cardiovascularly stable where blood loss or other causes of cardiovascular instability are not expected during surgery. However, the potential effects of NSAIDs on renal homeostasis are well recognized and renal ischaemia may result from systemic hypotension during surgery when NSAIDs have been administered. Therefore, NSAIDs should be delayed until such a time that the animal is normovolaemic and normotensive after anaesthesia and surgery in patients that are cardiovascularly unstable or when instability due to significant haemorrhage is expected. The use of perioperative NSAIDs in patients with concurrent chronic kidney disease (CKD) is also debated. Although NSAIDs have not been shown to hasten the progression of CKD or decrease longevity in cats with osteoarthritis (Gowan *et al.*, 2011; 2012), the effect of perioperative NSAIDs in cats and dogs with CKD is unknown and the authors advise delaying administration of NSAIDs until these patients are normally hydrated and normotensive. Another area of contention surrounding perioperative NSAID administration is their use in patients that have undergone gastrointestinal (GI) surgery where the negative effects of NSAIDs on healing of the GI tract might be detrimental (Luna *et al.*, 2007; Monteiro-Steagall *et al.*, 2013). In the absence of evidence to the contrary, it is recommended to avoid NSAID use in patients that have undergone significant GI trauma where delayed healing of the GI tract is likely to be clinically problematic. Administration of intravenous paracetamol might be an alternative option for additional analgesia alongside opioids in this patient group. Paracetamol is generally considered to be less detrimental to the GI tract than NSAIDs, although there are no data in dogs to support this statement. Paracetamol is contraindicated in cats. NSAIDs, through inhibition of platelet thromboxane A2 production, also have a well recognized effect of decreasing platelet aggregation (Luna *et al.*, 2007), although clinically this does not lead to overt bleeding in animals receiving NSAIDs over a prolonged time. It is not necessary to stop NSAID administration prior to surgery in healthy animals receiving chronic NSAID therapy. However, the perioperative administration of NSAIDs is probably unwise in animals with recognized disorders of haemostasis. In terms of decision making around which NSAID to choose for perioperative administration to cats and dogs, there are a number of factors to take into consideration. Be aware that not all NSAIDs are licensed for perioperative administration so it is imperative to check and select one that is licensed for this use. It is also important to consider ease of administration and whether there is an injectable preparation that may be easier to administer perioperatively than an oral tablet.

Opioids

Selection of the appropriate opioid for premedication is pivotal to adequate management of perioperative analgesia. The two most commonly administered licensed opioid drugs for premedication to cats and dogs are methadone and buprenorphine. This is because both drugs have a medium duration of action (methadone 4–5 hours, buprenorphine 6–8 hours) and therefore will provide a meaningful duration of action throughout the perioperative period in the majority of surgeries performed in veterinary practice. Pethidine, a licensed full mu agonist, provides good analgesic efficacy in cats and dogs but is short acting (60–90 minutes), necessitating frequent redosing in the perioperative period, which is disadvantageous. Butorphanol, a kappa agonist, provides inferior analgesia to both methadone and buprenorphine and its use as a premedicant prior to most surgical procedures is to be discouraged. Fentanyl, a short-acting full mu agonist opioid, is occasionally used for premedication, usually in combination with midazolam, for cardiovascularly unstable patients. In this instance the predominant role of the fentanyl is more commonly to provide sedation while limiting adverse events on the cardiovascular system rather than to provide analgesia. If analgesia is required it must be remembered that the duration of action of fentanyl is short after a single dose (10–20 minutes) and further top-ups will be necessary to provide sustained analgesia.

The use of opioids need not be confined to use in premedication; further opioids may be required to treat poorly controlled intraoperative nociception, recognized as difficulty in controlling depth of anaesthesia even with relatively high concentrations of inhalant agent. Methadone, administered as top-ups (0.1 mg/kg i.v.), fentanyl administered as a bolus dose (2–10 µg/kg) or continuous rate infusion (CRI) (5–10 µg/kg/h) will provide additional analgesia during invasive surgeries and will allow the concentration of inhalant agent required to maintain anaesthesia to be reduced (Simões et al., 2016). Dosing accuracy is important and a CRI should be given using controlled infusion apparatus. Care must be taken to support the respiratory system following intraoperative methadone or fentanyl administration, and it is recommended that respiratory function be monitored with capnography and ventilation supported with intermittent positive pressure ventilation if necessary. The other major side effect of methadone or fentanyl to be aware of following intraoperative administration is bradycardia, which can be managed by the administration of an anticholinergic if the low heart rate is having a negative impact on blood pressure. Buprenorphine has a longer onset of action than methadone and is not ideally suited to intraoperative administration for providing additional analgesia. Whether full mu agonists such as methadone should be administered after partial mu receptor agonists such as buprenorphine remains contentious; however, recent evidence in humans (Oifa et al., 2009) and dogs (Hunt et al., 2013) has challenged the concept of a negative interaction between full and partial mu agonist drugs suggesting that methadone administered after buprenorphine is efficacious.

Postoperative opioid selection depends on the anticipated pain level after surgery, with methadone the drug of choice for moderate to severe pain and buprenorphine reserved for use in patients experiencing mild pain or moderate pain if a multimodal approach to analgesia has been adopted. If analgesia with methadone is insufficient, a fentanyl CRI can be considered (1–5 µg/kg/h), with the rate adjusted according to pain score.

Local anaesthetics

Local anaesthetics can be utilized as part of a local or locoregional technique, or lidocaine can be used systemically.

Local anaesthetic techniques form a valuable adjunct to perioperative analgesic regimens and their use is encouraged whenever possible. Using a local anaesthetic technique can decrease the requirement for systemic analgesia for the duration of the block, which can be particularly advantageous in reducing the dose of systemic opioid required for adequate analgesia. An effective block may obviate the need for systemic opioids completely; for example administration of epidural morphine and bupivacaine for pelvic surgery may prevent the need for systemic opioids for the first 24 hours after surgery. Local anaesthetic blocks will also decrease the dose requirement for the inhalant agent during anaesthesia, i.e. exert a MAC sparing effect, which can be advantageous for the cardiovascular system. A large number of different local anaesthetic blocks are described dependent on the site of surgery. See Appendix 2 for more details about the different local anaesthetic techniques and appropriate drug choices and drug doses for blocks relevant for different types of surgery.

Lidocaine is a reversible blocker of sodium channels and has been used for many years to provide analgesia as part of local anaesthesia techniques. However, more recently it has been administered systemically to provide analgesia, although the mechanisms by which analgesia is provided are not fully understood (Lui and Ng, 2011). Similarly to the other adjunctive agents there is a limited evidence base to support administration of lidocaine systemically to small animals. Studies have investigated the antinociceptive effects of a lidocaine CRI in dogs undergoing surgery and found conflicting results, with one study showing that lidocaine blunted autonomic responses to surgery (Ortega and Cruz, 2011), and another showing no effect of lidocaine on autonomic responses (Columbano et al., 2012). Anecdotally, lidocaine is reported to be efficacious in the management of visceral pain although there is limited evidence to support this view. Doses of 50 μg/kg/min preceded by a loading dose of 2 mg/kg administered over 15 minutes are recommended in dogs; be aware that lidocaine will reduce the MAC of the inhalant agent so depth of anaesthesia should be monitored carefully when lidocaine is administered during surgery. Lidocaine infusions are not recommended for analgesia in cats due to negative effects on the cardiovascular system (Pypendop and Ilkiw, 2005).

Alpha-2 agonists

Alpha-2 agonists such as medetomidine and dexmedetomidine are widely used for premedication and as such contribute to perioperative analgesia. However, the analgesia from clinical doses of alpha-2 agonists is relatively short (10 μg/kg dexmedetomidine provides analgesia for approximately 45 minutes); therefore, dexmedetomidine or medetomidine must be given by a CRI to provide sustained analgesia. One study has investigated the postoperative analgesic effects of dexmedetomidine given by CRI in dogs after invasive surgery and showed similar analgesia was provided by a dexmedetomidine CRI at 1 μg/kg/h or morphine 0.1 mg/kg/h (Valtolina et al., 2009). However, a significant number of dogs in both groups required rescue analgesia with morphine highlighting the importance of pain scoring with any analgesic regimen. An experimental study in dogs compared the sedative and analgesic effects of dexmedetomidine alone using a neurophysiological model and found that doses of 3–5 μg/kg/h dexmedetomidine were required to provide analgesia in this model,

suggesting that doses higher than 1 μg/kg/h might be needed to provide significant analgesia in the absence of other analgesic drugs (van Oostrom et al., 2011). This study also clearly showed that it is not possible to obtain analgesia from alpha-2 agonists without concurrent sedation. Consideration must be given to the cardiovascular effects of alpha-2 agonists when deciding whether to use even a low-dose CRI in individual patients because the cardiovascular effects are still apparent. Infusions of alpha-2 agonists will also increase urine production; therefore, bladder management (taking dogs outside frequently to toilet or expressing the bladder) is important in dogs that receive an alpha-2 agonist CRI.

Ketamine

Ketamine is widely used as part of injectable anaesthesia protocols and will contribute to perioperative analgesia through antagonism of the N-methyl-D-aspartate receptor. More recently, the analgesic effects of subanaesthetic doses of ketamine have been recognized (Laskowski et al., 2011; Yang et al., 2014), whereby ketamine is administered as a CRI during surgery and postoperatively at doses ranging from 2–10 μg/kg/min. A few studies have been conducted in dogs investigating the analgesic effects of low-dose ketamine administered by CRI and found variable results about the efficacy of this intervention. Wagner et al. (2002) investigated the analgesic effects of 10 μg/kg/min ketamine administered intraoperatively followed by 2 μg/kg/min ketamine postoperatively in dogs undergoing forelimb amputation and found that pain scores were significantly lower in dogs that received ketamine compared with a group that did not receive a ketamine CRI. However, the difference in pain scores was numerically small and the biological relevance of this difference can be questioned. In contrast, Sarrau et al. (2007) found no effect on postoperative analgesic requirements between dogs undergoing mastectomy receiving either a high-dose or low-dose ketamine CRI and a control group that did not receive ketamine. In an experimental model, Bergadano *et al.* (2009) investigated the effect of a loading dose of ketamine (0.5 mg/kg i.v.) followed by a 10 µg/kg/min CRI on nociceptive withdrawal reflexes (NWR) in dogs and found minimal modulation of the NWR, suggesting that at the doses studied intravenous ketamine does not modulate spinal sensory processing. There are no clinical studies investigating the effects of a ketamine CRI on pain in cats. The conflicting data in dogs make it difficult to make evidence-based recommendations about the use of ketamine in the perioperative period in dogs and cats. In humans, ketamine is used specifically to reduce the requirement for perioperative opioids (Carstensen and Möller, 2010) and it is recommended that ketamine be used alongside opioids in dogs and cats. It is important that a loading dose is administered (e.g. 0.5 mg/kg) and infusion rates of 5–10 µg/kg/min ketamine are suggested. Pain scoring to confirm the efficacy of ketamine in the cases where it is used postoperatively is mandatory.

Example regimens
Castration and spay
These cases are generally considered 'routine' in veterinary practice and are generally performed on healthy, young animals. In these cases, perioperative analgesia should include preferably methadone (or buprenorphine) in the premedication. Recent evidence suggests that pain scores are lower for the first 8 hours after surgery in bitches undergoing ovariohysterectomy that received methadone for premedication compared with those that received buprenorphine (Shah *et al.*, 2018), supporting selection of methadone for premedication prior to ovariohysterectomy in dogs. In cats, there have been no studies that have directly compared the analgesic efficacy of buprenorphine and methadone in surgical models. There is good evidence in cats undergoing ovariohysterectomy and premedicated with acepromazine that butorphanol provides inadequate analgesia for the procedure with high pain scores reported in the postoperative period (Warne *et al.*, 2013; 2014).

NSAIDs can often be administered preoperatively in these cases as the animals are generally healthy, although in some cases there is a risk of haemorrhage and therefore administration should be delayed. There is no evidence to suggest that one NSAID is safer than another for perioperative administration (Hunt *et al.*, 2015b) and generally there is also no evidence to indicate that as a class of drug one NSAID preparation is more efficacious in terms of analgesia than another. The only study to show superior analgesia for one NSAID over another was conducted in cats undergoing ovariohysterectomy and showed robenacoxib to be superior to meloxicam (Kamata *et al.*, 2012). However, it is important to note that in this study pain scores were very low in all animals, so the clinical relevance of the lower pain scores in the robenacoxib group can be questioned.

In dogs undergoing castration 1 mg/kg lidocaine injected into each testicle has been shown to reduce the requirement for isoflurane and is a simple and cheap method of enhancing analgesia (McMillan *et al.*, 2012).

As the majority of neutering procedures are short, alpha-2 agonists may help to provide additional analgesia despite their short duration of action.

Simple fractures
There is evidence that methadone provides superior analgesia to buprenorphine in dogs undergoing orthopaedic surgery (Hunt *et al.*, 2013). The study by Hunt *et al.* (2013) supports the selection of methadone as the premedicant opioid for animals expected to experience moderate to severe surgical pain. Buprenorphine is more suitable for animals expected to experience mild pain during surgery or moderate pain if a multimodal analgesia technique employing local anaesthesia techniques is utilized.

Local or locoregional techniques should be used where possible in these cases; details of techniques can be found in Appendix 2.

Mass removal
Perioperative analgesia should be provided based on the site and extent of the mass to be

removed. There is good evidence in both animals and humans that the perioperative period can influence the likelihood of cancer recurrence and metastasis (Snyder and Greenberg, 2010). Acute pain and stress will increase the likelihood of recurrence at the site and metastases, and therefore the authors believe that good perioperative analgesia is imperative for these cases. Lidocaine, and the preoperative use of morphine and tramadol, has been shown to have a positive effect on outcome and survival in cancer patients (both animal and human); therefore, the authors believe that local anaesthetic techniques should be employed where possible in these cases to attempt to reduce local recurrence and metastases. There is some evidence that ketamine may increase the likelihood of metastasis and local recurrence and therefore other methods of analgesia should be preferentially employed in these cases (Melamed et al., 2003).

Ear procedures

In the authors' experience, animals undergoing even simple ear procedures experience high levels of nociceptive input; therefore, adequate perioperative analgesia should be provided for these cases. In animals undergoing total ear canal ablation local techniques have not been shown to increase analgesia over systemic opioids; however, the use of lidocaine in wound catheters has been shown to provide better analgesia than morphine (Buback et al., 1996; Wolfe et al., 2006).

References and further reading

Bergadano A, Andersen OK, Arendt-Nielsen L et al. (2009) Plasma levels of a low-dose constant-rate-infusion of ketamine and its effect on single and repeated nociceptive stimuli in conscious dogs. Veterinary Journal 182, 252–260

Berry SH (2016) Analgesia in the perioperative period. Veterinary Clinics of North America: Small Animal Practice 45, 1013–1027

Brondani JT, Loureiro Luna SP, Beier SL, Minto BW and Padovani CR (2009) Analgesic efficacy of perioperative use of vedaprofen, tramadol or their combination in cats undergoing ovariohysterectomy. Journal of Feline Medicine and Surgery 11, 420–429

Buback JL, Boothe HW, Carroll GL and Green RW (1996) Comparison of three methods for relief of pain after ear canal ablation in dogs. Veterinary Surgery 25, 380–385

Capner CA, Lascelles BD and Waterman-Pearson AE (1999) Current British veterinary attitudes to perioperative analgesia for dogs. Veterinary Record 145, 95–99

Carstensen M and Möller AM (2010) Adding ketamine to morphine for intravenous patient-controlled analgesia for acute postoperative pain: a qualitative review of randomized trials. British Journal of Anaesthesia 104, 401–406

Columbano N, Secci F, Careddu GM et al. (2012) Effects of lidocaine constant rate infusion on sevoflurane requirement, autonomic responses, and postoperative analgesia in dogs undergoing ovariectomy under opioid-based balanced anaesthesia. Veterinary Journal 193, 448–455

Credie RG, Teixeira Neto FJ, Ferreira TH et al. (2010) Effects of methadone on the minimum alveolar concentration of isoflurane in dogs. Veterinary Anaesthesia and Analgesia 37, 240–249

Gowan RA, Baral RM, Lingard AE et al. (2012) A retrospective analysis of the effects of meloxicam on the longevity of aged cats with and without overt chronic kidney disease. Journal of Feline Medicine and Surgery 14, 876–881

Gowan RA, Lingard AE, Johnston L et al. (2011) Restrospective case-control study of the effects of long-term dosing with meloxicam on renal function in aged cats with degenerative joint disease. Journal of Feline Medicine and Surgery 13, 752–761

Grape S and Tramèr MR (2007) Do we need preemptive analgesia for the treatment of postoperative pain? Best Practice and Research Clinical Anaesthesiology 21, 51–63

Gruet P, Seewald W and King JN (2013) Robenacoxib versus meloxicam for the management of pain and inflammation associated with soft tissue surgery in dogs: a randomized, non-inferiority clinical trial. BMC Veterinary Research 9, 92

Hunt JR, Attenburrow PM, Slingsby LS and Murrell JC (2013) Comparison of premedication with buprenorphine or methadone with meloxicam for postoperative analgesia in dogs undergoing orthopaedic surgery. Journal of Small Animal Practice 54, 418–424

Hunt JR, Dean RS, Davis GN et al. (2015b) An analysis of the relative frequencies of reported adverse events associated with NSAID administration in dogs and cats in the United Kingdom. Veterinary Journal 206, 183–190

Hunt JR, Knowles TG, Lascelles BD and Murrell JC (2015a) Prescription of perioperative analgesics by UK small animal veterinary surgeons in 2013. Veterinary Record 176, 493

Jakobsson JG (2014) Pain management in ambulatory surgery – a review. Pharmaceuticals (Basel) 7, 850–865

Kamata M, King JN, Seewald W et al. (2012) Comparison of injectable robenacoxib versus meloxicam for peri-operative use in cats: results of a randomised clinical trial. Veterinary Journal 193, 114–118

Katz J, Clarke H and Seltzer Z (2011) Review article: preventive analgesia: quo vadimus? Anaesthesia and Analgesia 113, 1242–1253

Kelly DJ, Ahmad M, Brull SJ (2001) Preemptive analgesia II: recent advances and current trends. Canadian Journal of Anesthesia 48, 1091–1101

Kissin I (2000) Preemptive analgesia. Anesthesiology 93, 1138–1143

Lascelles BDX, Capner CA and Waterman-Pearson AE (1999) Current British veterinary attitudes to perioperative analgesia for cats and small mammals. Veterinary Record 145, 601–604

Lascelles BD, Cripps PJ, Jones A and Waterman-Pearson AE (1998) Efficacy and kinetics of carprofen, administered preoperatively or postoperatively, for the prevention of pain in dogs undergoing ovariohysterectomy. *Veterinary Surgery* **27**, 568–582

Laskowski K, Stirling A, McKay WP and Lim HJ (2011) A systematic review of intravenous ketamine for postoperative analgesia. *Canadian Journal of Anesthesia* **58**, 911–923

Lui F and Ng KF (2011) Adjuvant analgesics in acute pain. *Expert Opinion on Pharmacotherapy* **12**, 363–385

Luna SP, Basilio AC, Steagall PV *et al.* (2007) Evaluation of the adverse effects of long-term oral administration of carprofen, etodolac, flunixin meglumine, ketoprofen, and meloxicam in dogs. *American Journal of Veterinary Research* **68**, 258–264

McMillan MW, Seymour CJ and Brearley JC (2012) Effect of intratesticular lidocaine on isoflurane requirements in dogs undergoing routine castration. *Journal of Small Animal Practice* **53**, 393–397

McQuay HJ (1995) Pre-emptive analgesia: a systematic review of clinical studies. *Annals of Medicine* **27**, 249–256

Melamed R, Bar-Yosef S, Shakhar G, Shakhar K and Ben-Eliyahu S (2003) Suppression of natural killer cell activity and promotion of tumor metastasis by ketamine, thiopental, and halothane, but not by propofol: mediating mechanisms and prophylactic measures. *Anesthesia and Analgesia* **97**, 1331–1339

Moiniche S, Kehlet H and Dahl JB (2002) A qualitative and quantitative systematic review of preemptive analgesia for postoperative pain relief: the role of timing of analgesia. *Anaesthesiology* **96**, 725–741

Monteiro-Steagall BP, Steagall PV and Lascelles BD (2013) Systematic review of nonsteroidal anti-inflammatory drug-induced adverse effects in dogs. *Journal of Veterinary Internal Medicine* **27**, 1011–1019

Nakamura T and Takasaki M (2001) Intrathecal pre-administration of fentanyl effectively suppresses formalin evoked c-Fos expression in spinal cord of rat. *Canadian Journal of Anesthesia* **48**, 993–999

Oifa S, Sydoruk T, White I *et al.* (2009) Effects of intravenous patient-controlled analgesia with buprenorphine and morphine alone and in combination during the first 12 postoperative hours: a randomized, double blind, four-arm trial in adults undergoing abdominal surgery. *Clinical Therapeutics* **31**, 527–541

Ortega M and Cruz I (2011) Evaluation of a constant rate infusion of lidocaine for balanced anaesthesia in dogs undergoing surgery. *Canadian Veterinary Journal* **52**, 856–860

Pypendop BH and Ilkiw JE (2005) Assessment of the haemodynamic effects of lidocaine administered IV in isoflurane-anaesthetized cats. *American Journal of Veterinary Research* **66**, 661–668

Sarrau S, Jordan J, Dupuis-Soyris F and Verwaerde P (2007) Effects of postoperative ketamine infusion on pain control and feeding behaviour in bitches undergoing mastectomy. *Journal of Small Animal Practice* **48**, 670–676

Shah M, Yates D, Hunt J and Murrell J (2018) A comparison between methadone and buprenorphine for perioperative analgesia in dogs undergoing ovariohysterectomy. *Journal of Small Animal Practice* **59**, 531–538

Simões CR, Monteiro ER, Rangel JP, NUnes-Junior JS and Campagnol D (2016) Effects of a prolonged infusion of fentanyl, with or without atropine, on the minimum alveolar concentration of isoflurane in dogs. *Veterinary Anaesthesia and Analgesia* **43**, 136–144

Slingsby LS and Waterman-Pearson AE (2000) The post-operative analgesic effects of ketamine after canine ovario-hysterectomy—a comparison between pre- or post-operative administration. *Research in Veterinary Science* **69**, 147–152

Snyder GL and Greenberg S (2010) Effect of anaesthetic technique and other perioperative factors on cancer recurrence. *British Journal of Anaesthesia* **105**, 106–115

Valtolina C, Robben JH, Uilenreef J *et al.* (2009) Clinical evaluation of the efficacy and safety of a constant rate infusion of dexmedetomidine for postoperative pain management in dogs. *Veterinary Anaesthesia and Analgesia* **36**, 369–383

van Oostrom H, Doornenbal A, Schot A, Stienen PJ and Hellebrekers LJ (2011) Neurophysiological assessment of the sedative and analgesic effects of a constant rate infusion of dexmedetomidine in the dog. *Veterinary Journal* **190**, 338–344

Wagner AE, Walton JA, Hellyer PW, Gaynor JS and Mama KR (2002) Use of low doses of ketamine administered by constant rate infusion as an adjunct for postoperative analgesia in dogs. *Journal of the American Veterinary Medical Association* **221**, 72–75

Warne LB, Beths T, Holm M and Bauquier SH (2013) Comparison of perioperative analgesic efficacy of methadone and butorphanol in cats. *Journal of the American Veterinary Medical Association* **243**, 844–850

Warne LN, Beths T, Holm M, Carter JE and Bauquier SH (2014) Evaluation of the peri-operative analgesic efficacy of buprenorphine, compared with butorphanol, in cats. *Journal of the American Veterinary Medical Association* **245**, 195–202

Wolfe TM, Bateman SW, Cole LK and Smeak DD (2006) Evaluation of a local anesthetic delivery system for the postoperative analgesic management of canine total ear canal ablation – a randomized, controlled, double-blinded study. *Veterinary Anaesthesia and Analgesia* **33**, 328–330

Yang L, Zhang J, Zhang Z *et al.* (2014) Preemptive analgesia effects of ketamine in patients undergoing surgery. A meta-analysis. *Acta Cirúrgica Brasileira* **29**, 819–825

Zanuzzo FS, Teixeira-Neto FJ, Teixeiro LR *et al.* (2015) Analgesic and antihyperalgesic effects of dipyrone, meloxicam or a dipyrone-meloxicam combination in bitches undergoing ovariohysterectomy. *Veterinary Journal* **205**, 33–37

Chapter 4

Chronic and osteoarthritic pain

Kate White and James Hunt

Ongoing pain in dogs and cats presents specific challenges in terms of diagnosis, evaluation of pain, and response to treatment. Persistent pain may result from ongoing inflammatory conditions, such as degenerative joint disease (Brown *et al.*, 2008) or neoplasia (Brown *et al.*, 2009), resulting in ongoing nociceptive and inflammatory pain; impingement on, or dysfunction of, neural tissue (Brisson, 2010; Plessas *et al.*, 2012) producing neuropathic pain; or maladaptive changes following tissue healing, akin to persistent post-surgical pain in humans (Katz and Seltzer, 2009), which may include aspects of continued inflammatory and neuropathic pain, although the authors are unable to identify any veterinary case reports of the latter in the literature. One or more mechanisms of central sensitization (see below) may be provoked by, and further contribute to, any of the above sources of persistent pain.

Musculoskeletal pain represents a significant disease burden in veterinary species, with 20% of adult dogs (Johnston, 1997) and over 22% of adult cats (Bennett *et al.*, 2012) demonstrating radiographic signs of degenerative joint disease (DJD). Effective management of pain in such conditions is imperative for the welfare of affected animals; dogs affected by osteoarthritis (OA) have been identified as experiencing decreased quality of life, compared with unaffected dogs (Wiseman-Orr *et al.*, 2006). The focus of this chapter will be managing chronic pain associated with osteoarthritis.

Peripheral components of pain
Nociceptive pain

Potentially tissue-damaging stimuli (heat, pressure, cold, chemical) are capable of activating specific ion channels (e.g. TRPV1, TRPA1) located within Aδ and C fibre nociceptor cell membranes, permitting the influx of sodium and calcium, and generating action potentials, which are transmitted to the dorsal horn of the spinal cord. At synapses with ascending projection neurones, primary afferent fibres release glutamate, which binds to ligand-gated sodium and calcium channels (AMPA, NMDA), causing postsynaptic depolarization and propagation of action potentials to the brainstem, from where autonomic responses to nociception are coordinated, and higher centres, where nociceptive transmissions are integrated to generate perception of the nature, location and intensity of the pain.

Inflammatory pain

Actual tissue damage, such as may be encountered within inflamed synovial joints, results in the liberation of inflammatory molecules from damaged cells, which may produce a state of **peripheral sensitization**, in which the altered cellular environment results in the recruitment of 'silent' (high threshold, inactive in uninjured tissue) nociceptors, augmented action potential generation in response to the application of suprathreshold stimuli (producing **hyperalgesia**), and generation of spontaneous action potentials (causing spontaneous pain). Ongoing inflammatory processes, such as OA, will maintain nociceptors in a state of hyperexcitability.

Neuropathic pain

Pain arising as a direct consequence of a lesion or disease affecting the somatosensory system is termed neuropathic pain (Treede *et al.*, 2008) and may arise from lesions in either the peripheral or central nervous system (CNS). Common examples of neuropathic pain producing pathologies in small animals include syringomyelia and spinal cord compressive disc lesions. It is important to note that neuropathic pain is not synonymous with central sensitization, the latter (described below) may result from high intensity of sustained nociceptive input owing to nociceptive, inflammatory or neuropathic sources of pain.

Central sensitization

The propensity of ascending neurones to relay nociceptive information to higher structures within the CNS is governed by the net effect of opposing facilitatory and inhibitory mechanisms, which act to regulate the excitability of spinal cord neurones. A number of these mechanisms are described here.

Facilitation of nociceptive transmission

Increased facilitation of nociceptive impulses within ascending neurones can be produced by repeated C fibre stimulation, as may be present during inflammatory states. One mechanism through which facilitation occurs involves the N-methyl-D-aspartate (NMDA) receptor. During normal states, the influx of calcium to postsynaptic neurones caused by the binding of glutamate to the NMDA receptor (calcium channel) is reduced by the presence of a magnesium ion within the channel pore. Ongoing depolarization of the postsynaptic membrane (e.g. frequent C fibre action potentials) results in removal of the magnesium blockade, and greatly increased calcium influx in response to glutamate binding (Nowak *et al.*, 1984). Postsynaptic facilitation has also been ascribed to synaptic release of substance P, tumour necrosis factor alpha, and prostaglandins. Increased central transmission in response to nociceptive stimulation contributes to the clinical phenomenon of hyperalgesia.

Access of non-nociceptive afferents to nociceptive dorsal horn cells

Non-nociceptive information, such as touching or stroking of the skin, is conveyed to the CNS via Aβ afferent fibres. Similar to nociceptive afferents, these fibres synapse with modality-specific ascending projection neurones; however, the specificity of sensory transfer is reliant on effective inhibitory interneurones, which prevent cross-talk between low threshold Aβ fibres and ascending nociceptive neurones (Schoffnegger *et al.*, 2008; Sandkuhler, 2009). A failure of inhibitory interneurone activity permits innocuous sensations to be misinterpreted as painful, a phenomenon termed **allodynia**.

Decreased endogenous inhibition of nociceptive information

C fibre nociceptive afferent input provokes a spino-bulbar-spinal reflex termed descending noxious inhibitory control (DNIC), which increases the activity in descending alpha-2 adrenergic and 5-HT neurones, resulting in decreased dorsal horn activity in response to noxious stimuli applied to distant sites. In a number of chronic pain conditions, including OA, decreased efficacy of DNIC has been reported, which has then normalized following successful joint replacement (Kosek and Ordeberg, 2000).

Glial cell activation

Non-neuronal peripheral and centrally located immune cells have been implicated in the maintenance of neuropathic pain through their release of cytokines, histamine and serotonin (Moalem and Tracey, 2006). Experimental inhibition of glial cells reduced the development of hyperalgesia associated with myositis in rats (Chacur et al., 2009).

Myofascial pain

Myofascial trigger points (MTrPs), defined as 'a hyperirritable spot in skeletal muscle that is associated with a hypersensitive palpable nodule in a taut band' (Dommerholt et al., 2006) may contribute to the overall pain experience of patients with musculoskeletal disease. In humans, such points exhibit characteristic ultrasonographic, electromyographic, biochemical and clinical features (Dommerholt et al., 2006; Shah et al., 2008; Sikdar et al., 2009). The presence of active MTrPs correlates with a higher intensity of ongoing pain in women with OA of the knee (Alburquerque-Garcia et al., 2015). There is no currently published work investigating the presence of MTrPs in animals with respect to validated pain scoring or objective measures of locomotor function; however, it is likely that, as in humans, they do represent further sources of pain beyond the joint and the nervous system.

Assessment of chronic pain

Dogs

The assessment of chronic pain in dogs is reliant upon subjective and objective measures reported by the owner. These will likely include changes in daily activities, behaviours and possibly lameness. Owners may observe changes such as aggression, withdrawal or mood changes and, in some cases, signs such as inappropriate elimination or lack of grooming. It may not be obvious on initial presentation that some of these signs are related to pain. A comprehensive and methodical history-taking and clinical examination are of the utmost importance.

There are a small number of pain assessment tools (PATs) (Figure 4.1) that can be used to help the owner and vet describe the maladaptive pain that the dog is experiencing and these can also help in monitoring the response to treatment. Pain assessment tools should ideally be able to cover the various domains of chronic pain, and include changes in movement, posture, and the emotional aspects.

Pain assessment tool	Validation and examples of use	Comments
Liverpool Osteoarthritis in Dogs questionnaire (LOAD)	(Walton et al., 2013)	• Owner questionnaire • 23 questions using a 5-point Likert scale • Questions cover lifestyle and mobility
Canine Brief Pain Inventory (CBPI)	(Brown et al., 2007)	• Owner questionnaire • 11 questions on an 11 point (0–10) numerical scale • Questions cover pain severity and pain interference

4.1 Pain assessment tools for maladaptive pain in dogs. QoL = quality of life. (continues) ▶

Pain assessment tool	Validation and examples of use	Comments
Helsinki Chronic Pain Index (HCPI)	(Hielm-Björkman et al., 2009)	• Owner questionnaire • 11 questions • Questions cover mood and mobility. Dogs experiencing ongoing painful conditions are differentiated from dogs without pain when they score greater than 12 on the HCPI
American College of Veterinary Surgeons Canine Orthopaedic Index	(Brown, 2013)	• Owner questionnaire • 16 questions using a 5-point Likert scale • Relating to four domains; stiffness, function, gait, and quality of life
Client Specific Outcome Measures (CSOM)	A patient-specific tool for all species; templates are available (Lascelles et al., 2008)	• Objective tool designed between owner and veterinary surgeon for each dog to assess measures to which the client can relate
Quality of Life Assessment (HRQL) Vetmetrica	(Reid et al., 2013)	• Web-based owner questionnaire • 46 questions • The outcome generates a QoL profile
Quality of Life Assessment (Yazbek)	(Yazbek and Fantoni, 2005)	• Owner questionnaire • 12 questions • QoL tool to assess pain secondary to cancer
End of trial questionnaires	(Hielm-Björkman et al., 2007)	• Can be used to assess satisfaction with trial or guessing what group the animal was in
Visual analogue scale (VAS)	(Hielm-Björkman et al., 2011)	• Useful low cost, basic observational tool • Some limitations for inexperienced owners
Numeric rating scale (NRS)	(Wiseman-Orr et al., 2006)	• Useful low cost, basic observational tool • VAS more sensitive than NRS
Simple descriptive scale	(Hielm-Björkman et al., 2003)	• Simple tool • 3–5 answers ranked on a severity scale

4.1 (continued) Pain assessment tools for maladaptive pain in dogs. QoL = quality of life.

Cats

The assessment of chronic pain in cats is particularly difficult; the signs of pain are subtle and can be difficult to describe. In addition, owners are typically less likely to seek veterinary advice in these cases, and it is likely that the options for treatment are considered very limited. A paucity of validated quality of life questionnaires or chronic OA questionnaires, and limited data about complementary treatments and disease-modifying agents or dietary supplements, which is often at best anecdotal, further hamper this, in contrast to the dog. Notwithstanding these challenges, the feline patient should not be deprived of options for addressing the pain. Figure 4.2 details the PATs that can be used for cats.

Physical examination

The environment for the examination is very important; a table with a comfortable soft, non-slip surface, away from other animals and with no places to escape (for cats) should be used, with an awareness that the examination/consultation can take considerable time to perform thoroughly.

Gently examine the animal with minimal restraint; this may require a stepwise approach, pausing regularly to allow the animal to move around and explore before resuming

Pain assessment tool	Examples of use	Comments
Client questionnaire of behavioural and lifestyle changes	(Bennett and Morton, 2009)	• Owner questionnaire for before and after (1 month of) therapy • Four domains: mobility, activity, grooming, temperament
Feline Musculoskeletal Pain Index (FMPI)	(Benito et al., 2013)	• Owner questionnaire • 21 questions covering activity, pain intensity and overall QoL
Client questionnaire of behavioural and lifestyle changes	(Slingerland et al., 2011)	• Owner questionnaire • 26 questions covering activities, lifestyle and behaviours • Based on Bennett and Morton (2009) and Lascelles et al. (2007)
Client Specific Outcome Measures (CSOM)	A patient-specific tool for all species; templates are available (Lascelles et al., 2007)	• Objective tool designed between owner and veterinary surgeon for each cat to assess measures to which the client can relate
Combination of CSOM & FMPI used before and after cessation of trial	(Gruen et al., 2014)	• Novel methodology to limit the placebo effect including a masked washout period
End of trial questionnaires	(Hielm-Björkman et al., 2007)	• Can be used to assess satisfaction with trial or guessing what group the animal was in
Visual analogue scale (VAS)	Has been used in acute pain in cats (Slingsby et al., 2001)	• Useful low cost, basic observational tool
Numeric rating scale (NRS)	Has been used in acute pain in cats (Ingwersen et al., 2012)	• Useful low cost, basic observational tool
Simple descriptive scale (SDS)	(Clarke and Bennett, 2006)	• Simple tool • 3–5 answers ranked on a severity scale

4.2 Pain assessment tools for maladaptive pain in cats. QoL = quality of life.

examination. A gentle, slow and thorough approach will also ensure a solid relationship of trust is established with the owner.

The evaluation should begin with a general examination before proceeding to a complete neurological and orthopaedic examination. In addition, the animal should undergo systematic myofascial palpation, with gentle pressure along the muscle bellies starting on the neck, working along the longitudinal muscles either side of the spinous processes, to the pelvic girdle and down each muscle mass. During the palpation it may be possible to locate myofascial trigger points; these discrete and usually longitudinal regions are hardened areas in the muscle belly, distinct from generalized muscle spasm.

A comprehensive history must also be taken to identify the signs of OA (Klinck et al., 2012). The use of a checklist or questionnaire for the owner to carefully consider the animal's behaviours and activity ensures no aspects are omitted. It is also worth questioning the owner about the personality of the cat or dog as this can affect the pain assessment both at home and in the hospital environment (Zeiler et al., 2014). There remains uncertainty as to whether the owner should be reminded of their previous answers or scoring when they revisit for follow-up (Muller et al., 2016). In all situations, it is important to consider the sensory and affective (emotional) aspects of pain. Questions for the owner should attempt to address both these domains.

Based on the history and clinical examination, further diagnostic imaging and haematological/biochemical evaluation may be necessary. If the aetiology is identifiable, a resolution may be possible, but in many cases long-term palliative treatments will be required. The use of a questionnaire at each visit will help to tailor the treatment plan and assess improvement or deterioration.

Treatment of chronic pain

Chronic pain has many different aetiologies and these should be considered when devising a treatment plan. The goal of treatment is the provision of effective analgesia with minimal side effects. Many different analgesics can be used and the agents are listed in Figures 4.3 (dogs) and 4.4 (cats), with suggested algorithms for approaches to treatment outlined in Figures 4.5 (dogs) and 4.6 (cats).

Drug	Dose	Comments
Carprofen	2–4 mg/kg orally q24h (or divided in two doses) for 5 days, then reduced to 2 mg/kg daily depending on clinical response	Indicated for musculoskeletal disorders and DJD
Cimicoxib	2 mg/kg orally q24h	Indicated for pain and inflammation of OA
Deracoxib	1–2 mg/kg orally q24h	Indicated for OA in USA No MA in UK
Etodolac	10–15 mg/kg orally q24h	Indicated for OA in USA No MA in UK
Firocoxib	5 mg/kg orally q24h	Indicated for OA in dogs Field trials limited to 90 days
Grapiprant	2 mg/kg orally q24h	Indicated for OA
Paracetamol (acetaminophen)	10–15 mg/kg orally q8–12h 10 mg/kg i.v. q12h	
Phenylbutazone	20 mg/kg orally q24h (preferably divided in two or three doses) for 7 days, then 10 mg/kg q24h (divided in two or three doses)	Indicated for OA, rheumatoid and other arthritic diseases
Prednoleucotropin (PLT) (cinchophen and prednisolone)	25 mg/kg cinchophen and 0.125 mg/kg prednisolone orally q12h	Indicated for OA, 14 day trial followed by 14 days free of treatment
Mavacoxib	2 mg/kg orally once then repeated 12 days later, then monthly for up to 6 months	Indicated for pain and inflammation of DJD
Meloxicam	0.2 mg/kg orally q24h on day 1, followed by 0.1 mg/kg orally	Indicated for pain and inflammation in chronic musculoskeletal disorders
Robenacoxib	1–2 mg/kg orally q24h	Indicated for pain and inflammation of chronic OA
Tepoxalin	10–20 mg/kg orally q24h on day 1 followed by 10 mg/kg orally q24h	Indicated for OA

4.3 Non-steroidal anti-inflammatory drugs (NSAIDs) and other anti-inflammatory and pain-relieving products for use in dogs with chronic maladaptive pain. Very few products have long-term market authorization (MA) and treatment must be closely supervised by a veterinary surgeon. Consult datasheets for further information. Use the lowest effective dose and a multimodal approach. All NSAIDs are capable of causing gastrointestinal signs and lesions, and hepatic and renal injury. Regular monitoring of patients is necessary. DJD = degenerative joint disease; OA = osteoarthritis.

Drug	Dose	Comments
Aspirin	10 mg/kg every third day	Used as an anti-thrombotic agent
Carprofen	N/A	Not recommended
Etodolac	N/A	Not recommended
Firocoxib	N/A	Not trialled in cats
Paracetamol (acetaminophen)	N/A	Contraindicated
Phenylbutazone	N/A	Not recommended
Prednisolone	0.5–1 mg/kg orally q24h	Do not administer NSAIDs concurrently
Meloxicam	0.1 mg/kg orally q24h on day 1, followed by 0.05 mg/kg orally	Indicated for pain and inflammation in chronic musculoskeletal disorders
Robenacoxib	1–2 mg/kg orally q24h (up to 6 days)	Indicated for pain and inflammation of chronic OA, may be suitable for longer term administration
Tepoxalin	12 mg/kg/day	No MA, but one study found tepoxalin was well tolerated compared with meloxicam particularly for urinary tract discomfort (Charlton *et al.*, 2013)
Tolfenamic acid	4 mg/kg orally q24h (up to 3 days)	Not indicated for chronic pain
Vedaprofen	0.5 mg/kg orally q24h (up to 3 days)	Not indicated for chronic pain

4.4 Non-steroidal anti-inflammatory drugs (NSAIDs) and other anti-inflammatory and pain-relieving products for use in cats with chronic maladaptive pain. Very few products have long-term market authorization (MA) and treatment must be closely supervised by a veterinary surgeon. Consult datasheets for further information. Use the lowest effective dose and a multimodal approach. All NSAIDs are capable of causing gastrointestinal signs and lesions, and hepatic and renal injury. Regular monitoring of patients is necessary. OA = osteoarthritis.

Non-steroidal anti-inflammatory drugs

NSAIDs remain the most popular medications for treating chronic pain in dogs and cats. They reduce the production of inflammatory prostaglandins by selective inhibition of the cyclooxygenase-2 (COX-2) enzyme producing a peripheral anti-inflammatory effect. Furthermore, these drugs will cause a reduced sensitization within the CNS. Several formulations have market authorization for long-term use in dogs; meloxicam is licensed for long-term use in cats in the UK and guidelines have been developed for long-term use of NSAIDs in cats (Sparkes *et al.*, 2010). Recent studies also suggest robenacoxib may be safe in cats (King *et al.*, 2015; King *et al.*, 2012). There are no controlled trials demonstrating superiority of one NSAID over another in OA, and there appears to be significant interpatient variability in terms of efficacy and side effects. In animals that show a lack of response to one NSAID, it is worth considering swapping to another. In cases where a swap is made it is suggested to allow a 5–7 day washout period between the drugs (Kukanich *et al.*, 2012). Sustained release formulations of NSAIDs are being developed and trialled.

Non-cyclo-oxygenase anti-inflammatory drugs

To attempt to reduce the potential for adverse events associated with the inhibition of COX enzymes, an EP4 prostaglandin receptor antagonist has been studied in client-owned dogs, which demonstrated improved pain relief compared with placebo (Derra *et al.*, 2016). Grapiprant is planned for release in the UK in early 2019.

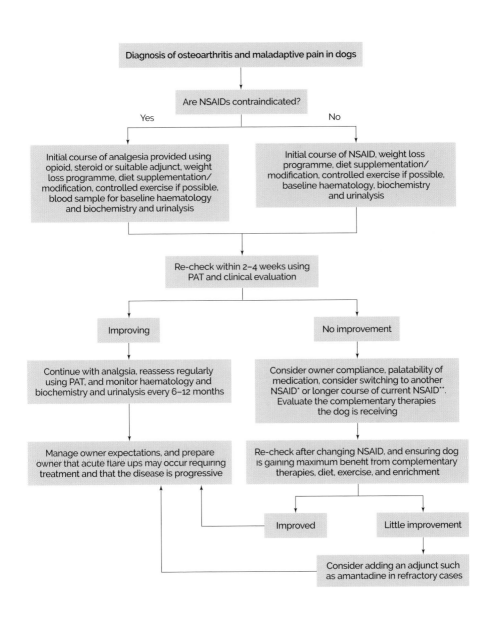

4.5 Decision-making algorithm for managing chronic pain in dogs. NSAID = non-steroidal anti-inflammatory drug; PAT = pain assessment tool. * = Bridging medication may be required for the washout period; ** = Re-evaluate diagnosis.

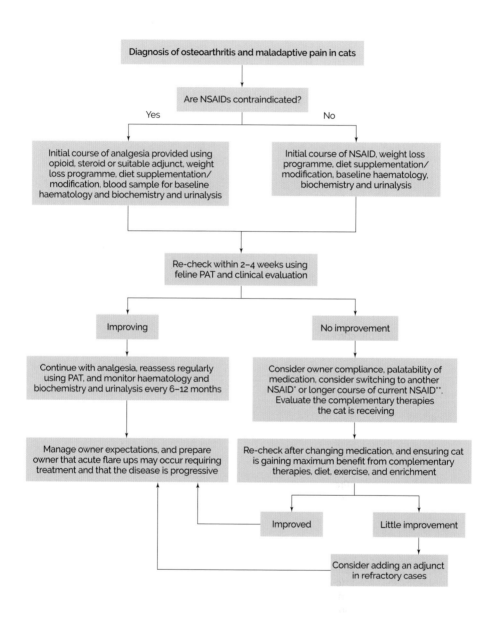

4.6 Decision-making algorithm for managing chronic pain in cats. NSAID = non-steroidal anti-inflammatory drug; PAT = pain assessment tool. * = Bridging medication may be required for the washout period; ** = Re-evaluate diagnosis.

Paracetamol

Paracetamol's mode of action is still to be completely described but it has peripheral and central actions, and is widely prescribed in humans for chronic pain, although evidence for efficacy is weak (Hunter and Ferreira, 2016). Currently, there is no strong evidence to support the use of paracetamol in OA in dogs, but it may be suitable for use as a bridging medication (between switching NSAIDs) or in some cases in conjunction with NSAIDs. Paracetamol is available as a licensed formulation in combination with codeine limited to a 5-day course. The licence states it should not be co-administered with NSAIDs; however, it may, as in humans, be safe to use in dogs in conjunction with NSAIDs. The recommended dosage is 33 mg/kg in two or three divided doses. It is also available as an injectable solution (10 mg/kg over 5 mins). Paracetamol should be avoided in cats.

Steroids

Steroids can be of use if the chronic pain has an inflammatory component, but are not a commonly used first-line treatment because of the side effects associated with long-term use. Paradoxically, it has also been shown that steroids can exacerbate neuropathic pain in some human conditions (McEwen and Kalia, 2010). A prednisolone and cinchophen (prednoluecotropin) combination is available for dogs with OA and can be efficacious in some patients where other modalities have failed to bring about an improvement. Prednisolone can also be effective in cats; the lowest possible effective dose should be used.

Opioids

Long-term administration of opioids in cases of chronic pain is uncommon because of the side effects caused by these drugs (constipation, anorexia, sedation, pupil dilation, euphoria). Liposome-encapsulated and sustained-release formulations, which allow for a slower release and fewer side effects, may be suitable for some patients and conditions. Opioids may be of use in conjunction with other modalities, especially for acute episodes of flare up. See Chapters 3 and 5 for more information about acute pain and pharmacology, respectively.

Tramadol

Tramadol is an atypical synthetic opioid that interacts with adrenergic, serotonin and opioid receptors (Kukanich and Papich, 2004). The opioid mechanisms of action can be attributed to both the interaction of the parent compound and its metabolite mono-O-desmethyltramadol (M1) at the mu opioid receptor, although the production of active M1 is variable between dogs and this may explain the variability in analgesia efficacy. Currently the evidence is weak to support its use in dogs or cats with OA. Following administration there is a large variability in uptake, particularly with the human sustained-release formulation. In one study tramadol has been shown to have a positive effect in dogs with OA (Malek et al., 2012) and may be useful in some cases of chronic pain. Tramadol can be used in cats, but administration is hampered by the seemingly unpleasant taste of the tablet and side effects such as dysphoria and agitation. The recommended dosage for dogs is 2–4 mg/kg two to four times a day and for cats 2–4 mg/kg twice a day. Tramadol alone is unlikely to be efficacious for treating chronic pain, but may be a useful drug for animals with chronic pain that experience a flare up. Tramadol should not be used in animals that have received a monoamine oxidase inhibitor.

Adjunctive treatments

Gabapentin

Gabapentin is an anticonvulsant drug with antinociceptive effects. It has been successfully used as a first-line treatment in animals with neuropathic pain (Grubb, 2010). The recommended initial dose is 2.5–10 mg/kg two to three times a day, and gradual increases in dose are less likely to result in the side effect of sedation. It can be useful in managing chronic pain especially in cats unable to tolerate long-term administration of NSAIDs (Robertson, 2008), and appears to be a safe drug to use that can be dosed to effect (Rychel, 2010). Doses can be increased up to 50 mg/kg two to three times daily. The drug is eliminated exclusively via the renal route, so care should be taken in patients with renal insufficiency and doses modified accordingly. Pregabalin is similar to gabapentin, both being structural analogues of gamma-aminobutyric acid (GABA) and is also thought to modulate the presynaptic calcium channels resulting in a reduction of presynaptic transmitter release.

Amantadine and memantine

Amantadine is a NMDA antagonist drug and can be useful in conjunction with NSAIDs in dogs with chronic OA pain that is refractory to NSAIDs alone (Lascelles *et al.*, 2008). Amantadine can also be used alone for treating chronic pain. The side effects include agitation, sedation and mild GI signs, and are usually self-limiting (Macfarlane *et al.*, 2014); the drug is well tolerated in the geriatric animal. The most commonly recommended dose is 3–5 mg/kg once a day, but 2–10 mg/kg two to three times daily has also been suggested (Pozzi *et al.*, 2006).

Memantine has also been used in cases where amantadine was unavailable, with similar efficacy. The dosage for memantine is 0.3–0.5 mg/kg once or twice daily, increasing to 1 mg/kg twice daily (Schneider *et al.*, 2009).

Amitriptyline

Amitriptyline is a tricyclic antidepressant used in humans for controlling neuropathic pain. The mechanism of action is thought to be via central opioid receptors and also as a noradrenaline and serotonin reuptake inhibitor. One small study has documented its use in treating neuropathic pain in dogs. The recommended dose is 0.25–2 mg/kg once a day to twice a day. It may be prescribed in cats as well, with variable effects; 3–4 weeks of treatment may be necessary before the benefit is seen. Tricyclic antidepressants should not be used with tramadol, St John's wort, and other drugs that inhibit serotonin and noradrenaline uptake.

The placebo effect

The placebo effect should also be considered when assessing a patient's response to treatment. Caregiver placebo effects, affecting both the owner and veterinary surgeon, are very common in dogs undergoing treatment for OA (Conzemius and Evans, 2012).

The multimodal approach to treating maladaptive pain

The owner needs to appreciate that OA is a lifelong condition that can be managed but not cured. The plan should include analgesia, joint protection and nutritional support, which can then facilitate strengthening, conditioning, and increased exercise. In addition to the aforementioned drugs, the non-pharmacological pain therapies including physiotherapy, hydrotherapy and acupuncture play a large role in ensuring patient comfort. These modalities are covered in Chapter 6B.

It is vitally important that the owner is educated about the positive impact that all the modalities can have on their pet.

Environmental enrichment and modification

Careful consideration should be given to the animal's everyday environment. Simple concepts such as providing soft comfortable bedding, appropriate siting of beds, food bowls and litter trays, and reducing slippery floors, steep steps and the necessity to jump will ensure aggravation of OA is reduced. Enrichment such as regular grooming, toys, and human–animal interaction will also ensure mental stimulation and improve the animal's well being. Owners can be reassured that stroking and patting will not cause further pain, but may be of benefit as a gentle form of massage that may go some way to breaking the maladaptive cycle of irritating somatosensory input that causes allodynia.

In cases with identified myofascial trigger points, an attempt to address the pain and discomfort associated with this additional strain is essential with either dry needling, therapeutic lasers, or physical/manual therapy. The treatment of MTrP is still in its infancy in veterinary medicine, but its importance in contributing to chronic pain is becoming more widely recognized.

Disease-modifying interventions

Diet modification

Nutraceuticals are food supplements that are thought to modify the disease process of degenerative joint disease. The evidence for their efficacy in the maladaptive pain of OA is limited, despite their being widely used. The main body of evidence shows a benefit of oral supplementation with omega-3 fatty acids found in some fish oils and green-lipped mussel (*Perna canaliculus*) extracts (Bui and Bierer, 2001; Roush et al., 2010). One study recommended a dosage of 20–50 mg/kg/day of green-lipped mussel extract as a loading dose (Hielm-Björkman et al., 2009). Some prescription foods include these extracts in their mobility-promoting diets. Other food supplements, such as glucosamine, chondroitin, elk velvet antlers, hydrolysed collagen and turmeric, have only anecdotal evidence.

Palmitoyl ethanolamide (PEA) is a fatty acid amide molecule that has shown analgesic effects in a blinded comparison with ibuprofen for the treatment of temporomandibular joint pain in humans (Marini et al., 2012), but there are presently no published studies in dogs or cats. A nutritional supplement containing PEA was launched in the UK in 2016 (Redonyl, Dechra).

More importantly, owners must address weight reduction in pets that are above their ideal bodyweight. It is worth explaining to owners that obesity is a chronic low level inflammatory state that can exacerbate OA through the adipokines released from white adipose tissue. A moderate weight loss can reduce pain scores in animals suffering from OA (Marshall et al., 2010) and weight loss alone has been shown to improve quality of life in dogs (German et al., 2012), but the welfare obligation to provide pain relief remains, and the provision of analgesia may be required to enable the animal to undertake more exercise and strengthen muscles in the first instance.

Exercise

The role exercise can play in the management of the condition must be stressed to owners. Exercise will assist with weight reduction in overweight animals, the strengthening of muscles, and go some way to reduce the muscle atrophy that accompanies OA. Furthermore, the emotive component that exercise provides is likely to be of benefit. Exercise is shown to have a significant benefit in chronic pain conditions (Bobinski et al., 2015). See Chapter 6.

Other disease-modifying agents

Polysulphated glycosaminoglycans

These disease-modifying agents are indicated for use in dogs with OA and are licensed in some countries for intramuscular administration twice weekly for 4 weeks. Concurrent NSAIDs should be avoided and PSGAGs must not be given to animals with bleeding disorders.

Pentosan polysulphate

This agent is available as an injectable for a course of four injections each a week apart. Studies show conflicting and inconsistent results (Read et al., 1996; Sandersoln et al., 2000).

Hyaluronan

This is a non-sulfated glycosaminoglycan with little evidence of a positive effect on the progression of osteoarthritis.

Emerging treatments

Nerve growth factor antibody treatment

Two studies have recently been published demonstrating an analgesic effect of intravenous administration of a canine nerve growth factor antibody to dogs (Webster et al., 2014; Lascelles et al., 2015).

Stem cells

Intra-articular introduction of adipose-derived stem cells has shown efficacy in canine OA for 6 months following injection (Black *et al.*, 2007; 2008).

Summary

All treatment plans should be tailored to the individual patient and should take the form of plan, treat, evaluate. The PLATTER acronym can be used to educate the team and owners of the steps and remind everyone of the continuous cycle of pain control (Epstein *et al.*, 2015) (Figure 4.7).

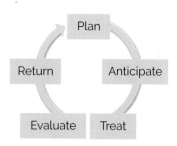

| **4.7** | PLATTER – acronym for the treatment of osteoarthritis in cats and dogs (Epstein *et al.*, 2015). |

References and further reading

Alburquerque-Garcia A, Rodrigues-de-Souza DP, Fernández-de-las-Peñas C and Alburquerque-Sendin F (2015) Association between muscle trigger points, ongoing pain, function, and sleep quality in elderly women with bilateral painful knee osteoarthritis. *Journal of Manipulative and Physiological Therapeutics* **38**, 262–268

Benito J, Hansen B, Depuy V *et al.* (2013) Feline musculoskeletal pain index: Responsiveness and testing of criterion validity. *Journal of Veterinary Internal Medicine* **27**, 474–482

Bennett D and Morton C (2009) A study of owner observed behavioural and lifestyle changes in cats with musculoskeletal disease before and after analgesic therapy. *Journal of Feline Medicine and Surgery* **11**, 997–1004.

Bennett D, Zainal Ariffin SM and Johnston P (2012) Osteoarthritis in the cat: 2. How should it be managed and treated? *Journal of Feline Medicine and Surgery* **14**, 76–84

Black LL, Gaynor J, Adams C *et al.* (2008) Effect of intraarticular injection of autologous adipose-derived mesenchymal stem and regenerative cells on clinical signs of chronic osteoarthritis of the elbow joint in dogs. *Veterinary Therapeutics* **9**, 192–200

Black LL, Gaynor J, Gahring D *et al.* (2007) Effect of adipose-derived mesenchymal stem and regenerative cells on lameness in dogs with chronic osteoarthritis of the coxofemoral joints: a randomized, double-blinded, multicenter, controlled trial. *Veterinary Therapeutics: Research in Applied Veterinary Medicine* **8**, 272–284

Bobinski F, Ferreira TAA, Córdova MM *et al.* (2015) Role of brainstem serotonin in analgesia produced by low-intensity exercise on neuropathic pain following sciatic nerve injury in mice. *Pain* **156**, 2595–2606

Brisson BA (2010) Intervertebral disc disease in dogs. *Veterinary Clinics of North America – Small Animal Practice* **40**, 829–858

Brown DC (2014) The Canine Orthopedic Index. Step 3: Responsiveness Testing. *Veterinary Surgery* **43**, 247–254

Brown DC, Boston RC, Coyne JC and Farrar JT (2007) Development and psychometric testing of an instrument designed to measure chronic pain in dogs with osteoarthritis. *American Journal of Veterinary Research* **68**, 631–637

Brown DC, Boston RC, Coyne JC and Farrar JT (2008) Ability of the canine brief pain inventory to detect response to treatment in dogs with osteoarthritis. *Journal of the American Veterinary Medical Association* **233**, 278–1283

Brown DC, Boston RC, Coyne JC and Farrar JT (2009) A novel approach to the use of animals in studies of pain: Validation of the canine brief pain inventory in canine bone cancer. *Pain Medicine* **10**, 133–142

Brown DC, Boston RC and Farrar JT (2013) Comparison of force plate gait analysis and owner assessment of pain using the canine brief pain inventory in dogs with osteoarthritis. *Journal of Veterinary Internal Medicine* **27**, 22–30

Bui LM and Bierer RL (2001) Influence of green lipped mussels (*Perna canaliculus*) in alleviating signs of arthritis in dogs. *Veterinary Therapeutics: Research in Applied Veterinary Medicine* **2**, 101–111

Chacur M, Lambertz D, Hoheisel U and Mense S (2009) Role of spinal microglia in myositis-induced central sensitisation: An immunohistochemical and behavioural study in rats. *European Journal of Pain* **13**, 915–923

Clarke S and Bennett D (2006) Feline osteoarthritis: a prospective study of 28 cases. *Journal of Small Animal Practice* **47**, 439–445

Conzemius MG and Evans RB (2012) Caregiver placebo effect for dogs with lameness from osteoarthritis. *Journal of the American Veterinary Medical Association* **241**, 1314–1319

Derra LR, Huebner M and Wofford J (2016) A prospective, randomized, masked, placebo-controlled multisite clinical study of grapiprant, an EP4 prostaglandin receptor antagonist (PRA), in dogs with osteoarthritis. *Journal of Veterinary Internal Medicine* **30**, 756–763

Dommerholt J, Bron C and Franssen J (2006) Myofascial trigger points: an evidence-informed review. *Journal of Manual and Manipulative Therapy* **14**, 203–221

Epstein ME, Rodanm I, Griffenhagen G *et al.* (2015) 2015 AAHA/AAFP pain management guidelines for dogs and cats. *Journal of Feline Medicine and Surgery* **17**, 251–272

German AJ, Holden SL, Wiseman-Orr ML *et al.* (2012) Quality of life is reduced in obese dogs but improves after successful weight loss. *Veterinary Journal* **192**, 428–434

Gowan RA, Baral RM, Lingard AE *et al.* (2012) A retrospective analysis of the effects of meloxicam on the longevity of aged cats with and without overt chronic kidney disease. *Journal of Feline Medicine and Surgery* **14**, 876–881

Gowan RA, Lingard AE, Johnston L *et al.* (2011) Retrospective case-control study of the effects of long-term dosing with meloxicam on renal function in aged cats with degenerative joint disease. *Journal of Feline Medicine and Surgery* **13**, 752–761

Grubb T (2010) Chronic neuropathic pain in veterinary patients. *Topics in Companion Animal Medicine* **25**, 45–52

Gruen ME, Griffith E, Thomson A, Simpson W and Lascelles BD (2014) Detection of clinically relevant pain relief in cats with degenerative joint disease associated pain. *Journal of Veterinary Internal Medicine* **28**, 346–350

Hielm-Björkman AK, Kapatkin AS and Rita HJ (2011) Reliability and validity of a visual analogue scale used by owners to measure chronic pain attributable to osteoarthritis in their dogs. *American Journal of Veterinary Research* **72**, 601–607

Hielm-Björkman AK, Kuusela E, Liman A *et al.* (2003) Evaluation of methods for assessment of pain associated with chronic osteoarthritis in dogs. *Journal of the American Veterinary Medical Association* **222**, 1552–1558

Hielm-Björkman AK, Reunanen V, Meri P and Tulamo RM (2007) Panax Ginseng in combination with brewers' yeast (Gerivet®) as a stimulant for geriatric dogs: a controlled-randomized blinded study. *Journal of Veterinary Pharmacology and Therapeutics* **30**, 295–304

Hielm-Björkman AK, Rita H and Tulamo RM (2009) Psychometric testing of the Helsinki chronic pain index by completion of a questionnaire in Finnish by owners of dogs with chronic signs of pain caused by osteoarthritis. *American Journal of Veterinary Research* **70**, 727–734

Hielm-Björkman AK, Tulamo R-M, Salonen H and Raekallio M (2009) Evaluating complementary therapies for canine osteoarthritis part I: Green-lipped mussel (*Perna canaliculus*). *Evidence-based Complementary and Alternative Medicine* **6**, 365–373

Hunter DJ and Ferreira ML (2016) Osteoarthritis: yet another death knell for paracetamol in OA. *Nature Reviews: Rheumatology* **12**, 320–321

Ingwersen W, Fox R, Cunningham G *et al.* (2012) Efficacy and safety of 3 *versus* 5 days of meloxicam as an analgesic for feline onychectomy and sterilization. *The Canadian Veterinary Journal* **53**, 257–264

Johnston SA (1997) Osteoarthritis. Joint anatomy, physiology, and pathobiology. *Veterinary Clinics of North America: Small Animal Practice* **27**, 699–723

Katz J and Seltzer Z (2009) Transition from acute to chronic postsurgical pain: risk factors and protective factors. *Expert Review of Neurotherapeutics* **9**, 723–744

King JN, Hotz R, Reagan EL *et al.* (2012) Safety of oral robenacoxib in the cat. *Journal of Veterinary Pharmacology and Therapeutics* **35**, 290–300

King JN, King S, Budsberg SC *et al.* (2015) Clinical safety of robenacoxib in feline osteoarthritis: results of a randomized, blinded, placebo-controlled clinical trial. *Journal of Feline Medicine and Surgery* **18**, 632–642

Klinck MP, Frank D, Guillot M and Troncy E (2012) Owner-perceived signs and veterinary diagnosis in 50 cases of feline osteoarthritis. *Canadian Veterinary Journal* **53**, 1181–1186

Kosek E and Ordeberg G (2000) Lack of pressure pain modulation by heterotopic noxious conditioning stimulation in patients with painful osteoarthritis before, but not following, surgical pain relief. *Pain* **88**, 69–78

Kukanich B, Bidgood T and Knesl O (2012) Clinical pharmacology of nonsteroidal anti-inflammatory drugs in dogs. *Veterinary Anaesthesia and Analgesia* **39**, 69–90

Kukanich B and Papich MG (2004) Pharmacokinetics of tramadol and the metabolite O-desmethyltramadol in dogs. *Journal of Veterinary Pharmacology and Therapeutics* **27**, 239–246

Laflamme D (1997) Development and validation of a body condition score system for dogs. *Canine Practice* **22**, 10–15

Landsberg GM, Denenberg S and Araujo JA (2010) Cognitive dysfunction in cats. A syndrome we used to dismiss as 'old age.' *Journal of Feline Medicine and Surgery* **12**, 837–848

Lascelles BDX, DePuy V, Thomson A *et al.* (2010) Evaluation of a therapeutic diet for feline degenerative joint disease. *Journal of Veterinary Internal Medicine* **24**, 487–495

Lascelles BDX, Gaynor JC, Smith ES *et al.* (2008) Amantadine in a multimodal analgesic regimen for alleviation of refractory osteoarthritis pain in dogs. *Journal of Veterinary Internal Medicine* **22**, 53–59

Lascelles BDX, Hansen BD, Roe S *et al.* (2007) Evaluation of client-specific outcome measures and activity monitoring to measure pain relief in cats with osteoarthritis. *Journal of Veterinary Internal Medicine* **21**, 410–416

Lascelles BDX, Knazovicky D, Case B *et al.* (2015) A canine-specific anti-nerve growth factor antibody alleviates pain and improves mobility and function in dogs with degenerative joint disease-associated pain. *BMC Veterinary Research* **11**, 101

Lascelles BDX and Robertson SA (2010) DJD-associated pain in cats. What can we do to promote patient comfort? *Journal of Feline Medicine and Surgery* **12**, 200–212

Macfarlane PD, Tute AS and Alderson B (2014) Therapeutic options for the treatment of chronic pain in dogs. *Journal of Small Animal Practice* **55**, 127–134

Malek S, Sample SJ, Schwartz Z *et al.* (2012) Effect of analgesic therapy on clinical outcome measures in a randomized controlled trial using client-owned dogs with hip osteoarthritis. *BMC Veterinary Research* **8**, 185

Marini I, Bartolucci ML, Bortolotti F, Gatto MR and Bonetti GA (2012) Palmitoylethanolamide *versus* a nonsteroidal anti-inflammatory drug in the treatment of temporomandibular joint inflammatory pain. *Journal of Orofacial Pain* **26**, 99–104

Marshall WG, Hazewinkel HA, Mullen D *et al.* (2010) The effect of weight loss on lameness in obese dogs with osteoarthritis. *Veterinary Research Communications* **34**, 241–253

McEwen BS and Kalia M (2010) The role of corticosteroids and stress in chronic pain conditions. *Metabolism* **59**, S9–15

McMillan CJ, Livingston CR, Clark PM *et al.* (2008) Pharmacokinetics of intravenous tramadol in dogs. *Canadian Journal of Veterinary Research* **72**, 325–331

Moalem G and Tracey DJ (2006) Immune and inflammatory mechanisms in neuropathic pain. *Brain Research Reviews* **51**, 240–264

Muller C, Gaines B, Gruen M *et al.* (2016) Evaluation of clinical metrology instrument in dogs with osteoarthritis. *Journal of Veterinary Internal Medicine* **30**, 836–846

Nowak L, Bregestovski P, Ascher P, Herbert A and Prochiantz A (1984) Magnesium gates glutamate-activated channels in mouse central neurones. *Nature* **307**, 462–465

Plessas IN, Rusbridge C, Driver CJ *et al.* (2012) Long-term outcome of Cavalier King Charles Spaniel dogs with clinical signs associated with Chiari-like malformation and syringomyelia. *Veterinary Record* **171**, 501

Pozzi A, Muir WW III and Traverso F (2006) Prevention of central sensitization and pain by N-methyl-D-aspartate receptor antagonists. *Journal of the American Veterinary Medical Association* **228**, 53–60

Read RA, Cullis-Hill D and Jones MP (1996) Systemic use of pentosan polysulphate in the treatment of osteoarthritis. *Journal of Small Animal Practice* **37**, 108–114

Reid J, Wiseman-Orr ML, Scott EM and Nolan AM (2013) Development, validation and reliability of a web-based questionnaire to measure health-related quality of life in dogs. *Journal of Small Animal Practice* **54**, 227–233

37

Robertson SA (2008) Managing pain in feline patients. *Veterinary Clinics of North America – Small Animal Practice* **38**, 1267–1290

Roush JK, Cross AR, Renberg WC *et al.* (2010) Evaluation of the effects of dietary supplementation with fish oil omega-3 fatty acids on weight bearing in dogs with osteoarthritis. *Journal of the American Veterinary Medical Association* **236**, 67–73

Rychel JK (2010) Diagnosis and treatment of osteoarthritis. *Topics in Companion Animal Medicine* **25**, 20–25

Sandersoln RO, Beata C, Flipo RM *et al.* Systematic review of the management of canine osteoarthritis. *Veterinary Record* **164**, 418–424

Sandkuhler J (2009) Models and mechanisms of hyperalgesia and allodynia. *Physiological Reviews* **89**, 707–758

Schneider BM, Dodman NH and Maranda L (2009) Use of memantine in treatment of canine compulsive disorders. *Journal of Veterinary Behavior: Clinical Applications and Research* **4**, 118–126

Schoffnegger D, Ruscheweyh R and Sandkühler J (2008) Spread of excitation across modality borders in spinal dorsal horn of neuropathic rats. *Pain* **135**, 300–310

Shah JP, Danoff JV, Desai MJ *et al.* (2008) Biochemicals associated with pain and inflammation are elevated in sites near to and remote from active myofascial trigger points. *Archives of Physical Medicine and Rehabilitation* **89**, 16–23

Sikdar S, Shah JP, Gebreab T *et al.* (2009) Novel applications of ultrasound technology to visualize and characterize myofascial trigger points and surrounding soft tissue. *Archives of Physical Medicine and Rehabilitation* **90**, 1829–1838

Slingerland L, Hazewinkel H, Meij B, Picavet P and Voorhout G (2011) Cross-sectional study of the prevalence and clinical features of osteoarthritis in 100 cats. *Veterinary Journal* **187**, 304–309

Slingsby LS and Waterman-Pearson AE (2001) Analgesic effects in dogs of carprofen and pethidine together compared with the effects of either drug alone. *Veterinary Record* **148**, 441–444

Sparkes AH, Heiene R, Lascelles BD *et al.* (2010) ISFM and AAFP consensus guidelines: long-term use of NSAIDs in cats. *Journal of Feline Medicine and Surgery* **12**, 521–538

Tolbert K, Bissett S, King A *et al.* (2011) Efficacy of oral famotidine and 2 omeprazole formulations for the control of intragastric pH in dogs. *Journal of Veterinary Internal Medicine* **25**, 47–54

Treede RD, Jensen TS, Campbell JN *et al.* (2008) Neuropathic pain: Redefinition and a grading system for clinical and research purposes. *Neurology* **70**, 1630–1635

Walton MB, Cowderoy E, Lascelles D and Innes JF (2013) Evaluation of construct and criterion validity for the 'Liverpool Osteoarthritis in Dogs' (LOAD) clinical metrology instrument and comparison to two other instruments. *PLoS ONE* **8**, e58125

Webster RP, Anderson GI and Gearing DP (2014) Canine Brief Pain Inventory scores for dogs with osteoarthritis before and after administration of a monoclonal antibody against nerve growth factor. *American Journal of Veterinary Research* **75**, 532–535

Wiseman-Orr ML, Scott EM, Reid J and Nolan AM (2006) Validation of a structured questionnaire as an instrument to measure chronic pain in dogs on the basis of effects on health-related quality of life. *American Journal of Veterinary Research* **67**, 1826–1836

Yazbek KVB, Fantoni, DT (2005) Validity of a health-related quality-of-life scale for dogs with signs of pain secondary to cancer. *Journal of the American Veterinary Medical Association* **226**, 1354–1358

Zeiler GE, Fosgate GT, van Vollenhoven E and Rioja E (2014) Assessment of behavioural changes in domestic cats during short-term hospitalisation. *Journal of Feline Medicine and Surgery* **16**, 499–503

Case example 1: Hip dysplasia

HISTORY AND PRESENTATION

Pilot, a 10-year-old male neutered Labrador Retriever, was diagnosed with hip dysplasia at 2 years of age when he underwent British Veterinary Association hip scoring. Since diagnosis, his owner has administered cod liver oil via his food. Two years ago, Pilot was presented to the veterinary surgery, as he exhibited increased stiffness during the mornings and was more reluctant to play with other dogs. At that time, meloxicam was prescribed for Pilot, who responded well to treatment and the owner reports that for a long time he was 'back to his old self'. The owner has telephoned to report that for the past 6 weeks Pilot has again shown increased morning stiffness and has been inappetant on one or two mornings a week.

Failure to respond appropriately to an NSAID administered at the licensed dose is an indication to re-examine the patient to assess for any additional musculoskeletal disease (ligament disruption, bone tumour growth) which could result in increased pain or disability. Inappetance in a patient administered NSAIDs should prompt re-examination as it may be a sign of gastrointestinal ulceration associated with treatment.

→ **CASE EXAMPLE 1 CONTINUED**

CLINICAL SIGNS AND SIGNS OF PAIN

Pilot's owner presents him to you for examination. He is bright, alert and responsive and you judge his body condition to be 6/9 (Laflamme, 1997). Chest auscultation and abdominal palpation are unremarkable. His heart sounds and peripheral pulses are synchronous with a rate of 120 bpm and he is panting continuously. His mucous membrane colour is pink and capillary refill time less than 1 second. The range of motion of both hips is reduced and, during extension of his hips, Pilot stops panting.

Signs of pain during physical examination are rarely overt in trained dogs. Most commonly pain is inferred from resistance to movement of joints and mild changes in behaviour (lip licking, discontinuing panting) in response to joint manipulation.

INVESTIGATIONS AND INITIAL TREATMENT

In instances where there is concern about treatment-related gastrointestinal adverse events, consider assessing faecal occult blood or serum urea/creatinine (disproportionate increase in urea may be related to gastrointestinal bleeding). Precautionary treatment for gastric ulceration is appropriate, based on history, and the authors would discontinue NSAIDs and administer omeprazole at 1 mg/kg twice daily for 7–10 days (Tolbert et al., 2011) before reinstating NSAID treatment. Inappetance may also be associated with pain; during the period of NSAID withdrawal the authors would prescribe a licensed paracetamol-containing product at the datasheet recommended doses (33.3 mg/kg three times daily). NSAID (including paracetamol) datasheets state that their prescription is contraindicated in the presence of gastrointestinal disorders; therefore, prescribing NSAIDs or paracetamol in such cases is 'off-licence' and a cost–benefit

analysis should be considered in consultation with the dog's owner.

Pilot's owner returns a week later and reports that his appetite has improved, but that he has been noticeably stiffer and slower to move out of his bed in the morning.

The improvement in Pilot's appetite is encouraging, but presents a dilemma – his musculoskeletal pain appears to benefit from NSAID treatment; however, this is potentially causing gastrointestinal adverse effects. In this circumstance, reintroducing the original NSAID, whilst continuing omeprazole and monitoring closely for further gastrointestinal effects, would seem reasonable; however, his owner reported that Pilot was doing less well than previously on the original NSAID and therefore switching to an alternative licensed NSAID could also be considered. To minimize risks associated with concurrent administration of NSAIDs, a washout period without NSAID treatment of 5–7 days is currently recommended (Epstein et al., 2015). There are no current methods of predicting response to a particular NSAID. In the case of concerns over efficacy in a patient, the authors would tend to replace non-coxib NSAIDs with coxibs, or *vice versa*. Monitoring response to treatment alterations can be challenging. The severity of OA-associated signs can wax and wane over time. Owners are more likely to present dogs when they become aware of an exacerbation of signs; therefore, improvements in the condition related to a natural waning in signs (regression to the mean) may be erroneously attributed to treatment. Client completed questionnaires such as the Helsinki Chronic Pain Index (Hielm-Björkman et al., 2009) or Canine Brief Pain Inventory (Brown et al., 2007) can be useful to track changes in levels of pain and disability. Quality of life questionnaires, such as that produced by Newmetrica (www.newmetrica.com), may be used to investigate how the dog's disease is affecting his experience of life. Collar-mounted accelerometers are increasingly affordable and may provide objective data on the amount and type of activity the dog engages in.

→

→ **CASE EXAMPLE 1 CONTINUED**

LONG-TERM MANAGEMENT

After discussing the options with Pilot's owner the decision was made to initiate treatment with robenacoxib at the licensed dosage, and continue omeprazole. The owner completed the Helsinki Chronic Pain Index (HCPI) weekly. After 4 weeks of treatment, Pilot's demeanour was still concerning to his owner, and the scores on HCPI were indicative of chronic pain (greater than 12) (Hielm-Björkman et al.,

2003). Considering that there may be a component of central sensitization to his disease, the decision was made to add (unlicensed) amantadine at 4 mg/kg daily (Lascelles et al., 2008) to the robenacoxib and omeprazole treatment. Pilot's demeanour improved after approximately 2 weeks of treatment and after 4 weeks his HCPI scores had reduced to the 6–11 range, suggesting present control of his pain. In the long term, weight loss should be advised for the dog to reach a target body condition score of 4 or 5 out of 9.

Case example 2: Degenerative joint disease

HISTORY AND PRESENTATION

Socks is a 13-year-old female neutered Domestic Shorthaired cat who has been fed a restricted phosphate diet since diagnosis of renal insufficiency during a geriatric health screen 12 months previously. Her owner is concerned as she has defecated next to her litter tray on three occasions over the past fortnight.

INVESTIGATIONS AND INITIAL TREATMENT

On examination Socks is bright, alert and responsive with a body condition score of 4 out of 9; her weight is unchanged since her previous check-up 6 months earlier. Her heart rate is 192, respiratory rate 28 and no goitre is palpable. Both kidneys feel small on abdominal palpation and her urinary bladder is moderately full. Crepitus is noted on flexion of both elbows and stifles.

While cognitive changes in older animals may be associated with loss of house training (Landsberg et al., 2010), medical causes, including pain preventing access to the tray

or effective posturing, need to be excluded. Given the crepitus noted in multiple joints it is likely that the Socks has degenerative joint disease (DJD), and a trial period of analgesia should be considered. NSAIDs have demonstrated efficacy in managing musculoskeletal pain in cats (Lascelles et al., 2007; Gruen et al., 2014) but owing to their effects on prostaglandin formation, require additional caution when prescribed to animals with renal disease that may be prone to dehydration. There is some evidence that cats with chronic renal disease and DJD, treated with low doses of meloxicam (median dose 0.02 mg/kg daily) do not experience increased morbidity or mortality relative to untreated renal disease in cats (Gowan et al., 2011; 2012), and also that renal disease does not increase the risk of adverse events associated with administration of the licensed dose of robenacoxib over a 28-day period (King et al., 2015). It is worth noting that none of the above studies have provided data on the effects of treatment of cats with proteinuric renal disease with NSAIDs in addition to angiotensin-converting ➡️

→ **CASE EXAMPLE 2 CONTINUED**

enzyme (ACE) inhibitors and, therefore, such drug combinations may still present an increased risk to renal homeostasis (Sparkes *et al.*, 2010).

Following a recent (within 1 month) assessment of biochemistry and haematology, urinalysis, and systolic arterial blood pressure, NSAID therapy could be prescribed as a trial analgesic with the informed consent of the owner. Client specific outcome measures (Lascelles *et al.*, 2007) and the feline musculoskeletal pain index (Benito *et al.*, 2013) could be utilized to monitor response to treatment; however, be aware that there may be a significant placebo effect associated with treatment (Gruen *et al.*, 2014).

LONG-TERM MANAGEMENT

Reassessment, to ascertain that the cat is not suffering acute adverse effects, is recommended after 5–7 days of treatment followed by a full re-examination including blood and urine analysis after 2–4 weeks and ongoing reassessment at 2–6 month intervals (Sparkes *et al.*, 2010).

A positive response to NSAID treatment suggests that analgesia should be continued; however, longer term adjuncts to management of feline musculoskeletal pain, including omega-3 fatty acid/green-lipped mussel/glucosamine-chondroitin containing feedstuffs or supplements (Lascelles *et al.*, 2010) may permit a reduction in NSAID dose without a detrimental effect on pain levels. Environmental modifications can further promote comfort and a recent review considers a number of important areas, including steps and ramps to reach favoured locations, multiple feeding, drinking and appropriately accessible toileting sites, and activities to engage mental stimulation (Bennett *et al.*, 2012).

Adjunctive analgesic drugs including gabapentin, tramadol, amantadine and amitriptyline may be considered for off-licence prescription in individual cases; however, there is presently little evidence regarding their effectiveness or safety in feline musculoskeletal pain (Lascelles and Robertson, 2010).

Chapter 5

Pharmacological treatment of pain

Federico Corletto and Colette Jolliffe

In recent years there has been increased recognition of the importance of analgesia for veterinary patients. This has been accompanied by the development and licensing of several analgesic drugs for veterinary use. There is a good evidence base regarding the use, safety and efficacy of licensed drugs; research into non-licensed drugs, which may be used according the Cascade, continues. Veterinary surgeons (veterinarians), therefore, have a relatively wide range of treatment options to prevent and alleviate pain.

Analgesia use in practice

Opioids

Opioids are widely used in human and veterinary practice to provide analgesia. Although they have many side effects, these are rarely significant in veterinary patients, so opioids are usually safe even for sick animals.

Mechanism of action

Opioids act on opioid peptide receptors, which are part of the endogenous endorphin/enkephalin-mediated analgesia system. Analgesia is mediated by receptors in the brain and spinal cord, and sometimes elsewhere, for example in joints, where receptors are upregulated in response to inflammation. There are three main types of opioid receptors: the delta (DOP), the kappa (KOP), and the mu opioid peptide receptors (MOP). The most important type for analgesia is the MOP receptor. Opioid receptors are situated both pre- and post-synaptically, for example, in the dorsal horn of the spinal cord. Agonism of an opioid receptor results in hyperpolarization of the neurone, which decreases cell excitability, reducing propagation of the action potential and onward neurotransmitter release.

Metabolism and excretion

Most opioids are metabolized by the liver, the exception being remifentanil, which has a very short duration of action due to metabolism by esterase enzymes in plasma. Some opioids have active metabolites and the analgesic effect may depend on hepatic biotransformation; for example, in humans much of the analgesic effect of morphine is due to one of its metabolites, morphine-6-glucuronide. The duration of action of opioids may be increased in animals with hepatic dysfunction so the dosing interval should be increased (based on

BSAVA Guide to Pain Management in Small Animal Practice. Edited by Ian Self. ©BSAVA 2019

individual pain assessment). Animals with hepatic encephalopathy may be more sensitive to the sedative effects of opioids, and a lower than normal dose may be appropriate.

Adverse effects

These are mediated by opioid receptors in the central nervous system and throughout the body. Adverse effects are less likely to occur if the animal is experiencing pain at the time of opioid administration.

Respiratory system: Opioids can increase the threshold at which arterial CO_2 levels trigger ventilation, and decrease the threshold at which hypoxaemia triggers ventilation. This respiratory depression has historically prevented the prescription of opioids to animals, and it is a real problem in human anaesthesia. Fortunately, veterinary patients are less prone to respiratory depression than humans, and it is very unlikely to happen when conscious dogs or cats are given opioids at clinical doses. Respiratory depression may occur with overdose, or when opioids are combined with other respiratory depressant drugs, for example, during sedation or general anaesthesia. Monitoring (pulse oximetry, capnography) will detect this problem, and supplementation of oxygen and controlled ventilation may be necessary to counteract the respiratory depression. For example, controlled ventilation may be necessary during general

anaesthesia when a fentanyl infusion is used to provide analgesia. In the author's [CJ] opinion, administration of opioids to dyspnoeic animals is not contraindicated, and can be helpful due to analgesic and sedative effects.

Opioids depress the cough centre and are antitussive. They have been licensed for this purpose (e.g. butorphanol tablets for cough prevention in dogs). Prevention of cough is useful for some procedures such as bronchoscopy, but it should be remembered that coughing is sometimes required to aid clearance of the respiratory tract, so coughing should not be prevented for more than a few hours in animals with wet/productive coughs. Opioids often cause panting in dogs (see 'Thermoregulation').

Circulatory system: Opioids increase vagal tone and may cause bradycardia, respiratory sinus arrhythmia and even second-degree atrioventricular block or other bradyarrhythmias. In the author's [CJ] experience, this is most likely to occur in animals with existing high vagal tone, such as fit animals or brachycephalic breeds, during general anaesthesia when full MOP agonists are used. An example would be an anaesthetized working Springer Spaniel that has received methadone as part of the pre-anaesthetic medication. Usually, the reduction in heart rate is compensated for by an increase in stroke volume, maintaining cardiac output. If the

Opioids and intracranial disease

Respiratory depression may occur after administration of opioids in mentally depressed animals with intracranial disease, for example, following head trauma, or as a result of space-occupying intracranial lesions. In these patients, decreased ventilation and the resulting increased arterial CO_2 levels may cause a further increase in intracranial pressure, worsening neurological status and potentially lead to brain herniation and Cushing's triad (hypertension, bradycardia and respiratory disturbances due to pressure on the brainstem and catecholamine release). Opioids can be used in patients with intracranial disease, but low doses should be used and titrated to effect, and the patient's neurological status and vital signs should be carefully monitored. If respiratory depression occurs, the opioid could be antagonized, or the patient anaesthetized, the trachea intubated and the lungs ventilated to achieve normocapnia. Sedation due to opioids may also interfere with neurological assessment. Patients with head trauma or intracranial disease may experience severe pain so other forms of analgesia, including multimodal analgesia, should be considered, especially if opioids cannot be used.

Opioids for pregnancy, Caesarean section, lactating mothers and very young animals

There is very little published in the veterinary literature on analgesia for these patient groups. In humans and laboratory animals, chronic opioid use during pregnancy can have adverse effects on the progeny. However, short-term opioid use during pregnancy is unlikely to be detrimental to the fetuses and may be necessary on welfare grounds (Mathews, 2005).

Opioids given to the dam during parturition or as part of an analgesia strategy for Caesarean section may result in sedation and respiratory depression in the newborns due to penetration of the placental barrier by the drug. While some authors recommend the use of opioids as pre-anaesthetic medication, it may be preferable to postpone the use of opioids in the dam until after the birth of the young to optimize their viability, and to consider other means of providing analgesia for the dam (e.g. local anaesthetic techniques). Use of buprenorphine preoperatively for Caesarean section is listed as a contraindication on the datasheet. Most anaesthetists agree that short-term use of an opioid to provide analgesia to the dam following Caesarean section is acceptable.

Opioids are secreted in milk and their use is not recommended (according to most datasheets) during lactation. However, is important to treat pain in a nursing mother otherwise she may demonstrate aggressive or aversive behaviour towards her offspring. It seems sensible to use drugs that are less likely to cross into the milk, for example, those with low lipid solubility such as morphine. However, methadone has been used in lactating humans with no detrimental effect on the baby. If opioids are used in lactating mothers, drug administration could be timed to avoid nursing at the time of peak plasma concentration, and the dam and offspring should be monitored for adverse effects. The epidural or intrathecal routes of administration might be appropriate in some cases.

Most drugs are not safety tested on young animals (less than 6–8 weeks old) and therefore the manufacturers recommend caution in their use in such patients. Young animals are likely to be more sensitive to the sedative effect of opioids, and very young animals (less than 6 weeks old) may be slower to metabolize these drugs. Therefore, use of low doses given to effect is recommended (see 'Clinical use').

The cost-benefit analysis of using opioids in these cases and the above circumstances should be considered; the datasheet of the particular opioid formulation should be checked; and informed written consent to use drugs off licence, or unlicensed drugs, should be obtained from the owner.

heart rate is very low (less than about 30 beats per minute) and/or there is a suspicion of reduced cardiac output (usually assessed by measuring blood pressure), then the bradycardia can be treated using an anticholinergic drug (atropine 20–40 µg/kg i.v. or glycopyrronium 5–10 µg/kg i.v.). If alpha-2 agonists have also been used then administration of atipamezole can be considered instead of using anticholinergic drugs. In this case, the patient may become more lightly anaesthetized, requiring additional anaesthetic administration, for example, increasing the vaporizer setting.

Some opioids cause histamine release, which can lead to urticaria, but also sometimes vasodilation with or without hypotension and tachycardia. This is common following pethidine administration so it should not be administered intravenously. Morphine can also cause histamine release.

Central nervous system: Opioids can cause sedation, dysphoria and euphoria. Sedation can be useful when opioids are used as part of pre-anaesthetic medication or in a sedative combination. The sedative effect is synergistic with that of other sedatives (e.g. acepromazine or alpha-2 agonists). Sedation may be an unwanted effect in hospitalized animals that require high levels of analgesia for several days, as their appetite and mobility may be impaired, and it is more difficult to assess their mental status. In this case, use of multimodal analgesia and careful titration of the dose of opioid is required. Sometimes opioids can cause dysphoria, characterized by abnormal behaviour, agitation, vocalization and appearing to 'see things', in both dogs and cats. This is less likely to happen at appropriate doses, in combination with sedative agents or if the animal is in pain at the time of drug administration. Cats in particular may experience euphoria, demonstrating purring, kneading with their paws and affectionate behaviour. In the author's [CJ] experience this is often seen following buprenorphine administration in cats, making buprenorphine a useful drug to improve feline well being and compliance while hospitalized.

Thermoregulation: Opioids affect thermoregulation, probably by resetting the hypothalamic 'thermostat', and can cause hyperthermia in cats, and hypothermia in dogs. The effect of opioids on temperature in an individual may also depend on ambient temperature and the degree of mobility. Hyperthermia in cats has been demonstrated following administration of hydromorphone, morphine, buprenorphine and butorphanol (Posner *et al.*, 2010), and also non-opioid anaesthesia-related drugs (Posner *et al.*, 2007). It is likely to occur with other opioids. The aetiology is not well understood, but the increase in temperature does not seem to be of clinical significance and is self-limiting. Opioid administration should be considered as a differential diagnosis for hyperthermia in cats.

Dogs may become hypothermic after administration of opioids, especially when they pant, which is a common effect of opioid administration in this species (Monteiro *et al.*, 2008). This is probably due to opioid-induced resetting of the hypothalamic thermoregulatory threshold, resulting in activation of cooling mechanisms (panting), to reach the lower set temperature. Attempts to warm the animal are likely to result in resumption of panting (Adler *et al.*, 1988). Panting may be a sign of pain in dogs, so this can be confusing, emphasizing the importance of proper pain assessment.

Ocular effects: Opioids tend to cause miosis in dogs and mydriasis in cats. Mydriasis may result in increased light sensitivity and decreased visual acuity, and possibly contributes to clinical signs of dysphoria. It may last longer than the analgesic effect of the opioid (up to 12 hours following methadone administration (Slingsby *et al.*, 2016)). Apart from this, the changes in pupil size are of little clinical significance. Several opioids (pethidine, fentanyl, butorphanol and morphine) have been documented to cause decreased tear production, and regular corneal lubrication is indicated for patients at risk of corneal ulceration when receiving opioids.

Urinary system: Opioids cause urine retention by increasing urethral sphincter tone and detrusor muscle relaxation (Baldini *et al.*, 2009). Epidurally administered opioids are often thought to generate a higher incidence of this problem compared with other routes, but a recent report demonstrated that epidural morphine administration was not associated with urine retention (defined as no urination within 24 hours), and that urine retention can also occur following parenteral opioid administration (Peterson *et al.*, 2014). Urine retention usually resolves without treatment. It is unlikely to result in complications such as bladder rupture unless the bladder wall is weak, for example, following trauma, cystotomy or in the presence of neoplasia. In these situations, an indwelling catheter can be used to prevent urine retention.

A separate effect of opioids is decreased urine output, possibly due to an arginine vasopressin-mediated effect. This may make assessment of volume status using urine output more complicated in animals receiving opioids (Anderson and Day, 2008).

Gastrointestinal system: Opioids can stimulate the chemoreceptor trigger zone (CRTZ) (situated outside the blood–brain barrier), to cause emesis, and the vomiting centre (within the blood–brain barrier) to have an antiemetic effect (Blancquaert *et al.*, 1986). Whether the CRTZ or the vomiting centre is affected first depends on the lipophilicity of the drug, dose, and route of administration. Morphine, which is hydrophilic, administered at low doses intramuscularly or subcutaneously frequently causes vomiting within 5 minutes of injection since it crosses the blood–brain barrier slowly and therefore influences the CRTZ before the vomiting centre. The incidence of vomiting and signs of nausea can be reduced by prior administration of maropitant or acepromazine (Koh *et al.*, 2014). Opioids that are likely to cause vomiting should be avoided in some patients, for example, those with an oesophageal foreign body, increased intracranial pressure or a fragile eye at risk of rupture.

Opioids may increase the incidence of gastro-oesophageal reflux (GOR) during anaesthesia due to effects on cardiac sphincter tone. Pethidine has been shown to reduce the incidence of GOR compared with morphine (Wilson *et al.*, 2007).

Opioids delay gastric emptying and increase gut transit time, which may result in constipation with prolonged administration. Pyloric sphincter tone is increased, and this may affect the ease of entering the duodenum during endoscopy in dogs. In the author's [CJ] experience, a clinical dose of opioid included in the pre-anaesthetic medication does not adversely affect this procedure, although evidence from recent studies is contradictory. Since opioids can cause contraction of the sphincter of Oddi in humans, there is a belief that they should be avoided in veterinary patients with pancreatitis or biliary tract obstruction. In humans and cats, the bile duct merges with the pancreatic duct before entering the duodenum, so the sphincter of Oddi controls flow of bile and pancreatic juice into the duodenum. In dogs, the sphincter of Oddi only controls flow through the bile duct, which is separate from the pancreatic duct, so that effects on the sphincter of Oddi are probably irrelevant in dogs with pancreatitis. There is little evidence in humans and none in cats and dogs that opioids have a deleterious effect when used to control pain due to pancreatitis or biliary tract disease. There is no evidence that pethidine is superior to other opioids for these conditions, and longer-acting opioids (e.g. methadone, buprenorphine), or those that can be administered by intravenous infusion (e.g. morphine, fentanyl), probably benefit these patients more than pethidine.

Prevention, reduction or reversal of adverse effects

Many of these adverse effects (emesis, histamine release, dysphoria, panting) can be reduced or prevented by administration of acepromazine. This should be given before the opioid to reduce the incidence of emesis. If necessary, adverse effects of opioids can be reversed by administration of a MOP antagonist such as naloxone at a dose of 0.002–0.04 mg/kg intravenously, intramuscularly or subcutaneously. This will also antagonize the analgesic effects of the opioid, so another analgesic strategy should be implemented. Naloxone has a short duration of action, and re-administration may be necessary after 30 to 60 minutes. Adverse effects of opioids may also be reduced by administration of a partial MOP agonist such as buprenorphine, or a mixed agonist/ antagonist such as butorphanol, which may maintain some analgesia but antagonize the unwanted effect.

Different effects of opioids at the receptors

Different opioids may have different effects at the opioid receptors and some may have effects at more than one type of opioid receptor (Figure 5.1).

Effect	Activity at receptor	Comments	Examples	
			Drug	**Receptor**
Full agonist (high efficacy)	Dose-dependent effect	Maximal effect achieved at high dose Suitable for treating moderate to severe pain	Fentanyl	MOP
Partial agonist (low efficacy)	Dose-dependent effect to a certain dose Acts as agonist and antagonist at the same receptor type	Maximal effect is never achieved despite increased dose Suitable for treating mild to moderate pain	Buprenorphine	MOP
Antagonist	No effect	Competes with agonist at receptor resulting in reversal (antagonism) of agonist effect	Naloxone	MOP
Mixed agonist/ antagonist	Agonist at one receptor type, antagonist at another receptor type	Can be used to reverse (antagonize) effects at one receptor type while still exerting an effect at a different receptor type	Butorphanol	KOP (agonist), MOP (antagonist)

5.1 Classification of drugs acting on opioid receptors. KOP = kappa opioid peptide receptor; MOP = mu opioid peptide receptor.

The term 'potency' can cause confusion. It refers to the dose of a drug needed to achieve a desired effect. For example, a commonly used analgesic dose of buprenorphine is 0.02 mg/kg. The same dose of methadone is unlikely to alleviate pain, approximately ten times the dose would be needed for this (about 0.2 mg/kg methadone). This means that buprenorphine is more potent than methadone, but it does not mean that buprenorphine provides better analgesia than methadone. In fact, since methadone is a full MOP agonist and buprenorphine is a partial MOP agonist, better analgesia is likely to be achieved using methadone when appropriate doses are used (methadone has higher efficacy).

Clinical use of opioids

Factors influencing drug choice include:

- Availability
- Licensing
- Familiarity
- Patient history (previous opioid use)
- Suitability for chosen route of administration
- Dosing interval/suitability for intravenous infusion

- Likely degree of pain experienced by the animal
- Likelihood of adverse effects
- Concurrent illness.

Pre-anaesthetic medication

Opioids may be combined with other sedatives such as acepromazine, alpha-2 agonists and benzodiazepines in pre-anaesthetic medication for any procedure. They are particularly useful for painful procedures or when pain due to pre-existing conditions is likely, for example, radiography of a patient with osteoarthritis. For geriatric or sick patients (for whom the cardio-vascular effects of acepromazine or alpha-2 agonists are undesirable) they can be used as the sole pre-anaesthetic agent. They enhance the sedative effect of the other drugs, reduce injectable and inhalant anaesthetic require-ments, and provide pre-emptive analgesia.

Intraoperative analgesia

The opioid used as part of the pre-anaesthetic medication may be adequate for intraoperative analgesia, especially if used as part of a multimodal analgesia strategy. However, additional opioids may be required during the procedure, for example, if the initial opioid has worn off, if there is intense surgical stimulation, or as part of a balanced anaesthesia technique aiming to reduce inhalation agent requirements and mitigate the effects of anaesthesia on the circulatory system. Opioids can be administered intramuscularly, as an intravenous bolus or as an intravenous infusion. Adverse effects such as apnoea, respiratory depression or bradycardia may occur (less likely if the drug is administered intramuscularly, but the onset of analgesia will be delayed). Ideally, the patient's ventilation should be monitored using capnography, and intermittent positive-pressure ventilation (IPPV) may be required. Bradycardia may be treated using glycopyrronium 5–10 μg/kg or atropine 20–40 μg/kg intravenously if the patient becomes hypotensive.

To ensure that the patient is comfortable during the recovery period, it may be wise to administer a long-acting opioid (e.g. methadone or buprenorphine) prior to discontinuation of the anaesthetic if the analgesia provided by the pre-anaesthetic medication is likely to be waning. For example, the author [CJ] often administers a second dose of methadone intramuscularly 3–4 hours after the pre-anaesthetic medication.

Postoperative analgesia and analgesia for hospitalized patients

Opioids should be used as part of a multimodal analgesia strategy. Ideally, pain assessment should be an integral part of the use of opioids. The aims of pain assessment are to identify when an animal is in pain, to try and quantify the pain, to assess the degree and duration of effect of the analgesic agents used, and to enable opioids to be used to effect, i.e. to increase or decrease the dose or dosing interval as required for the patient, or to give an additional dose (top-up) if the initial dose is not adequate. The onset, effects and duration of the drug may vary with dose and route of administration. The response of the individual animal to the opioid may vary due to differences in sensitivity to the drug, duration of the drug effect, occurrence of adverse effects, and the influence of disease (e.g. hepatic or renal disease) on the action and duration of the drug. In particular, cats can demonstrate marked individual variation in the effect and duration of different opioids. Intravenous infusions are useful for providing sustained analgesia without the need for repeated injections in the postoperative period.

Intravenous infusions

Intravenous infusions are useful for providing intra- and postoperative analgesia. Compared with repeated intramuscular or intravenous doses of analgesics, they provide a relatively constant plasma concentration of the analgesic drug, which should result in a stable plane of analgesia. A syringe driver or volumetric fluid pump must be used to ensure accurate dosing. Infusions can be easily titrated to effect, usually starting with an intravenous bolus (a similar dose to that which will be infused per hour) to ensure adequate plasma levels are reached, then beginning the infusion and increasing or decreasing the dose as required, according to regular patient assessment. For example, a bolus of 0.1 mg/kg of morphine can be followed by an intravenous infusion of 0.1 mg/kg/hour. Additional boluses may be given during the infusion, for example, if a patient receiving 0.1 mg/kg/hour morphine seems painful, an intravenous bolus of 0.1 mg/kg could be administered, and the infusion rate increased to 0.2 mg/kg/hour.

It has become common practice to mix several different analgesic drugs together in a bag of fluids and administer the mixture intra- or postoperatively. Typical mixtures are morphine or fentanyl mixed with lidocaine and ketamine (MLK or FLK, see table below). In the author's [CJ] opinion, it is preferable to administer the drugs separately, with the advantage that the

▶

Intravenous infusions *continued*

individual drugs can be titrated to effect, and one or more of the infusions can be discontinued as the patient improves, or if it experiences side effects caused by one of the drugs.

Drug	Loading dose (i.v.)	Maintenance dose (i.v.)	Comment/adverse effects
MLK: Morphine Lidocaine Ketamine	Dog: 0.1–0.2 mg/kg 1 mg/kg 0.5 mg/kg **Cats: leave out lidocaine**	0.1 mg/kg/h 2 mg/kg/h 0.6 mg/kg/h	Add to 250 ml saline: • 25 mg morphine • 500 mg lidocaine • 150 mg ketamine • Remove appropriate volume from saline bag first • Infuse at 1 ml/kg/h during surgery • Post-surgery adjust up or down depending on patient comfort • Sedation is common
FLK: Fentanyl Lidocaine Ketamine	Dog: 0.5–3 µg/kg i.v. 1 mg/kg i.v. 0.5 mg/kg i.v. **Cats: leave out lidocaine**	3 µg/kg/h (0.003 mg/kg/h) 2 mg/kg/h 0.6 mg/kg/h	Add to 250 ml saline: • 750 µg (0.75 mg) fentanyl • 500 mg lidocaine • 150 mg ketamine • Remove appropriate volume from saline bag first • Infuse at 1 ml/kg/h during surgery • Post-surgery adjust up or down depending on patient comfort • Sedation is common. Be aware of the potential for respiratory depression

Individual drugs

Figure 5.2 provides an explanation of drug classes, suggested doses and particular adverse effects for each drug. All of the drugs discussed below are Schedule 2 Controlled Drugs in the UK (must be stored in a locked cabinet and detailed records of supply and use must be kept), except buprenorphine (Schedule 3), butorphanol and codeine.

Methadone: Methadone is licensed in several countries as an analgesic in cats (i.m.) and dogs (i.v., i.m. and s.c.). It is a full MOP agonist and also an *N*-methyl-D-aspartate (NMDA) receptor antagonist. It is unlikely to cause vomiting or histamine release and is the opioid most commonly used by the authors. The doses recommended in Figure 5.2 are lower than

those licensed, but the authors have found them to be effective. Since absorption from the subcutis is slow and variable, yielding low plasma levels, intravenous or intramuscular administration is recommended (Ingvast-Larsson *et al.*, 2010). Onset of action is 10–15 minutes by intravenous or intramuscular injection. Duration of action is 2–4 hours in dogs and up to 6 hours in cats. Methadone can be used by intravenous infusion at the same dose rates as morphine. It can be used to supplement analgesia during general anaesthesia by intravenous or intramuscular injection or intravenous infusion. Intravenous boluses during general anaesthesia may cause apnoea and marked bradycardia, this may be prevented by injecting very slowly (over at least 5 minutes) or by using the intramuscular route instead.

Class	Route of administration	Dose range and frequency		Adverse effects	Comments
		Dogs	Cats		
Buprenorphine					
Partial MOP agonist	i.m., i.v., oral transmucosal route in cats	20 µg/kg q6–8h. Give an additional 10 µg/kg after 3–4 hours if necessary	20 µg/kg q6–8h. Repeat the same dose after 2 hours if necessary	Euphoria in cats, occasional dysphoria in dogs	Multidose vial unsuitable for oral transmucosal administration, causes hypersalivation
Butorphanol					
KOP agonist, MOP antagonist	i.v. or i.m.	0.1–0.4 mg/kg q1–2h			Good sedative, poor analgesic
Fentanyl					
Full MOP agonist	i.v. bolus	1–2 µg/kg q20min		Apnoea, brady-cardia, possible hypotension	If used during general anaesthesia. Not licensed in cats
	i.v. infusion	5–20 µg/kg/hour during anaesthesia 2–5 µg/kg/hour in conscious patients			
	Transcutaneous patch	2–5 µg/kg/hour. Change every 3 days			Not licensed
Methadone					
Full MOP agonist, NMDA receptor antagonist	i.m.	0.2–0.5 mg/kg q2–4h	0.2–0.5 mg/kg q2–6h	Dysphoria	Licensed in dogs and cats
	i.v.	0.1–0.3 mg/kg q 2–4h	0.1–0.3 mg/kg q2–6h		
	i.v. infusion	0.1–0.3 mg/kg/hour. start with an i.v. bolus of 0.1–0.3 mg/kg injected over about 5 minutes			
Morphine					
Full MOP agonist	i.v. infusion	0.1–0.3 mg/kg/hour. start with an i.v. bolus of 0.1–0.3 mg/kg injected over about 5 minutes		Vomiting, histamine release	Not licensed
	i.v.	0.1–0.3 mg/kg q2–4h			
	i.m.	0.2–0.5 mg/kg q2–4h			
	Epidural injection	0.1 mg/kg		Pruritus has been reported	Use preservative-free morphine
Pethidine					
Full MOP agonist	i.m.	3–5 mg/kg q1–2h		Histamine release, pain on injection	Do not administer intravenously. Bradycardia less likely
Remifentanil					
Full MOP agonist	i.v. infusion	0.05–0.2 µg/kg/minute			Not licensed. Bolus dose unnecessary

5.2 Commonly used opioids. Doses provided are those used by the authors. KOP = kappa opioid peptide receptor; MOP = mu opioid peptide receptor; NMDA = N-methyl-D-aspartate.

Morphine: Morphine is not currently licensed in veterinary species and it may be difficult to justify its use via the Cascade since other full MOP agonists are licensed. Morphine can cause vomiting; this effect is not dose- or route-dependent (see above). It can also cause histamine release when injected intravenously, and should be administered slowly to minimize the risk of histamine-related adverse effects. The authors frequently use morphine by intravenous infusion or by epidural injection.

The use of morphine as an intravenous infusion has been extensively researched in dogs, and it is widely used in dogs and cats to provide a constant level of analgesia to animals in severe pain. An infusion rate of 0.12 mg/kg/hour morphine has been shown to give equivalent analgesia to that achieved with repeated intravenous boluses of 1 mg/kg every 4 hours in dogs (Lucas *et al.*, 2001). In that study, two of the dogs in the repeated bolus group had periods of semi-consciousness; none of the dogs in the infusion group experienced this. The infusion can be titrated to effect, starting with an intravenous bolus to ensure adequate plasma levels are reached, then beginning the infusion at the low end of the dose range and increasing the dose if required. After the infusion is discontinued, the terminal half-life is less than 40 minutes (Guedes *et al.*, 2007).

Morphine is hydrophilic and does not cross cell membranes easily. This property is exploited when morphine is administered by epidural injection since the drug remains within the epidural space, providing analgesia for up to 24 hours, probably by acting on MOP receptors on the spinal nerve roots. Epidurally injected morphine also tends to spread forwards independent of the volume used, and has been shown to provide analgesia as far cranially as the forelimb (Valverde *et al.*, 1989). Only preservative-free morphine should be injected into the epidural space, and knowledge of anatomy, contraindications and complications is required. It can be used alone, diluted in sterile saline to a maximum volume of about 0.2 ml/kg, or mixed with a local anaesthetic agent. When used as the sole agent, it provides analgesia only, not local anaesthesia. A single dose of morphine, usually 0.1 mg/kg, can provide analgesia for up to 24 hours with fewer side effects than parenterally administered opioids.

Buprenorphine: Buprenorphine is a partial MOP agonist licensed in dogs and cats for treatment of mild to moderate pain. It has a slow onset of action due to slow receptor binding, high affinity for MOP receptors and a long half-life, resulting in a longer duration of action than most opioids. The exact onset and duration of action is not clear, since the many studies on this subject have conflicting results, probably due to different study designs, doses, routes of administration, nociceptive stimuli, concurrent drug administration and also marked individual variation (especially in cats). Reported times for onset and duration of action in cats are 15 to 60 minutes (Steagall *et al.*, 2013), and 6 to 12 hours respectively (Robertson *et al.*, 2003; Slingsby *et al.*, 2016). Duration of action in dogs is considered to be around 6 hours (Shih *et al.*, 2008), although one study reported a duration of action of 16 hours (Ko *et al.*, 2011). This emphasizes the importance of pain assessment clinically. The high receptor affinity means that naloxone may not fully antagonize its effects.

Absorption of buprenorphine following subcutaneous injection is variable and results in poor analgesia (Steagall *et al.*, 2006). In cats, it can be administered by the oral transmucosal route, avoiding the need for injections. This is because the alkaline pH of feline saliva facilitates the absorption of the drug across the oral mucous membrane, with absorption similar to that achieved by the intramuscular route. However, there is conflicting evidence on the quality of analgesia when buprenorphine is given by this route. Therefore, the intramuscular or intravenous routes are the most reliable.

In dogs, buprenorphine can be used to treat mild to moderate pain; a full MOP agonist is more suitable for treating severe pain (Hunt *et al.*, 2013). In cats, buprenorphine has been shown to be more effective than morphine (Stanway *et al.*, 2002), although a later study disagreed with this finding (Robertson *et al.*, 2003). It may not be suitable for treating acute, severe pain due to its long onset of action. It has fewer side effects than other opioids although it can cause dysphoria in dogs. It frequently causes euphoria in cats, and can be used to improve cooperation in some feline patients.

Buprenorphine has a bell-shaped dose–response curve in some species (in theory it could antagonize its own effect at higher doses), so practitioners are often reluctant to use it to effect. However, the plateau of the curve occurs at doses much higher than those used clinically (0.5 mg/kg in rats, Dum and Herz, 1981). Therefore, the bell-shaped curve is not clinically relevant and supplemental doses can be given (and are licensed).

Buprenorphine can be used to partially antagonize the effects of a full MOP agonist. For example, if a patient is dysphoric or over-sedated following the administration of a MOP agonist, buprenorphine can be administered to reduce these unwanted effects while still providing some analgesia. This is called sequential analgesia and has been demonstrated in humans and in rabbits sedated with fentanyl/fluanisone (Flecknell et al., 1989).

Fentanyl: Fentanyl is a full MOP agonist with a rapid onset and short duration of action at the doses commonly used clinically. The doses recommended in Figure 5.2 are lower than the licensed doses, but the authors have found them to be effective. It is highly lipid soluble, and resolution of its effects may be due to redistribution rather than metabolism. At higher doses it may accumulate. It is currently licensed for dogs as a 50 µg/ml injectable solution for intravenous bolus or infusion (its short duration of action limits its usefulness by the intramuscular route). Fentanyl transdermal patches (unlicensed) have been used in both dogs and cats, and can provide analgesia for several days.

The injectable solution can be used in both dogs and cats as a co-induction agent and to provide intra- and postoperative analgesia. Onset of action is less than 5 minutes when administered as a bolus, making fentanyl very useful for providing analgesia in response to surgical stimulation intraoperatively. If surgical stimulation is sustained, an intravenous infusion can be administered, and the dose rate titrated to effect; additional boluses can be given as necessary. Concerns about accumulation of fentanyl during infusion seem to be unfounded based on a study that assessed the pharmacokinetics of a 10 µg/kg intravenous bolus followed by an infusion of 10 µg/kg/hour for up to 4 hours (Sano et al., 2006). During general anaesthesia, administration of a fentanyl bolus or infusion can cause bradycardia, respiratory depression or even apnoea. It is advisable to discontinue fentanyl infusion at least 20 minutes before the end of anaesthesia to avoid respiratory depression in the recovery period. Respiratory depression is very unlikely to occur in conscious patients.

Fentanyl patches have been widely used to provide long-term analgesia in dogs and cats although they are unlicensed. An area of relatively immobile skin, for example, at the dorsal or lateral thorax should be clipped and

Use of full MOP agonists following buprenorphine administration

If an appropriate dose of buprenorphine does not achieve the required analgesic effect, a full MOP agonist can be administered. It is still not clear if adjustment of the dose of the full agonist is required, and if so, whether an increase or decrease of the dose is appropriate. Whatever course of action is chosen, it is unlikely to harm the patient. Trial therapy with the usual dose of the full MOP agonist seems sensible; supplemental doses can be administered if necessary. Alternatively, the full MOP agonist could be administered in small intravenous increments until analgesia is achieved. In this situation it is also important to use multimodal analgesia as some types of pain may respond better to other classes of analgesics than to opioids. If use of a full MOP agonist for intraoperative analgesia is anticipated, for example, epidural morphine injection or fentanyl infusion, it makes sense to use a full MOP agonist in the pre-anaesthetic medication rather than buprenorphine.

cleaned with water. The skin should be allowed to dry, the patch applied firmly and covered with an adhesive dressing. An Elizabethan collar may be required to prevent the animal licking or removing the patch. In the time since most of the veterinary studies have been published, the type of patch has been changed from a liquid gel patch to one with the drug contained in an adhesive matrix. Therefore, it is unknown whether the matrix type patches confer similar pharmacokinetics in animals. The rate of absorption from the patch to the skin depends on the surface area of the patch; several sizes are available, and patches may be partially covered to reduce the surface area in contact with the skin if required. Absorption also depends on skin perfusion, which is influenced by factors such as skin thickness, skin and ambient temperature, volaemic status and degree of vasoconstriction. Care must be taken if a patient is being actively warmed that the patch is not over-warmed as this has been shown to result in high plasma fentanyl concentrations, with the possibility of over-sedation and/or severe respiratory depression. The uptake of fentanyl is slow; onset of analgesia is about 24 hours in dogs or 12 hours in cats and therefore the patch should be applied the day before elective surgery, or another means of analgesia provided for the first 12 to 24 hours. Variable uptake means that, in some patients, adequate analgesia is not achieved with a patch alone, emphasizing the importance of regular pain assessment. Analgesia can be supplemented with another opioid (e.g. methadone) if required and multimodal analgesia is recommended. The duration of use of a single patch application is about 72 hours from the time of application, bearing in mind that adequate analgesic levels will not be reached for the first 12 to 24 hours. Although absorption from the patch declines rapidly after 3 days of use, a used fentanyl patch still retains a significant amount of fentanyl, which could be harmful to a human if ingested (Reed *et al.*, 2011). If planning to discharge a patient with a fentanyl patch attached, careful consideration of the risks should be made; for example, are there other animals or children in the household who could be at risk, and will the client ensure safe and appropriate use of the patch? It is wise to obtain signed, informed consent from the client. After use, the patch should be removed and folded inwards while wearing gloves, and returned to the practice for appropriate disposal, or the animal should return to the clinic for proper removal and disposal of the patch.

Remifentanil: Remifentanil is an unlicensed, ultra-short-acting full MOP agonist. Its onset and duration of action are less than 60 seconds, meaning that it is only suitable for intravenous infusion, no bolus is required, and the dose rate is rapidly titratable. The very short duration of action is due to its metabolism in plasma by esterase enzymes. The main indication is for intraoperative analgesia in patients with liver dysfunction. Since its effects resolve almost as soon as it is discontinued, it is imperative that analgesia is provided with another opioid for the postoperative period.

Pethidine: Pethidine (meperidine) is a full MOP agonist that has been licensed in dogs and cats for many years. Because it was originally developed as an anticholinergic agent, it causes less bradycardia than other opioids and may be useful in patients whose cardiac output is rate dependent, for example, paediatric patients or those with cardiac disease. Pethidine causes histamine release and should not be administered intravenously. Since it is less potent than other opioids, a large volume is required for intramuscular injection. Intramuscular injection of pethidine is painful. These factors, and its short duration of action (30 to 120 minutes) make it unsuitable for providing sustained analgesia, but is it useful as a sedative or pre-anaesthetic medication in selected cases. Its metabolite, norpethidine (which is renally excreted), can cause central nervous system stimulation and seizures. This is unlikely to occur except in overdose or in animals with severe renal dysfunction. Pethidine can be a contributor to serotonin toxicity (see textbox later), and should not be used with other drugs that increase serotonin concentrations.

Butorphanol: Butorphanol is a KOP agonist and a MOP antagonist. There is conflicting evidence, but most anaesthetists agree that butorphanol is a good sedative but a poor analgesic. Its usefulness as an analgesic is also limited by its short duration of action, which is about 30 minutes in dogs, and probably about 60 minutes in cats. Butorphanol is useful for antagonizing unwanted effects of MOP analgesics (e.g. dysphoria), while maintaining some analgesia, and can be titrated to effect for this purpose.

Codeine: Codeine is a full MOP agonist and is licensed in dogs in the UK in combination with paracetamol (acetaminophen) for oral administration. Codeine has very low oral bioavailability in dogs, but an active metabolite, codeine-6-glucuronide, is formed after oral administration, which may provide analgesia. There is very little research on codeine in cats and it cannot be recommended in this species.

Non-steroidal anti-inflammatory drugs

Non-steroidal anti-inflammatory drugs (NSAIDs) include many drugs used to provide analgesia, decrease inflammation and control fever. Licensed products for use in dogs and cats include: carprofen, cimicoxib, firocoxib, ketoprofen, mavacoxib, meloxicam, robenacoxib, and tolfenamic acid. Considering that acute and chronic and persistent nociceptive pain have an inflammatory component in the vast majority of cases, NSAIDs play a vital role in providing perioperative and long-term analgesia. They are also effective in treating certain types of cancer pain.

Mechanism of action

NSAIDs are non-narcotic and their mechanism of action consists mainly of peripheral inhibition of the activity of cyclo-oxygenase enzyme (COX-1 and COX-2), and thus of tissue prostaglandin (PG) biosynthesis, but there is increasing evidence that NSAIDs may also have a central mechanism of action, mostly supported clinically by the fact that anti-inflammatory and analgesic effects are unrelated (Björkman, 1995; Cashman, 1996; Vane and Botting, 1997; Burian and Geisslinger, 2005). Prostaglandins act peripherally as proinflammatory mediators, promoting oedema formation, sensitization of nociceptors and hyperalgesia. Proposed central mechanisms of action include interference with the descending nociceptive control system, either mediated by a direct effect on prostaglandin production, or by interference with endogenous opioid peptides, the serotoninergic mechanisms or NMDA receptors and excitatory amino acids (Vanegas *et al.*, 2010). NSAIDs also interfere with the mechanisms of cell adhesion, including leukocytes, platelets and tumour cells. Specific mechanisms of interference with cell adhesion and their clinical relevance depend on the class of NSAIDs considered (Cronstein *et al.*, 1994; Ulrich *et al.*, 2006; Silver and Lillich, 2016).

While older NSAIDs were COX-1 selective or poorly selective COX inhibitors, modern NSAIDs have greater selectivity towards COX-2, with diarylimidazol derivatives (coxibs) currently having the greatest selectivity.

COX-1 and COX-2 are membrane-associated enzymes, with COX-1 traditionally considered the 'housekeeping' isoform responsible for physiological production of PGs, and COX-2 the inductive isoform whose activity is increased in pathological conditions. More recent evidence has demonstrated that this distinction is simplistic, and both COX-1 and COX-2 have physiological and pathological roles. The quantity and quality of prostanoid produced by COXs depends on the tissue and the triggering stimulus; thus the nature of the cells present in the inflammatory site affects the profile of PG production (Kay-Mugford *et al.*, 2000; Wilson and Chandrasekharan, 2004; Sessions *et al.*, 2005).

Indications, contraindications and clinical use

NSAIDs are weakly acidic, highly protein-bound compounds, and generally have good oral bioavailability. Timing of administration with respect to anaesthesia, duration of treatment, and contraindications are specific to each drug, and this should be considered when administering NSAIDs. Interestingly, different formulations of the same active drug may have slightly different contraindications; therefore, it is essential to ensure the drugs are used within the terms of their marketing authorization.

For all NSAIDs, a clinical response following oral administration is generally seen within 7–10 days of starting treatment. However, response to injectable NSAIDs is far quicker. If clinical improvement is apparent, the dose can be reduced to a minimum effective dose (if specified on the datasheet), while if improvement is not apparent, the treatment should be discontinued. Transient gastrointestinal side effects are not uncommon immediately after starting the therapy and, while generally self-limiting, the treatment may need to be interrupted if they are severe or persistent. NSAIDs should not be used concomitantly with steroids, other NSAIDs or nephrotoxic medications. If a switch of NSAID is deemed necessary, a 24-hour treatment-free period must be respected, with the notable exception of mavacoxib, which requires a 1-month treatment-free period before administering any other NSAID.

While response to NSAIDs may be variable, especially when treating chronic pain, failure of a specific NSAID to provide analgesia does not imply that all NSAIDs will be ineffective. Individual variability in disposition, local conditions of the inflammatory site, and sensitivity to side effects may partly explain variability in response to NSAIDs. Most studies performed comparing NSAIDs demonstrated equal efficacy and not superiority. In terms of frequency of gastrointestinal side effects, NSAIDs with greater COX-2 selectivity are more likely to be tolerated. When switching NSAID, it is important to respect the prescribed washout period.

A very common reason for NSAID failure in chronic and persistent pain, for example osteoarthritis, is lack of owner compliance. The owner may find it difficult to resist the temptation to stop the therapy as soon as the clinical signs improve, resulting in their relapse. In the setting of persistent pain such as

osteoarthritis the underlying inflammatory process is always present, thus should be continuously treated. Clinical evidence suggests that continuous therapy with the lowest effective dose is more effective than pulse therapy. The minimal effective dose can be identified by tapering the administered dose once clinical improvement is apparent (Sparkes *et al.*, 2010).

Although many NSAIDs can be administered prior to an anaesthetic according to their license, other restrictions of their use must be considered when planning perioperative administration: hypotension, hypovolaemia, and dehydration are all absolute contraindications to NSAID administration; hepatic and renal compromise may be absolute or relative contraindications depending on the drug considered. The clinical condition of the animal and the likelihood of adverse events (hypotension, hypovolaemia) occurring in the perioperative period should be considered when choosing the timing of NSAID administration. Although many studies demonstrated a pre-emptive analgesic effect of various NSAIDs administered prior to surgery in dogs and cats, this was in most cases demonstrated using NSAIDs as the sole analgesic during surgery (Lascelles *et al.*, 1998; Horstman *et al.*, 2004; Bergmann *et al.*, 2007; Bufalari *et al.*, 2012; Kim *et al.*, 2015; Nir *et al.*, 2016). If other analgesic interventions are incorporated in the anaesthetic protocol (e.g. perioperative opioids, locoregional anaesthesia), as it happens in a real-life scenario, the different impact of pre- *versus* postoperative administration is likely to be less relevant (Nir *et al.*, 2016). Pre-emptive administration has been linked to a post-analgesic sparing effect in many prospective studies in humans and in a recent meta-analysis, and the safety of carprofen administered prior to anaesthesia has been demonstrated in normortensive and hypotensive healthy dogs under experimental conditions (Boström *et al.*, 2002). On the other hand, renal function was temporarily impaired in healthy dogs that received carprofen prior to anaesthesia, if dehydration was induced by administration of furosemide (Surdyk *et al.*,

2012). To minimize the risk of post-anaesthetic renal complications, and considering the fact that a multimodal analgesic protocol should always be preferred to a single-agent one, the author [FC] prefers to administer NSAIDs at the end of surgery, unless hypotension or hypovolaemia have occurred, in which case NSAID administration is postponed, for an interval of time that is judged on a case-by-case basis. Although the beneficial effect of NSAIDs may be slightly reduced, this is offset by the decreased risk of complications. If it is decided to administer NSAIDs preoperatively, it is imperative to ensure that this is in agreement with the manufacturer's indications, and minimize the risk of hypotension by using appropriate monitoring and interventions. Concurrent administration of drugs that may compromise renal autoregulation and decrease blood pressure (for example ACE inhibitors) is an independent factor that increases the risk of renal injury during anaesthesia, and it should be considered an absolute contraindication for pre-anaesthetic NSAID administration.

Adverse effects

The most relevant side effects of NSAIDs depend mainly on PG inhibition, and include renal (azotaemia, in more severe cases papillary necrosis) and gastrointestinal (vomiting, diarrhoea, melaena, and ulcerations, more frequently pyloric and duodenal) toxicity. PGs have a cytoprotective effect in the stomach and gastrointestinal system. In the kidney, PGs play an important role in regulating renal blood flow, especially in the presence of hypotension. PGs are also involved in central nervous system function, embryo implantation, placental development and platelet aggregation. Despite the role of COX-2 in maintaining homeostasis, it seems that greater inhibition of COX-2 over COX-1 (i.e. use of 'coxibs') may confer greater safety to NSAIDs, at least concerning gastrointestinal side effects (Lobetti and Joubert, 2000; Parton et al., 2000; Dowers et al., 2006; Frendin et al., 2006; Craven et al., 2007; Wooten et al., 2008; Gowan et al., 2011; Mullins et al., 2012; Surdyk et al., 2012; Monteiro-Steagall et al., 2013; Surdyk et al., 2013; Snow et al., 2014).

Long-term use: Many studies have been performed to investigate efficacy of long-term NSAID administration, mostly in animals with osteoarthritis. Safety and tolerability are considered secondary outcomes in most studies, and this results in a significant difference in definition, incidence and severity of side effects reported. A review of reported side effects suggest that on larger samples, the incidence of side effects is about 3–5% for most NSAIDs, with greater incidence in elderly animals and when small samples were considered (Luna et al., 2007; Monteiro-Steagall et al., 2013).

The safety of long-term administration of carprofen (full dose) has been investigated for periods up to 84 days, demonstrating an improvement of lameness, which was greater in dogs that had been lame for less than 6 months; side effects requiring interruption of the treatment were observed in approximately 3% of dogs, with diarrhoea and vomiting being most common, and liver toxicosis being observed in two dogs (Lipscomb et al., 2002; Mansa et al., 2007).

Efficacy and safety of mavacoxib and carprofen (full dose, not minimum effective dose) have been compared in dogs with oestheoarthritis for a period of 134 days, with both drugs improving clinical signs of the disease. Adverse effects, mostly transient gastrointestinal side effects, were observed in approximately half of the dogs, and approximately 2.5% of the dogs were excluded from the study due to severe side effects possibly linked to the treatment (sepsis in a mavacoxib-treated dog, gastrointestinal ulcerations in two carprofen-treated dogs) (Payne-Johnson et al., 2015).

Clinical efficacy and tolerability of cimicoxib administered for 30 days has been investigated in dogs with osteoarthritis, demonstrating improved locomotion, but the study was not designed to draw robust conclusions on side effects (Murrell et al., 2014).

Efficacy and adverse events after robenacoxib or carpofen administration for 12 weeks in dogs with osteoarthritis have been compared, demonstrating similar efficacy.

Transient diarrhoea or vomiting were reported in 23% and 24% of dogs receiving robenacoxib and carprofen, respectively. Serious hepatic adverse effects occurred in both groups in 1.5% of dogs; however, in all cases pre-existing liver disease was suspected (Reymond et al., 2011).

Efficacy and tolerability of firocoxib and carprofen administered for 30 days have been compared demonstrating a greater improvement of lameness scores with firocoxib, with incidence of adverse effects (anorexia, diarrhoea, emesis, polydipsia) being 20% and 31% for firocoxib and carprofen, respectively (Pollmeier et al., 2006).

Most studies in cats investigate the efficacy and safety of long-term treatment with meloxicam and focus the attention on particular subgroups of animals: cats with ostheoarthritis and chronic renal failure. The only side effects noticed in 4% of cats with ostheoarthritis treated with meloxicam (0.01–0.03 mg/kg) for a mean period of 5.8 months was gastrointestinal upset, and the efficacy was judged as good or excellent in 85% of cases. Two studies investigated the effect of meloxicam administration on progression of renal disease in cats, both demonstrating that administration of a low dose is safe in cats with stable chronic kidney disease, and even suggesting that administration of meloxicam may slow down progression of the renal condition, possibly because of its anti-inflammatory effect. Although this is very promising, use of meloxicam in cats with renal disease should be cautious and based on a risk–benefit analysis and owner informed consent, as this condition is a contraindication according to the manufacturer (Lascelles et al., 2001; Gunew et al., 2008; Gowan et al., 2011; 2012; Guillot et al., 2013).

Individual drugs
Figure 5.3 details clinical use of NSAIDs in specific conditions.

Robenacoxib: In cats, robenacoxib is 500 times more selective towards COX-2 than COX-1; in dogs it is 140 times more selective. Peak plasma concentration occurs 1 hour after subcutaneous administration and 30 minutes after oral administration; it is highly protein bound and undergoes liver metabolism. Its terminal half-life is short after subcutaneous administration (1.2 h in dogs, 1.1 h in cats), with longer persistence in inflamed tissues. In experimental models of osteoarthritis in dogs, robenacoxib demonstrated quicker penetration, higher concentration, and longer permanence in inflamed joints compared with healthy ones. Excretion is biliary (70% in cats, 65% in dogs) and renal. Gastrointestinal side effects are fairly common in cats (vomiting), and common in dogs. Robenacoxib must be taken without food (at least 30 minutes before or after a meal), otherwise oral bioavailability will be significantly decreased (King et al., 2010; Schmid et al., 2010; Silber et al., 2010; Pelligand et al., 2014; Borer et al., 2016).

Tolfenamic acid: Tolfenamic acid is a preferential COX-2 inhibitor; maximum plasma concentration occurs 2 hours after subcutaneous and intramuscular administration and 1 hour after oral administration in dogs, and after 1 hour in cats, as per the summary of product characteristics. It highly binds to plasma proteins. Its elimination half-life is approximately 6.5 hours in dogs, and it is subject to significant enterohepatic recirculation. Metabolites are excreted in the urine. Maximum concentration in exudate and transudate is achieved in 4.5 hours or more (McKellar et al., 1994b).

Mavacoxib: Mavacoxib is a COX-2 selective NSAID, characterized by a very slow clearance and large volume of distribution, resulting in a terminal half-life of 8 to 39 days in dogs, although in a small proportion of dogs it may exceed 80 days. Oral bioavailability is approaching 90% if mavacoxib is administered with food. The peculiar pharmacokinetics of this drug allows for monthly dosing after an initial administration at 2 weeks apart; therefore, this drug may be indicated when daily dosing is difficult due to the dog's temperament or owner's compliance (Cox et al., 2010; 2011; Vilar et al., 2013; Lees et al., 2014; Walton et al., 2014; Payne-Johnson et al., 2015).

Species	Route	Dosing	Duration	Pre general anaesthetic	Recommended for use?					Min. age	Other
					Cardiac	Renal	Liver	GI	Pregnancy		
Carprofen											
Dog	i.v., s.c.	4 mg/kg q24h 2 mg/kg q12h	Single	Y	N	N	N	N	N	6 weeks, use with caution	Contraindicated in animals with hypotension, hypovolaemia, dehydration
Dog	Orally	4 mg/kg q24h 2 mg/kg q12h	5 days postoperative	N	N	N	N	N	N		
Dog	Orally	2–4 mg/kg q24h	Long term with regular monitoring	N	N	N	N	N	N		Dose can be reduced after 7 days if a response is seen
Cat	i.v., s.c.	4 mg/kg	Single	Y	N	N	N	N	N		Not licensed in cats for repeated administration
Cimicoxib											
Dog	Orally	2 mg/kg q24h	3–7 days postoperative 6 months (OA), or longer with monitoring	Y	Care	Care	Care	N	N	10 weeks (use with caution up to 6 months)	Contraindicated in animals with hypotension, hypovolaemia, dehydration Common transient GI signs
Firocoxib											
Dog	Orally	5 mg/kg q24h	90 days, longer if monitoring (OA) 3 days postoperative	Y	Care	Care	Care	N	N	10 weeks or 3 kg	Contraindicated in animals with hypotension, hypovolaemia, dehydration

5.3 Clinical use of non-steroidal anti-inflammatory drugs (NSAIDs) in specific conditions. GA = general anaesthesia; GI = gastrointestinal; OA = osteoarthritis; PLE = protein-losing enteropathy. (continues)

Species	Route	Dosing	Duration	Pre general anaesthetic	Recommended for use?					Min. age	Other
					Cardiac	Renal	Liver	GI	Pregnancy		
Ketoprofen											
Dog and cat	Orally, i.v., i.m., s.c.	1 mg/kg q24h	Max. 5 days for acute pain	N	N	N	N	N	N	6 weeks, use with caution	Contraindicated in animals with hypotension, hypovolaemia, dehydration
Dog	Orally	0.25 mg/kg q24h	30 days for chronic pain	N	N	N	N	N	N		
Mavacoxib											
Dog	Orally	2 mg/kg, repeated after 14 days and then monthly	6.5 months to avoid accumulation if slow metabolism (7 doses)	N	N	N	N	N	N	12 months or 5 kg	Haematology and biochemistry to be checked before starting treatment. Contraindicated also in PLE
Meloxicam											
Dog	i.v., s.c.	0.2 mg/kg	Single (postoperative pain)	Y	N	N	N	N	N	6 weeks	Contraindicated in animals with hypotension, hypovolaemia, dehydration
Dog	s.c.	0.2 mg/kg	Single, followed by oral dosing (musculo-skeletal pain)	N	N	N	N	N	N		
Dog	Orally	0.1 mg/kg q24h	Daily (acute and chronic pain)	N	N	N	N	N	N		Adjust dose for chronic treatment
Cat	s.c.	0.3 mg/kg	Single (acute pain)	Y	N	N	N	N	N	6 weeks or 2 kg	No oral follow up with high s.c. dose
Cat	s.c.	0.2 mg/kg	Single, followed by orally for 4 days	Y	N	N	N	N	N		Postoperative pain

5.3 (continued) Clinical use of non-steroidal anti-inflammatory drugs (NSAIDs) in specific conditions. GA = general anaesthesia; GI = gastrointestinal; OA = osteoarthritis; PLE = protein-losing enteropathy. (continues)

Species	Route	Dosing	Duration	Pre general anaesthetic	Recommended for use?					Min. age	Other
					Cardiac	Renal	Liver	GI	Pregnancy		
Meloxicam continued											
Cat	Orally	0.05 mg/kg q24h	For up to 4 days after s.c. injection of 0.2 mg/kg	N	N	N	N	N	N	6 weeks or 2 kg	Postoperative pain
Cat	Orally	0.05 mg/kg q24h	No limit, following an initial dose of 0.1 mg/kg	N	N	N	N	N	N		For chronic musculo-skeletal disorders. Discontinue after 14 days if no response
Robenacoxib											
Dog	s.c.	2 mg/kg	Single	Y	Y	Y	Y	N	N	2 months or 2.5 kg	Contraindicated in animals with hypotension, hypovolaemia, dehydration
Dog	Orally	1 mg/kg q24h	No limit – toxicity investigated up to 6 months	N	Y	Y	N	N	N		Adjust to lowest effective dose for long-term treatment. Monitor liver enzymes before, and then at 2, 4, 8 weeks after therapy, then after 3–6 months. Care if hypotension, hypovolaemia or dehydration
Cat	s.c.	2 mg/kg	Single, followed up by orally	Y	Y	Y	Y	N	N	4 months or 2.5 kg	
Cat	Orally	1 mg/kg q24h	Up to 2 days after surgery	N	Y	Y	Y	N	N		

5.3 (continued) Clinical use of non-steroidal anti-inflammatory drugs (NSAIDs) in specific conditions. GA = general anaesthesia; GI = gastrointestinal; OA = osteoarthritis; PLE = protein-losing enteropathy. (continues)

Species	Route	Dosing	Duration	Pre general anaesthetic	Recommended for use?					Min. age	Other
					Cardiac	Renal	Liver	GI	Pregnancy		
Robenacoxib continued											
Cat	Orally	1 mg/kg q24h	Up to 6 days	Y	Y	Y	Y	N	N	4 months or 2.5 kg	Only to be used with butorphanol prior to GA. Care if hypotension, hypovolaemia or dehydration
Tolfenamic acid											
Dog	i.m., s.c.	4 mg/kg	Single; can be repeated once after 24 hours or treatment continued orally	Y	N	Y chronic; N acute	N	N	N	6 weeks, use with caution. Do not use if less than 7 kg	For perioperative pain or acute pain. Do not use in dehydrated, hypovolaemia, or hypotensive animals
Dog	Orally	4 mg/kg q24h	3 days, can be repeated every 7 days	N	N	Y chronic	N	N	N	6 weeks, use with caution	Treatment longer than 3 months must be under veterinary supervision
Cat	s.c.	4 mg/kg	Single administration	N	N	Y	N	N	N		Licensed for treatment of respiratory infections in association with antimicrobials
Cat	Orally	4 mg/kg q24h	3 days	N	N	Y chronic	N	N	N		

5.3 (continued) Clinical use of non-steroidal anti-inflammatory drugs (NSAIDs) in specific conditions. GA = general anaesthesia; GI = gastrointestinal; OA = osteoarthritis; PLE = protein-losing enteropathy.

Ketoprofen: Ketoprofen is a racemic mixture, preferentially inhibiting COX-1, mostly because of the activity of the S(+) enantiomer. The drug is characterized by a very short half-life (1.2 h), but prolonged COX-1 inhibition in exudate, thus presenting inflammatory tissue selectivity, similarly to robenacoxib, but without COX-2 selectivity (Lees *et al.*, 2003; Pelligand *et al.*, 2014).

Carprofen: Carprofen is a racemic mixture, with a preferential COX-2 inhibitory effect, but it is believed that other mechanisms of action may be involved in its anti-inflammatory and analgesic effects. Carprofen can be detected in inflammatory fluid within 2 hours and peaks at 7 hours after intravenous administration. Its half-life in the dog is about 8 hours and oral bioavailability is greater than 90%, while in the cat the half-life is considerably longer, explaining the reduced safety margin in this species. Differently from ketoprofen and robenacoxib, carprofen does not present inflammatory tissue selectivity. Hepatopathy of variable severity has been reported in dogs treated with carprofen (McKellar *et al.*, 1994a; Clark *et al.*, 2003; Taylor *et al.*, 2007; Messenger *et al.*, 2016).

Meloxicam: Meloxicam is a selective COX-2 inhibitor. It has an oral bioavailability in excess of 90%, and peak plasma concentration is achieved in approximately 8 hours in dogs and 3 hours in cats after oral administration. Administration with food may result in a delay in oral absorption. Its elimination half-life is approximately 24 hours both in the cat and the dog, with the majority of the metabolites excreted in the faeces. Meloxicam is also formulated as an oromucosal spray, which may make administration easier in some dogs (Montoya *et al.*, 2004; Carroll *et al.*, 2011).

Firocoxib: Firocoxib is a selective COX-2 inhibitor, with an oral bioavailability of 37% after administration to fasted dogs. Administration with food does not affect bioavailability, but will delay absorption. Peak plasma concentration is achieved 1.25 hours after oral administration to fasted dogs, and the elimination half-life is 7.8 hours. Metabolism is hepatic and metabolites are eliminated in the bile. Steady state concentration is achieved after 3 days of dosing, according to the summary of product characteristics and further research (Pollmeier *et al.*, 2006; Ryan *et al.*, 2010).

Cimicoxib: Cimicoxib is a very selective COX-2 inhibitor. Oral bioavailability is 44%, and it is not significantly affected by feeding status. Time to peak plasma concentration is 2.25 hours and the elimination half-life is 1.4 hours, with the major metabolite being eliminated in bile, and its glucuronide conjugate in urine. Population pharmacokinetics in dogs has identified slow metabolizers, with the half-life twice as long in some cases. Despite the short half-life, clinical trials have determined that once daily administration is clinically appropriate (Grandemange *et al.*, 2013; Kim *et al.*, 2014; Murrell *et al.*, 2014; Schneider *et al.*, 2015).

Grapiprant: This is a new non-COX inhibiting NSAID. It targets the EP4 prostaglandin receptor, which is the primary mediator of canine osteoarthritis pain and inflammation.

Local anaesthetics

The pharmacology of local anaesthetics is relevant because of their local effect and systemic absorption from the site of administration after performing a locoregional technique, and because of the systemic effects and disposition of lidocaine after intravenous administration.

Although modern local anaesthetics are safer than their predecessors, they are not devoid of side effects, and severe adverse reactions are still possible, although rare. It is therefore crucial to understand the pharmacology and toxicity of these compounds and to choose the dose, volume and concentration in view of the desired effects.

It is necessary to point out, before further discussing local anaesthetics, that currently there are only two licensed formulations for cats and dogs (lidocaine with adrenaline and procaine with adrenaline), and the licence terms limit their use to nerve blocks, paravertebral nerve blocks and local infiltration.

Structure–activity relationship

Local anaesthetics typically consist of a hydrophilic amine domain and a hydrophobic domain, separated by an ester or amide linkage. They are synthetic derivatives of cocaine, the first compound used for its local anaesthetic properties. The local anaesthetics currently used are mostly amides, as esters are more likely to cause allergic reactions. Amide anaesthetics are considerably more stable than esters, and they can even be autoclaved. As a rule of thumb, local anaesthetics whose name contains an 'i' before the 'caine' suffix have an amide linkage (lidocaine, bupivacaine, ropivacaine) (Tucker and Mather, 1979; Aguirre *et al.*, 2012; Becker and Reed, 2012).

Local anaesthetics are chiral compounds, therefore exist as stereoisomers, and the two enantiomers may present different pharmacokinetic and pharmacodynamic characteristics. Bupivacaine, for example, is the racemic mixture of two enatiomers (R(+) and S(–)), one of which (S(–)) is marketed as levobupivacaine) and presents less cardiotoxicity. Similarly, ropivacaine is an S-enantiomer (Aguirre *et al.*, 2012; Becker and Reed, 2012; Patel and Sadoughi, 2014).

While ester anaesthetics are metabolized by pseudocholinesterase, amide anaesthetics require extensive liver metabolism. The rate of removal from the site of injection is crucial for delivering the drug to the systemic circulation and the site of metabolism (and toxicity); therefore, addition of a vasoconstrictor in the formulation increases the duration of action and reduces systemic toxicity (Braid and Scott, 1966; Miranda *et al.*, 2016). Similarly, the total dose of anaesthetic administered affects the duration of action and the risk of toxicity.

Local anaesthetics block nerve conduction by reversibly binding to the voltage-gated sodium channels in the nerve, with greater affinity for the channel in the active state. The site of action is intracellular, and the ionized water-soluble formulation is converted to the un-ionized lipid soluble formulation which is able to cross cell membranes, because of the difference between the anaesthetic pK and the pH of tissues. The greater the pK of the local anaesthetic, the smaller the un-ionized fraction will be at body pH, delaying the onset of action. Infected and inflamed tissue has a lower pH and greater perfusion than normal tissue, so the effect and duration of action of local anaesthetics may be decreased, to the point of making them ineffective in the event of local infiltration (Scholz, 2002; Becker and Reed, 2006; Paganelli and Popescu, 2015).

The pH of local anaesthetic solutions is generally low; therefore, they may cause an intense burning sensation at the site of injection, and this could be relevant in conscious, sedated, or lightly anaesthetized animals. Alkalinization of local anaesthetic solutions with bicarbonate may reduce the burning sensation and reduce the onset time of the effect, increasing the un-ionized form, although excessive alkalinization will result in precipitation (Englesson, 1974; Tucker, 1986; Patel and Sadoughi, 2014).

Perineural administration

Sodium channel blockade reduces the excitability of the cell membrane, thus affecting the ability of the cell to depolarize. When a critical number of sodium channels are blocked in a nerve fibre, propagation of electrical signals stops. For myelinated fibres, a minimum of three Ranviers' nodes have to be blocked to stop propagation of electrical signals; however, incomplete blockade of more nodes may still be effective, provided that the concentration of the anaesthetic used is not too low, in which case the block becomes inconsistent.

The larger the nerve fibre, the more anaesthetic is needed to block conduction, and blockade of unmyelinated fibres requires more anaesthetic compared with myelinated fibres of the same diameter. Clinically, blockade caused by local anaesthetics shows a differential onset according to fibre diameter and type, first affecting nociception, then thermal sensation, and finally motor function. This is because nociception is transmitted by C fibres (unmyelinated, but very small) and Aδ fibres (myelinated, and of small diameter), while motor fibres are myelinated and considerably larger. Recovery of function follows the reverse order, with nociceptive fibre function returning last. The profile of differential recovery depends on the concentration and the anaesthetic molecule used, with lower concentrations having less effect on motor function, and some anaesthetics (bupivacaine, levobupivacaine and ropivacaine) presenting a more evident differential effect on motor and sensory fibres during the offset period (Aguirre *et al.*, 2012).

Duration of action of local anaesthetics depends mostly on their protein binding, with increased protein binding resulting in longer duration of action, because of a slower clearance from the administration site. Unfortunately, a high degree of protein binding also results in more anaesthetic binding to non-specific sites in the tissue adjacent to the nerve to be anaesthetized, with a slower onset of action. Administration of larger doses will prolong the duration of action, and also result in a faster onset. Addition of vasoconstrictors (generally adrenaline 1:100000–1:200000) prolongs the duration of action of local anaesthetics by decreasing their clearance, and the effect is more relevant for those with a short duration of action (i.e. prilocaine, lidocaine). While most local anaesthetics at clinical doses cause vasodilation, ropivacaine causes vasoconstriction, which explains its longer duration of action (Aguirre *et al.*, 2012; Becker and Reed, 2006).

Epidural administration

When administered epidurally, the main site of action of local anaesthetics is the nerve roots leaving the spinal cord, where the meninges taper off and the anaesthetic can easily reach the nerve. Part of the local anaesthetic, especially if administered at high concentrations, will penetrate the meninges and reach the spinal cord. The arachnoid membrane accounts for 90% of the resistance to drug migration. Transmeningeal uptake may also be promoted by addition of vasoconstrictors, which reduce systemic absorption, therefore maintaining a high concentration of drug in the epidural space that drives the uptake. The effect is less pronounced for ropivacaine, because of its intrinsic vasoconstrictor effect. The preferential extramedullary site of action can be exploited,

using specific combinations of volume and concentration, to cause segmental anaesthesia, therefore affecting only the nerves bathed by the local anaesthetic. The result is a 'belt' of anaesthesia, with minimally affected sensory and motor function cranially and caudally to the site of administration. The local anaesthetic is removed from the epidural space mostly by venous drainage and systemic absorption, distribution in the epidural fat and transmeningeal uptake, but also by exiting the spinal canal via the intervertebral foramen. The larger the volume of drug administered, the longer the duration of action (Burm, 1989; Feldman *et al.*, 1997; Clement *et al.*, 1999; Rose *et al.*, 2007; Ratajczak-Enselme *et al.*, 2007; O'Donohoe and Pandit, 2012; Siafaka, n.d.).

Subarachnoid 'spinal' administration

The site of action and the disposition of local anaesthetics administered in the subarachnoid space (spinal, subarachnoid or intrathecal anaesthesia) are considerably different from those of epidurally administered anaesthetics, as the anaesthetic is administered within the cerebrospinal fluid (CSF). The sites of action for drugs injected in the subarachnoid space are both the spinal cord and the nerve roots. Since all neural structures are exposed to the local anaesthetic, they are all affected by the block, resulting in sensory, motor and autonomic blockade. To some extent, this could be considered a 'temporary chemical cordectomy', although the extent of penetration into the spinal cord and nerve roots will depend on the amount and concentration of drug used.

The disposition of drugs administered intrathecally is still poorly understood, but possible mechanisms could be epidural diffusion, spinal cord diffusion, and bulk removal by CSF turnover. Regardless of the exact mechanism, the duration of action of intrathecal anaesthetics is considerably shorter than epidural administration and depends on the total amount of drug administered and, to some extent, on its concentration, with lower concentrations having a shorter effect (Clement *et al.*, 1999; Rose *et al.*, 2007; Sarotti *et al.*, 2011; Sarotti *et al.*, 2013; De Gennaro *et al.*, 2014).

Other routes

Other commonly used routes of administration for local anaesthetics are intra-articular, intrapleural and intraperitoneal. While there is little concern in terms of systemic toxicity after intra-articular administration, the absorption rate from the pleural and peritoneal space is significant, resulting in potentially toxic concentrations if large doses are administered. In cats, intraperitoneal administration of 2 mg/kg bupivacaine 0.5% did not result in systemic toxicity with peak plasma concentration occurring 30 minutes after administration, and had an elimination half-life of approximately 5 hours, suggesting that this dose and route of administration for bupivacaine may be safe, at least in the presence of a normal peritoneum. The major concern after intra-articular administration is chondrotoxicity. Studies in humans have demonstrated that this risk is significant for repeated administrations and infusions, while it is less clinically relevant after single administration. *In vitro* studies have demonstrated dose- and time-dependent chondrotoxicity for all local anaesthetics. A study in dogs has demonstrated chondrotoxicity for both lidocaine and bupivacaine after single administration with steroids in the shoulder joint (Aguirre *et al.*, 2012; Di Salvo *et al.*, 2014, 2015; Sherman *et al.*, 2015).

Liposomal bupivacaine

A liposomal bupivacaine formulation has been licensed by the US Food and Drug Administration for use in dogs undergoing cranial cruciate surgery. Liposomal bupivacaine has been licensed for use in humans since 2011, as a single dose local infiltration analgesic technique. After infiltration in soft tissues at the end of surgery, bupivacaine is slowly released from the vesicular liposomes, resulting in sustained analgesia for several days. In practical terms this is equivalent to continuous infusion of local analgesics using a wound soaking catheter, but without the possible catheter-related complications. This method of administration does not allow the exploitation of one of the most relevant advantages of local anaesthesia: preventive analgesia, which can be achieved only with pre-incisional administration (Chahar and Cummings, 2012; Viscusi *et al.*, 2014; Joshi *et al.*, 2015; Aratana, 2016; Lascelles and Kirkby Shaw, 2016).

Intravenous lidocaine

Unlike other local anaesthetics, lidocaine can be safely administered as an intravenous infusion due to its limited toxicity, at least in dogs. In cats, the margin of safety is smaller; therefore, there is a greater risk of side effects. While its use as an antiarrhythmic or its role in ischaemic reperfusion injury and shock are not the subject of this handbook, intravenous lidocaine infusion can be used to provide perioperative analgesia in the hospitalized animal. Lidocaine's efficacy in treating neuropathic pain has been reported in humans since the 1980s, in particular to treat post-herpetic, diabetic and chemotherapy-induced neuropathy. Its efficacy is supported by a Cochrane review (Kranke *et al.*, 2015). The most plausible mechanism of action of lidocaine in this setting is the blockade of sodium channels, reducing ectopic firing of damaged nerves and neurons. Injured fibres and neurons are more sensitive to lidocaine at low doses because of the characteristic upregulation of sodium channels observed after the injury. The response to lidocaine administration may be variable, depending on the type of sodium channel that is upregulated, as lidocaine is more effective in blocking tetrodotoxin-resistant sodium channels compared with tetrodotoxin-sensitive ones, with the former being mostly upregulated in nerves after injury. The analgesic and minimum alveolar concentration (MAC) sparing effect of systemic lidocaine has been demonstrated in the dog, although currently there are no systematic studies investigating its efficacy in treating neuropathic pain syndromes, and the current evidence is limited to case reports, expert opinion, and the known efficacy in human beings. Unfortunately, the use of intravenous lidocaine infusions to treat neuropathic pain is limited to the hospital setting; until a few years ago, mexiletine was available as an oral alternative to continue therapy at home in dogs that had a positive response to lidocaine. Despite this no longer being a possibility, a positive response to lidocaine infusion is still an invaluable tool to diagnose neuropathic pain, in view of utilizing other drugs inhibiting or blocking sodium channels. In a clinical setting, lidocaine infusion plays a big role, at least in dogs, in the control of pain syndromes that are poorly responsive to opioids and NSAIDs. The commonly used protocol suggests a loading dose of 1–2 mg/kg, followed by a continuous infusion of 2–3 mg/kg/h. Commonly observed side effects are sedation and reduced appetite, but they are generally mild and self-limiting, and rarely require discontinuation of the therapy, especially in the presence of neuropathic pain (Galer *et al.*, 1996; Jolliffe *et al.*, 2007; Hutson *et al.*, 2015; Papapetrou *et al.*, 2015; Przeklasa-Muszyńska *et al.*, 2016).

Transdermal administration

Lidocaine can also be delivered transdermally using a patch, which is licensed to treat postherpetic neuralgia (PHN) pain in humans. The drug transferred to the skin is believed to induce local analgesia by inhibiting spontaneous discharge of injured small nociceptive fibres (C and Aδ), without significantly affecting the function of large sensory fibres, therefore preserving sensation. While lidocaine patches are an effective treatment for PHN pain in human patients, they appear less effective in treating neuropathic pain of different origin. The role of lidocaine patches in treating postoperative pain in humans is still controversial, with a few studies and case reports reporting some efficacy, and meta-analyses suggesting that the overall effect is negligible.

Systemic absorption is minimal, and not sufficient to support a systemic effect of the drug. Studies in dogs and cats have demonstrated minimal systemic absorption, as in humans, and suggested that the patch may deliver lidocaine for up to 2 days after application on intact skin in dogs, and up to 3 days in cats. A recent study suggests that absorption may be greater if the patch is applied directly over a skin incision in dogs.

Currently the author [FC] is not aware of any prospective study or even case report supporting the efficacy of lidocaine patches in providing analgesia in dogs and cats, despite the products being available and having been used for many years (Meier *et al.*, 2003; Burch *et al.*, 2004; Weiland *et al.*, 2006; Ko *et al.*, 2007; Weil *et al.*, 2007; Ko *et al.*, 2008; Saber *et al.*, 2009; Gilhooly *et al.*, 2011; Bai *et al.*, 2015; Joudrey *et al.*, 2015).

Toxicity

Cardiovascular and neurological toxicity are major side effects secondary to systemic absorption or administration of local anaesthetics. At high concentrations, local anaesthetics also affect potassium and calcium channels, and this could further contribute to systemic toxicity (Nakahira *et al.*, 2016).

The most common causes of severe systemic toxicity are accidental intravascular administration and rapid systemic absorption after administration of large doses of anaesthetics. Neurological signs of toxicity are depression and twitching, progressing to generalized seizures (Cox *et al.*, 2003; Beecroft and Davies, 2016). Toxic doses after intravenous administration have been well characterized in dogs, suggesting an acute neurological toxicity occurring for doses of bupivacaine and ropivacaine greater than 2–3 mg/kg, and greater than 10 mg/kg for lidocaine (Feldman *et al.*, 1989).

Cardiovascular toxicity presents as progressive cardiovascular depression, with arrhythmias, including tachycardia, ventricular tachycardia and ventricular fibrillation. In a continuous intravenous infusion model, the cumulative dose that caused cardiovascular collapse was 21 mg/kg for bupivacaine, 27 mg/kg for levobupivacaine, 42 mg/kg for ropivacaine and 127 mg/kg for lidocaine. While all dogs in the lidocaine group could be resuscitated, mortality rates were 50% for bupivacaine, 30% for levobupivacaine, and 10% for ropivacaine overdose. This study also neatly demonstrates that cardiotoxicity is affected by stereoselectivity, as levobupivacaine appears to be less toxic than bupivacaine (Groban *et al.*,

2001). It should be appreciated that the dose was a cumulative dose administered over a significant amount of time and not as a rapid bolus. For comparison, another study reported a single rapid intravenous bolus of 11 mg/kg of bupivacaine to cause severe cardiovascular depression in dogs (Liu *et al.*, 1983).

A study in cats demonstrated that, in a model of continuous intravenous infusion, neurotoxicity occurred at 12 mg/kg for lidocaine and 4 mg/kg for bupivacaine. The cardiotoxic dose was found to be 47 mg/kg for lidocaine and 18 mg/kg for bupivacaine. While all cats in the lidocaine group could be resuscitated, 2/10 cats in the bupivacaine group could not (Chadwick, 1985).

It should be pointed out that these toxic doses are all obtained administering the drug intravenously, thus they represent the clinical scenario of accidental intravenous administration of a supra-clinical dose of local anaesthetic, not the uncomplicated use in locoregional anaesthesia (Aprea *et al.*, 2011).

Published data about toxic intravenous doses should be taken with a pinch of salt, as the rate of absorption from tissues should be taken into account in a clinical setting, and therefore the current suggested maximum dose is likely to be fairly conservative, as demonstrated by clinical studies in humans. The risk of toxicity probably is greater in smaller animals, as a relatively small increase in the administered volume results in a greater increase of the amount of drug administered on the basis of body mass (Rosenberg *et al.*, 2004).

In the event of toxicity, intravenous infusion of a lipid emulsion has been shown to dramatically improve haemodynamic side effects of bupivacaine overdose in experimental settings, and there are case reports describing its successful clinical use in veterinary medicine (Feldman *et al.*, 1991; Weinberg *et al.*, 2003; O'Brien *et al.*, 2010). It is widely used in humans, although recently its efficacy and safety have been questioned (O'Brien *et al.*, 2010; Picard and Meek, 2016; Rosenberg, 2016). Lipid rescue protocols reported in veterinary medicine suggest infusing 1.5 ml/kg Intralipid 20% over 10–30 minutes, and repeating this if necessary

(Weinberg *et al.*, 2003). If lipid rescue is not available, symptomatic treatment (anti-convulsants, antimuscarinics, antiarrhythmics, inotropes, vasopressors and fluids) can be attempted to control clinical signs while the toxic drug is cleared by the body (Aprea *et al.*, 2011).

Alpha-2 agonists

Alpha-2 agonists such as medetomidine and dexmedetomidine (its active enantiomer) are widely used in small animal practice for sedation and pre-anaesthetic medication. They also have analgesic properties. They bind to alpha-2 adrenergic receptors in the cerebral cortex and locus coeruleus of the brain, causing sedation, analgesia and a reduction in sympathetic tone, and in the dorsal horn of the spinal cord, causing analgesia. The mechanism of analgesia is complex and not well understood. Agonism of alpha-2 receptors in peripheral and pulmonary blood vessels causes vasoconstriction, hypertension, reflex bradycardia and decreased cardiac output. Other effects include hypothermia, decreased gastrointestinal motility, diuresis and hyperglycaemia. All these effects are dose-dependent, and can be antagonized using atipamezole, although this also removes any analgesic effect.

Because of their sedative and cardiovascular effects, alpha-2 agonists are unsuitable for use as the primary or sole analgesic, but may provide additional analgesia when used as part of an anaesthetic protocol. They act synergistically with opioids. The analgesic effect is of a shorter duration than the sedative effect, and requires higher plasma concentrations. They may be useful for treating neuropathic pain (Murrell and Hellebrekers, 2005).

Clinical use

Inclusion of alpha-2 agonists as part of the sedation or pre-anaesthetic protocol may provide additional analgesia for the patient. However, because of the cardiovascular effects of these drugs, they are usually reserved for healthy patients without cardiac disease.

Low-dose intravenous infusions are useful intraoperatively as part of a balanced anaesthesia technique to reduce anaesthetic requirements and postoperatively to provide titratable sedation and analgesia. Dexmedetomidine infusion (1 μg/kg/hour) has been shown to be as effective to a morphine infusion (0.1 mg/kg/hour) for providing analgesia following major surgery in dogs without adverse effects (Valtolina *et al.*, 2009). Dogs receiving dexmedetomidine in this study had lower heart rates and higher diastolic blood pressure than dogs receiving morphine, but these were still within acceptable ranges. The cardiovascular effects of an infusion are less severe than those that occur following intravenous or intramuscular injection of a bolus dose. Suggested doses for clinical use are 1–3 μg/kg/hour for medetomidine and 0.5–2 μg/kg/hour for dexmedetomidine, although the dose can be adjusted to achieve the desired effect. To achieve an appropriate plasma concentration of the drug quickly, an initial intravenous bolus is usually recommended. The aim should be a calm patient that can still function normally, i.e. eat, drink and ambulate, unless more profound sedation is required. Volumes used are very small so the solution must be diluted carefully, and an infusion pump or syringe driver should be used.

In locoregional anaesthesia, addition of alpha-2 agonists to the local anaesthetic solution significantly prolongs the duration of effect. For example, a technique for sciatic and femoral nerve blocks using dexmedetomidine (0.1 μg/kg for each block) combined with bupivacaine has been described (Bartel *et al.*, 2016). Only preservative-free solutions should be used for epidural or spinal anaesthesia.

NMDA receptor antagonists

N-methyl-D-aspartate (NMDA) receptors are located in the brain and spinal cord. Activation occurs after repeated or widespread input from afferent neurones carrying nociceptive signals (temporal and spatial summation). NMDA receptor activation results in prolonged depolarization of second order dorsal horn neurones, a phenomenon known as 'wind-up', which can result in remodelling of the central nervous system and ultimately alter the animal's perception of future painful and non-painful stimuli (central sensitization). Drugs that antagonize NMDA receptors are analgesic and can also help prevent central sensitization, secondary hyperalgesia and chronic pain.

Ketamine

Ketamine is a dissociative anaesthetic and analgesic that antagonizes NMDA receptors in the central nervous system. It also acts at other receptors including opioid receptors, and inhibits serotonin and dopamine reuptake. Ketamine is now a Schedule 2 Controlled Drug in the UK and must be kept in a locked cupboard with detailed records of its acquisition and use.

Effects: Ketamine's properties and uses vary with dose. At doses greater than 5 mg/kg intravenously or intramuscularly it can be used to induce dissociative anaesthesia, at lower doses it can be used as part of a sedation protocol, and at very low doses (0.5–1 mg/kg) it is an effective somatic analgesic. Because of its adverse effects (dysphoria, excitement, increased muscle tone, seizures in dogs), ketamine should not be used alone except at very low doses, and it is usually combined with an alpha-2 agonist or benzodiazepine for this reason. It can cause increased salivation and nausea. Ketamine has several beneficial effects compared with other induction agents: it maintains cardiac output and blood pressure due to its sympathomimetic effects with little effect on blood vessels. It also causes bronchodilation, preserves laryngeal reflexes and patients usually breathe well. However, ketamine increases cerebral blood flow and cerebral oxygen demand, which may result in increased intracranial pressure. Used alone, it increases intraocular pressure. In dogs, ketamine is metabolized in the liver (norketamine is an active metabolite) and excreted in urine; in cats, it is mostly excreted unchanged in urine and therefore its effects may be prolonged in cats with renal insufficiency.

Clinical use:

Sedation and anaesthesia induction: If used as part of the sedation or induction protocol prior to painful procedures, ketamine probably contributes significantly to analgesia and helps prevent central sensitization. Ketamine (combined with a benzodiazepine) can be a good choice for trauma patients because of its beneficial cardiorespiratory and analgesic properties, but it is not usually recommended for head trauma patients. It should be avoided in patients with intracranial disease, hypertrophic cardiomyopathy, or severe ocular trauma.

Intraoperative analgesia: Ketamine can be administered by intravenous infusion (5–20 µg/kg/min) or by intermittent intravenous boluses during anaesthesia (0.5–1 mg/kg). After a bolus it is quite common to see transient apnoea or a change in respiratory pattern. Ketamine infusion has been shown to reduce inhalant anaesthetic requirements.

Postoperative analgesia: Ketamine can be administered as a low-dose intravenous infusion (2–10 µg/kg/min) to provide analgesia in the postoperative period. Adverse effects are rarely seen at such low doses. Wagner *et al.* (2002) demonstrated that following forelimb amputation, dogs receiving ketamine (10 µg/kg/min intraoperatively followed by 2 µg/kg/min for 18 hours postoperatively) had lower pain scores at 12 and 18 hours post-surgery compared with dogs that did not receive ketamine. They were perceived by their owners to be more active at home 3 days after surgery. Similar results have been reported in humans and there is evidence in humans that use of low-dose ketamine reduces postoperative opioid requirement after major surgery. There is limited evidence regarding the optimal duration of ketamine infusion, but the authors usually use it for at least 24 hours postoperatively. For day patients it can be used intraoperatively, and postoperatively until the patient is discharged.

Treatment of chronic pain: Although not evidence-based, some anaesthetists recommend using ketamine to 'break the pain cycle' in animals experiencing chronic pain and hyperaesthesia. Options include a one-off subcutaneous or intravenous injection of a low dose of ketamine (0.5 mg/kg), or admitting the animal for a day to administer a low-dose intravenous ketamine infusion.

Amantadine

Amantadine is an NMDA receptor antagonist available as an oral capsule or syrup, which can be administered at home by owners. It may be useful for treating chronic pain. Research is limited, but the recommended dose is 3–5 mg/kg q24h in dogs and cats (Siao *et al.*, 2011; Norkus *et al.*, 2015c). Amantadine has been shown to improve activity in dogs with osteoarthritis when combined with meloxicam (Lascelles *et al.*, 2008), and it has been successfully used to treat neuropathic pain in a dog (Madden *et al.*, 2014). It is renally excreted. Anecdotally, it has been reported that amantadine can cause vomiting in dogs.

Nitrous oxide

Nitrous oxide has long been used as an analgesic and anaesthetic-sparing agent in humans and animals. It is an NMDA receptor antagonist, and its intraoperative use has been shown to reduce post-surgical opioid requirements and chronic pain in humans (Stiglitz *et al.*, 2010; Chan *et al.*, 2011). It is a gas that can be mixed with oxygen during anaesthesia, typically a 30:70 or 50:50 oxygen:nitrous oxide mix. Use of an oxygen analyser or a pulse oximeter is required when it is used in a circle system due to the potential for delivery of low oxygen concentrations to the patient. Nitrous oxide accumulates in gas-filled cavities and is contraindicated in patients with gastric dilatation and volvulus, pneumothorax and similar conditions. It is also contraindicated for patients with intracranial disease. Nitrous oxide causes a reduction in DNA synthesis, temporary bone marrow changes, and neurological symptoms. Theatre pollution with nitrous oxide must be avoided by use of proper scavenging; it should not be used during mask or chamber inductions.

Antidepressants

Antidepressants are often used as part of multimodal analgesia in the management of chronic, neuropathic and persistent pain, in some cases with good results (Mehta *et al.*, 2015; Moore *et al.*, 2015).

The antidepressant most used in veterinary medicine to manage pain is probably amitriptyline, a tricyclic antidepressant (TCA), despite not being licensed for use in dogs and cats. The veterinary TCA licensed for use in dogs is clomipramine, which shares most of the pharmacological properties that may be relevant to pain management.

TCAs with tertiary amine structure (amitriptyline and clomipramine) inhibit reuptake of noradrenaline and serotonin, but they are also mild NMDA antagonists, antimuscarinics, voltage-gated sodium channel blockers, alpha-1 adrenergic receptor and H1 histamine receptor antagonists, and activate descending inhibitory pathways. They also inhibit the NF-κB pathway, which is involved in promoting and maintaining neuroinflammation (Lenkey *et al.*, 2006; Rahimi *et al.*, 2012; Zychowska *et al.*, 2015). Clomipramine is more effective in promoting serotonin reuptake. Their mechanism of action on nociception can be explained in many different ways. Interestingly, most of the pathways involved in neuropathic, chronic and persistent pain are affected by tertiary amine TCAs, which makes these drugs very interesting in this setting.

Amitriptyline (1–2 mg/kg orally q24h) has been shown to be an effective treatment for severe recurrent idiopathic cystitis in cats, likely in part because of the behavioural effects, but also because of the effect on neuropathic pain, as this condition is a well known visceral pain syndrome, and the direct effect of increasing bladder capacity by relaxing bladder smooth muscles via stimulation of alpha adrenergic receptors (Westropp and Buffington, 2004; Chew *et al.*, 2016).

Despite the pharmacokinetics of amitriptyline having been well characterized in dogs (Norkus *et al.*, 2015a; 2015b), there are only case reports relating to its use in a clinical setting to treat neuropathic pain, within a multimodal therapy approach (Mathews, 2008; Cashmore *et al.*, 2009; Moore, 2016). The pharmacokinetic study has even raised the question that the current dose (1–2 mg/kg orally q12–24h) may be too low, considering the rapid metabolism of this drug by dogs.

Although in principle TCAs should be effective in the treatment of painful syndromes with a strong neuropathic component, for example, inflammatory bowel disease, feline interstitial cystitis, spinal cord injuries, traumatic peripheral nerve injury, syringohydromyelia, neoplastic nerve injury and paraneoplastic neuropathies and diabetic neuropathy, no large trials have been published to support their efficacy in treating these conditions in small animals.

Possible side effects of TCAs are sedation, tachycardia and, at very high doses, arrhythmias. It is paramount to avoid using TCAs in concomitance with drugs that affect the serotoninergic system, in particular tramadol, as the combination could precipitate serotonin toxicity (see 'Serotonin toxicity').

Steroids

Glucocorticoids are powerful anti-inflammatory drugs, and thus effective in treating inflammatory pain. Glucocorticoids bind to a dedicated cytoplasmic receptor, then translocate to the nucleus, where they cause upregulation or downregulation of glucocorticoid-responsive genes. Their anti-inflammatory action is mainly due to inhibition of the activity of phospholipase A2 (mediated by increased transcription of lipocortin), and therefore of prostaglandins production, but suppression of other pro-inflammatory mediators and non-genomic mechanisms also play an important role (Rhen and Cidlowski, 2005; Ayroldi *et al.*, 2012).

The role of glucocorticoids in perioperative analgesia has been investigated in humans, with particular emphasis on the risk of side effects *versus* potential benefits. Administration of a single dose of glucocorticoid (dexamethasone 0.1–0.2 mg/kg) has not been associated with increased risk of infection or delayed wound healing, and provided variable opioid sparing effect (Romundstad *et al.*, 2004; Waldron *et al.*, 2013).

Data are lacking in dogs about the analgesic effects of glucocorticoids and, despite dexamethasone being licensed as an anti-inflammatory (but not for perioperative analgesia), only the clinical efficacy of prednoleucotropin (PLT) has been documented (McKellar *et al.*, 1991).

The efficacy and tolerability of PLT, a combination of cinchophen and prednisolone, is also confirmed anecdotally and by direct clinical experience. Cinchophen is an NSAID, with a non-specific COX-inhibiting effect. PLT is licensed for the treatment of osteoarthritis in dogs, and it is contraindicated in pregnancy, severe renal disease, congestive heart failure, hepatitis, and concurrent diuretic therapy. It should not be used with other steroids and NSAIDs. Side effects of PLT are those typical of steroids and NSAIDs, and include polyuria/polydypsia/polyphagia, fat redistribution, immunosuppression, and gastrointestinal upset. The manufacturer's indications state that an initial 14-day treatment period should be followed by a 14-day treatment-free interval, before continuing with further treatment. The equivalent of 0.06 mg/kg of prednisolone should be administered twice daily with food. The dose should be tapered at the end of a treatment period, as for steroid therapy.

Tramadol

Tramadol is a MOP agonist with weak receptor affinity. It also inhibits serotonin and noradrenaline reuptake by spinal cord neurones, providing analgesia by enhancement of descending antinociceptive pathways at the spinal level. It is metabolized in the liver with several active metabolites potentially being produced and excreted in urine. In humans, tramadol can lower the seizure threshold and, while this has not been investigated in veterinary patients, it may be wise to avoid tramadol in animals with a history of seizures. There is some evidence in humans and dogs that tramadol or other serotonin reuptake inhibitors can increase the risk of gastro-duodenal ulceration in patients taking

NSAIDs, or those prone to this problem. This may be prevented by the administration of famotidine or omeprazole to reduce gastric acid production (KuKanich, 2013). (See 'Serotonin toxicity'.)

In humans, tramadol is metabolized to an active metabolite (O-desmethyl tramadol or ODM). ODM is a high affinity MOP agonist and is 200 times as potent as tramadol. Dogs produce only small amounts of ODM and lack of this metabolite may explain the variations in efficacy reported in this species. Indeed, a significant proportion of dogs may not respond at all. Analgesia associated with tramadol in dogs may be primarily due to its serotonin and noradrenaline reuptake inhibition. Cats produce more active metabolites and analgesia is likely due to opioid receptor agonism, and opioid-related adverse effects may occur. In cats, the duration of action is longer, so that twice daily dosing is appropriate (Pypendop and Ilkiw, 2008). Tramadol used alone is not suitable for treating severe pain (Benitez *et al.*, 2015), but it may be useful in combination with NSAIDs.

Tramadol has become popular as it can be given orally at home by the owners. It is useful when NSAIDs are contraindicated (e.g. if the patient is receiving corticosteroids), or if outpatients require analgesia in addition to that provided by NSAIDs. The usual recommended dose is 2–5 mg/kg twice (cats) or three times (dogs) daily by mouth.

Sustained release tramadol tablets are available for human use; however, these are unsuitable for dogs due to poor absorption and short duration of action (Giorgi *et al.*, 2012). Their use has not been investigated in cats.

Serotonin toxicity

Serotonin toxicity may occur if drugs that increase serotonin concentrations are overdosed or administered together. Reported veterinary cases have been due to overdose, rather than drug combinations. Examples include St John's wort, foods containing high levels of tryptophan (e.g. cheese), tramadol, pethidine, fentanyl, chlorpheniramine, selective serotonin ▶

<table>
<tr><td>

Serotonin toxicity *continued*

reuptake inhibitors (e.g. fluoxetine), monoamine oxidase inhibitors (e.g. selegiline) and tricyclic antidepressants (e.g. amitriptyline). The syndrome is characterized by clinical signs of autonomic hyper-reactivity, neuromuscular signs and altered mental status (e.g. diarrhoea, tachycardia, hypertension, hyperthermia, tremor, rigidity and seizures). The severity can range from mild clinical signs to death. Treatment is mainly supportive and involves discontinuation of the inciting drug.

</td></tr>
</table>

Tapentodol

Tapentodol is a MOP agonist and noradrenaline reuptake inhibitor, which has similarities to tramadol. It does not require metabolism to an active metabolite in humans, and it has minimal effect on serotonin reuptake, which reduces the risk of serotonin toxicity. It has been shown to be antinociceptive in dogs in an experimental study; in the same study tramadol showed no antinociceptive properties (Kogel *et al.*, 2014). However, oral bioavailability is poor in dogs (Giorgi *et al.*, 2012) and further research is needed before recommendations regarding clinical use can be made.

One potential disadvantage of tapentodol is its legal category, which is a Schedule II Controlled Drug in the UK. This means it must be kept in a locked cupboard with detailed records of its acquisition and use.

Paracetamol

Pharmacology

Paracetamol is a unique drug in that, while it does share similarities with NSAIDs, is not a strong anti-inflammatory. Chemically, paracetamol is a phenol, its protein binding is negligible, and it easily crosses cell membranes. Paracetamol inhibits prostaglandin synthetase activity by interfering with its peroxidase site, whose activity is necessary for the cyclooxygenase site to produce prostaglandins. Paracetamol is generally more effective in inhibiting COX-2, and is anti-inflammatory only in mild to moderate inflammatory states, when the COX-2 pathway is activated in preference to COX-1 (Graham *et al.*, 2013). In severe inflammatory states, where peroxidase levels are particularly high, paracetamol is less efficient in inhibiting COX-2. In this setting, coxibs are more effective, as their activity is peroxidase independent (Anderson, 2008).

Paracetamol, like NSAIDs, works both centrally and peripherally inhibiting prostaglandin synthesis, but its antinociceptive effects are also due to interference with the serotoninergic, endogenous opioids, and endocannabinoid systems. Interaction with the nociceptive effects of substance P and glutamate has also been hypothesized (Graham *et al.*, 2013). The only licensed preparation of paracetamol contains paracetamol and codeine and is licensed for use in the dog only (Pardale-V, NOAH, 2016). Although the Pardale-V datasheet states not to use it with NSAIDs, paracetamol and NSAIDs are often used in combination in human analgesia, and generic paracetamol (intravenous or oral) is often combined with NSAIDs in dogs.

Side effects and toxicity

The main advantage of paracetamol compared with conventional NSAIDs is its better gastrointestinal tolerance, and lesser nephrotoxicity. The main metabolite of paracetamol in dogs is its glucuronide conjugate, which is excreted in the urine. The half-life of paracetamol is only 0.96 hours in the dog (KuKanich, 2010), and experimental studies failed to identify toxicity after administration of 100 mg/kg (Savides *et al.*, 1984). Due to impaired glucuronidation capabilities, cats rely on sulphate conjugation alone to eliminate paracetamol in the urine, resulting in an increased risk of toxicity. Hepatic toxicity is mainly caused by a reactive metabolite, which is conjugated with glutathione, depleting its stores; risk of toxicity directly correlates with the extent of hepatic glutathione depletion and therefore indirectly with the glucuronidation capabilities of the species.

Clinical use and contraindications

The only licensed preparation of paracetamol contains paracetamol and codeine and is licensed for use in the dog only (NOAH, 2016). The licence allows treatment for up to 5 days, and concurrent use of other NSAIDs is contraindicated. The dose indicated in the datasheet is up to approximately 30 mg/kg of paracetamol and 0.75 mg/kg of codeine, administered every 8 hours. Administration in a clinical setting is usually started at 10 mg/kg of paracetamol and, although the licence does not mention this and there is no study suggesting that at this lower dose the treatment can be administered for longer periods, it is plausible that due to the mechanisms of toxicity (glutathione depletion), administration can be extended for longer than 5 days, especially when the drug is used in terminally ill animals. Use of the licensed preparation is contraindicated in animals with hepatic and renal disease, dehydrated, hypovolaemic and hypotensive animals, or when gastrointestinal ulceration or bleeding is possible, although the authors often use generic paracetamol (intravenous or oral) in patients with gastrointestinal ulceration or renal issues. Interestingly, there is no contraindication for use in pregnancy, or concurrent use of steroids, which are two major areas where NSAIDs are contraindicated, and animals could benefit from paracetamol/codeine administration (NOAH, 2016). Clinical evidence supporting the efficacy of analgesia is limited, and one investigation suggested that both paracetamol/codeine and tramadol are inadequate if used as the sole analgesic after a tibial plateau levelling osteotomy (Mburu et al., 1988; Benitez et al., 2015).

Gabapentin

Many antiepileptic drugs are effective in treating neuropathic pain in humans (Eisenberg et al., 2007). The hypothesized mechanism of action is blockade of sodium and calcium channels. Blockade of sodium or calcium channels stabilizes cell membranes of damaged nerves, decreasing the chances of spontaneous depolarization at the site of injury, which is one of the mechanisms sustaining neuropathic pain (Taylor et al., 1998).

Of the antiepileptics used in humans to treat neuropathic pain, the most commonly used one in dogs and cats is gabapentin. Despite its common use, especially in dogs, the evidence supporting its analgesic effect is limited to a small number of studies and case reports.

Mechanism of action and disposition

The analgesic mechanism of action of gabapentin and pregabalin is mediated by binding to the N-type voltage-gated calcium channel, inhibiting the release of excitatory neurotransmitters mediated by calcium influx.

The pharmacokinetics of gabapentin have been characterized in Greyhounds. After oral administration of 10 or 20 mg/kg, bioavailability was 80%, the time to peak plasma concentration was 1.3 and 1.5 hours, and the terminal half-life was 3.25 and 3.41 hours, respectively. Gabapentin is metabolized to N-methyl-gabapentin in dogs. In contrast to the case in humans, it seems that gabapentin gastrointestinal absorption is not affected by the dose administered. Based on the effective plasma concentration in humans, administration of an oral dose of 10–20 mg/kg every 8 hours should be appropriate in dogs (KuKanich and Cohen, 2011). Oral bioavailability of gabapentin in cats is high (88%), with a time to peak plasma concentration of approximately 100 minutes. Based on the pharmacokinetic parameters, oral dosing with 8 mg/kg every 6 hours should result in a plasma concentration similar to that effective in humans (Siao et al., 2010).

The pharmacokinetics of pregabalin after single dosing has been reported in the dog, although there are no clinical reports about the efficacy of this drug in treating pain (Salazar et al., 2009).

Clinical use

Oral administration of 10 mg/kg of gabapentin to dogs twice a day did not affect post-operative analgesia in dogs that underwent thoracolumbar disc surgery (Aghighi et al., 2012). Oral administration of 5 mg/kg did not affect postoperative pain after forelimb amputation (Wagner et al., 2010). On the other hand, administration of 10 mg/kg of gabapentin twice a day to dogs that underwent a mastectomy reduced postoperative morphine requirements compared with a control group (Crociolli et al., 2015). Use of gabapentin has also been suggested to manage neuropathic pain in dogs with Chiari-like malformation (Rusbridge and Jeffery, 2008). Interestingly, there is no evidence supporting the use of gabapentin to relieve the pain associated with degenerative joint disease and osteoarthritis, despite this probably being the setting where the drug is mostly used in veterinary medicine. Clinical trials in humans have demonstrated that gabapentin is effective in treating neuropathic pain, and it is likely that this should also be the case in veterinary medicine. The side effects related to gabapentin administration in dogs are relatively mild (sedation) and transient, and it is fair to question whether this drug is widely used because of its limited side effects, rather than because of evidence supporting its use in animals with osteoarthritis pain.

There are more publications supporting the use of gabapentin in cats, particularly as part of a multimodal approach to analgesia in cats undergoing major surgical procedures or after major musculoskeletal trauma (6.5–20 mg/kg two to three times a day), and responding inadequately to conventional analgesics (Vettorato and Corletto, 2011; Lorenz et al., 2012; Steagall and Monteiro-Steagall, 2013). Investigators failed to demonstrate an effect of gabapentin on isoflurane MAC and on thermal threshold in cats (Pypendop et al., 2010; Reid et al., 2010). Single reports of successful control of orofacial pain in cats have also been published (Rusbridge et al., 2010).

How to use analgesic agents in special circumstances

There is little information on the safety of the use of analgesics in special circumstances, such as for pregnant or lactating patients, for Caesarean section, for very young or very old animals, and those with renal disease. This can make provision of analgesia for these patients difficult, potentially resulting in inadequate analgesia and unnecessary suffering. Figures 5.4 and 5.5 summarize the available data and give the authors' recommendations in such circumstances.

Analgesia for patients with liver disease

Patients with liver dysfunction or hepatic encephalopathy can respond differently to drugs compared with healthy patients. Many patients with liver disease have hepatocellular damage (resulting in increases in alanine amino transferase and alkaline phosphatase) without liver dysfunction, and therefore carry no special considerations regarding administration of analgesics. To decide which patients with liver disease will process drugs differently (e.g. slower metabolism resulting in longer duration of action), it is necessary to try and assess the liver's metabolic function. Patients with low plasma concentrations of albumin, glucose, urea and clotting factors, and high ammonia, may have difficulty metabolizing drugs. Patients with increased bile acid concentrations may have decreased metabolic function, but raised bile acids can also be seen in patients with biliary tract obstruction. Patients with hepatic encephalopathy are likely to have decreased metabolic function, in addition they may be more sensitive to the sedative effects of drugs such as opioids. Use of some NSAIDs is contraindicated in patients with hepatic disease according to the datasheets (see Figure 5.3).

	Paediatric	Geriatric	Pregnant	Caesarean	Lactating
Opioids					
	No safety data available. Use low doses to effect	May be more sensitive to sedative effects, prolonged duration of action possible	Short-term use unlikely to harm fetuses, long-term use associated with fetal withdrawal syndrome	Offspring at risk of respiratory depression/sedation, consider delaying administration until neonates are delivered	In humans, low levels pass into milk, unlikely to be harmful to offspring, prevent feeding at time of peak plasma concentrations
NSAIDs					
	Consider individual licences, as there are significant differences	May be more sensitive to side effects, especially during chronic treatment. Use minimum effective dose	No safety data available. Use only if necessary, considering that all products are contraindicated in pregnancy	Do not use prior to Caesarean section, use cautiously if necessary after Caesarean section	Not licensed due to absence of safety data availability. Use with caution and if necessary
Paracetamol (dogs only!)					
	Use in animals younger than 6 weeks may involve additional risk	Use in older animals may involve additional risk	Can be used	Can be used	Can be used
Local anaesthetics					
	Can be used – there is greater risk of overdose due to the small size	Can be used	Can be used, provided hypotension is not caused that may compromise placental blood flow	Can be used, provided arterial blood pressure is monitored and hypotension treated	Can be used
Tramadol					
	No data in paediatric dogs and cats, widely used in children	May be more sensitive to sedative effects	Possibly teratogenic but limited data in humans	No data, unlikely to be required	In humans low levels pass into milk, unlikely to be harmful to offspring, prevent feeding at time of peak plasma concentrations
Antidepressants					
	No data in paediatric dogs and cats	No data in dogs and cats. May be more sensitive to sedative effects	No data in dogs and cats. In humans SSRIs are considered safe. Some TCAs have been linked to birth defects. MAOIs are contraindicated	No data, see pregnancy column	See pregnancy column

5.4 Analgesic considerations for special patient populations. MAOI = monoamine oxidase inhibitor; SSRI = selective serotonin reuptake inhibitor; TCA = tricyclic antidepressant. (continues)

	Paediatric	Geriatric	Pregnant	Caesarean	Lactating
Gabapentin	No data in paediatric dogs and cats. May be more sensitive to side effects	No data in dogs and cats. May be more sensitive to side effects	No data in dogs and cats. Use of gabapentin in humans has been linked to preterm birth	See pregnancy column	No data in dogs and cats. Gabapentin may pass in small amounts into the milk, unlikely to be harmful, but may cause sedation
Ketamine	Duration of action may be prolonged in neonates, low-dose infusion unlikely to be harmful	Suitable for use	May increase uterine tone, potential for abortion. No data on use of low-dose infusion	Avoid – causes fetal depression, neonates less likely to breathe spontaneously. No data on low-dose infusion	Ketamine passes into milk in cattle, and is detectable 48 hours after a single iv. dose. No data on low-dose infusion
Amantadine	No data	Possible prolonged duration of action if there is renal impairment	Possibly teratogenic but limited data in humans	No data	No data
Alpha-2 agonists	Avoid in neonates because of cardiovascular effects. Effects of low-dose infusion not known, unlikely to be harmful	Avoid high doses because of cardiovascular effects, effects of low-dose infusion not known, unlikely to be harmful	Avoid – may decrease uterine blood flow and cause fetal hypoxaemia, possible risk of abortion	Avoid – may decrease uterine blood flow, cause fetal hypoxaemia and increase fetal mortality	Avoid – in humans alpha-2 agonists pass into breast milk

5.4 (continued) Analgesic considerations for special patient populations. MAOI = monoamine oxidase inhibitor; SSRI = selective serotonin reuptake inhibitor; TCA = tricyclic antidepressant.

Renal disease	Liver disease
Opioids	
Norpethidine is renally excreted, accumulation could cause seizures in animals with severe renal disease	Prolonged duration of action or accumulation possible Patients with hepatic encephalopathy more sensitive to sedation Morphine may be less effective due to decreased production of active metabolites (dogs)
NSAIDs	
Consider individual licences, use in case of chronic nephropathy is controversial, and should be judged according to risk–benefit analysis. Do not use in acute renal disease or in animals at risk of acute renal disease	Most are contraindicated in animals with liver disease, some can be used with caution in animals with liver disease
Paracetamol (dogs only!)	
Contraindicated, but it is commonly used with caution as it is probably safer than non-steroidal anti-inflammatory drugs	Contraindicated
Local anaesthetics	
Can be used, provided hypotension is avoided	Can be used
Tramadol	
Active metabolites excreted in urine, possible prolonged duration of action (cats)	Longer duration of action possible Decreased production of active metabolite may lead to reduced efficacy (cats)
Antidepressants	
No data in dogs and cats, use with caution	No data in dogs and cats, use with extreme caution
Gabapentin	
No data in dogs and cats. Duration of action may be prolonged	No data in dogs and cats. Duration of action may be prolonged and side effects more evident
Ketamine	
Renally excreted in cats, possible prolonged duration of action or accumulation	Metabolized by the liver in dogs, possible prolonged duration of action or accumulation
Amantadine	
Renally excreted, prolonged duration of action possible	No data
Alpha-2 agonists	
May reduce renal blood flow Reversible Effects of low-dose infusion not known, unlikely to be harmful	May reduce liver blood flow Prolonged duration of action or accumulation possible Reversible Effects of low-dose infusion not known, unlikely to be harmful

5.5 Analgesic considerations for patients with renal and hepatic disease.

Example regimens

Lens luxation and glaucoma

Analgesia for enucleation in a healthy young Jack Russell Terrier due to lens luxation and glaucoma is detailed in Figure 5.6.

Ear flush

Analgesia for an elderly Cocker Spaniel with chronic otitis externa for an ear flush (outpatient) is detailed in Figure 5.7.

Exploratory laparotomy

Analgesia for an uncooperative cat with triaditis undergoing exploratory laparotomy for liver and intestinal biopsies (inpatient) is detailed in Figure 5.8.

Perioperative period	Drugs and protocol	Comments
Pre-anaesthetic medication	Methadone 0.3 mg/kg i.m., medetomidine 5 µg/kg i.m., carprofen 4 mg/kg s.c.	Good analgesia from methadone (possibly enhanced by the medetomidine) and carprofen. Moderate sedation, anti-inflammatory effect
Intraoperative analgesia	Fentanyl 2 µg/kg i.v. if there is reaction to surgical stimulation, repeat as necessary	May cause transient apnoea and bradycardia
Local anaesthetic technique	Retrobulbar block or splash block using bupivacaine	Excellent analgesia for 6–8 hours but possibility of failure of block or patchy block
Postoperative analgesia	Consider methadone 0.3 mg/kg i.m. at the end of procedure if this is around 4 hours after pre-anaesthetic medication. Pain checks every 2 hours initially, with methadone repeated every 2–4 hours if painful	Additional opioid may not be required due to the retrobulbar block and carprofen. Retrobulbar block should wear off after 6–8 hours, pain checks should be scheduled for this time
Analgesia at home	Carprofen 2 mg/kg orally q12h for 3 days	

5.6 Recommended analgesic protocol for enucleation in a healthy young Jack Russell Terrier.

Perioperative period	Drugs and protocol	Comments
Pre-anaesthetic medication	Methadone 0.3 mg/kg i.m.	Good analgesia from methadone, mild sedation
Intraoperative analgesia	Ketamine 0.5 mg/kg i.v. as co-induction or after induction	Good analgesia for chronic pain. May cause transient change in ventilation pattern
Local anaesthetic technique	Consider auriculotemporal and great auricular nerve blocks using lidocaine or bupivacaine	Some dogs with otitis are very reactive during ear procedures due to severe chronic pain and may shake their heads despite being deeply anaesthetized; nerve blocks will prevent this
Postoperative analgesia/ analgesia at home	Non-steroidal anti-inflammatory drugs or paracetamol 10 mg/kg q8–12h	Paracetamol can be used concurrently with steroids

5.7 Recommended analgesic protocol for an ear flush in an elderly Cocker Spaniel with chronic otitis externa.

Perioperative period	Drugs and protocol	Comments
Pre-anaesthetic medication	Methadone 0.3 mg/kg i.m., ketamine 5 mg/kg i.m., medetomidine 10 µg/kg i.m.	Good analgesia and profound sedation from this drug combination enabling i.v. catheter placement and reduction of anaesthetic agent requirements
Intraoperative analgesia	Fentanyl 2 µg/kg i.v. if there is reaction to surgical stimulation, repeat as necessary or convert to infusion at 5–10 µg/kg/minute. Ketamine infusion 10 µg/kg/minute	May cause transient apnoea and bradycardia
Local anaesthetic/regional analgesia technique	Consider an epidural injection of 0.1 mg/kg preservative-free morphine. Infiltration of laparotomy incision with bupivacaine	Epidural morphine provides good analgesia for up to 24 hours, but there is possibility of failure of administration
Postoperative analgesia	Consider methadone 0.3 mg/kg i.m. at the end of procedure if this is around 4 hours after pre-anaesthetic medication. Pain checks every 2 hours initially, then every 4 hours as the patient improves, with methadone repeated every 2–4 hours if painful. Ketamine infusion at 5 µg/kg/min. Non-steroidal anti-inflammatories if still painful	Consider changing to buprenorphine after 24 hours (to avoid interaction with morphine epidural). A single dose of NSAID is unlikely to cause a problem even if liver function is decreased, but avoid if the patient has a coagulopathy

5.8 Recommended analgesic protocol for an uncooperative cat with triaditis undergoing exploratory laparotomy for liver and intestinal biopsies.

References and further reading

Adler MW, Geller EB, Rosow CE and Cochin J (1988) The opioid system and temperature regulation. *Annual Review of Pharmacology and Toxicology* **28**, 429–449

Aghighi SA, Tipold A, Piechotta M, Lewczuk P and Kästner SB (2012) Assessment of the effects of adjunctive gabapentin on postoperative pain after intervertebral disc surgery in dogs. *Veterinary Anaesthesia and Analgesia* **39**, 636–646

Aguirre JA, Votta-Velis G and Borgeat A (2012) Practical pharmacology in regional anesthesia. In: *Essentials of Regional Anesthesia*, ed. A Kaye, R Urman and N Vadivelu, pp. 121–156. Springer, New York

Anderson BJ (2008) Paracetamol (acetaminophen): mechanisms of action. *Pediatric Anesthesia* **18**, 915–921

Anderson MK and Day TK (2008) Effects of morphine and fentanyl constant rate infusion on urine output in healthy and traumatized dogs. *Veterinary Anaesthesia and Analgesia* **35**, 528–536

Aprea F, Vettorato E and Corletto F (2011) Severe cardiovascular depression in a cat following a mandibular nerve block with bupivacaine. *Veterinary Anaesthesia and Analgesia* **38**, 614–618

Aratana (2016) NOCITA® (bupivacaine liposome injectable suspension) [online]. Available from: http://www.aratana.com/wp-content/uploads/2016/08/NOCITA-Prescribing-Information.pdf

Ayroldi E, Cannarile L, Migliorati G *et al.* (2012) Mechanisms of the anti-inflammatory effects of glucocorticoids: genomic and nongenomic interference with MAPK signaling pathways. *The FASEB Journal* **26**, 4805–4820

Bai Y, Miller T, Tan M, Law LS-C and Gan TJ (2015) Lidocaine patch for acute pain management: a meta-analysis of prospective controlled trials. *Current Medical Research and Opinion* **31**, 575–581

Baldini G, Bagriy H, Aprikian A and Carli F (2009) Postoperative urinary retention: anesthetic and perioperative considerations. *Anesthesiology* **110**, 1139–1157

Bartel AKG, Campoy L, Martin-Flores M *et al.* (2016) Comparison of bupivacaine and dexmedetomidine femoral and sciatic nerve blocks with bupivacaine and buprenorphine epidural injection for stifle arthroscopy in dogs. *Veterinary Anaesthesia and Analgesia* **43**, 435–443

Becker DE and Reed KL (2006) Essentials of local anesthetic pharmacology. *Anesthesia Progress* **53**, 98–109

Becker DE and Reed KL (2012) Local anesthetics: review of pharmacological considerations. *Anesthesia Progress* **59**, 90–102

Beecroft C and Davies G (2016) Systemic toxic effects of local anaesthetics. *Anaesthesia and Intensive Care Medicine* **17**, 1–3

Benitez ME, Roush JK, McMurphy R, KuKanich B and Legallet C (2015) Clinical efficacy of hydrocodone-acetaminophen and tramadol for control of postoperative pain in dogs following tibial plateau leveling osteotomy. *American Journal of Veterinary Research* **76**, 755–762

Bergmann HM, Nolte I and Kramer S (2007) Comparison of analgesic efficacy of preoperative or postoperative carprofen with or without preincisional mepivacaine epidural anesthesia in canine pelvic or femoral fracture repair. *Veterinary Surgery* **36**, 623–632

Björkman R (1995) Central antinociceptive effects of non-steroidal anti-inflammatory drugs and paracetamol. *Acta Anaesthesiologica Scandinavica Suppl.* **103**, 1–44

Blancquaert J-P, Lefebvre RA and Willems JL (1986) Emetic and antiemetic effects of opioids in the dog. *European Journal of Pharmacology* **128**, 143–150

Borer LR, Seewald W, Peel JE and King JN (2016) Evaluation of the dose-response relationship of oral robenacoxib in urate crystal-induced acute stifle synovitis in dogs. *Journal of Veterinary Pharmacology and Therapeutics* **10**, 148–157

Boström IM, Nyman GC, Lord PF *et al.* (2002) Effects of carprofen on renal function and results of serum biochemical and hematologic analyses in anesthetized dogs that had low blood pressure during anesthesia. *American Journal of Veterinary Research* **63**, 712–721

Braid DP and Scott DB (1966) Effect of adrenaline on the systemic absorption of local anaesthetic drugs. *Acta Anaesthesiologica Scandinavica* **10**, 334–346

Bufalari A, Maggio C, Cerasoli I, Morath U and Adami C (2012) Preemptive carprofen for peri-operative analgesia in dogs undergoing tibial plateau leveling osteotomy (TPLO): A prospective, randomized, blinded, placebo controlled clinical trial. *Schweizer Archiv für Tierheilkunde* **154**, 105–111

Burch F, Codding C, Patel N and Sheldon E (2004) Lidocaine patch 5% improves pain, stiffness, and physical function in osteoarthritis pain patients. *Osteoarthritis and Cartilage* **12**, 253–255

Burian M and Geisslinger G (2005) COX-dependent mechanisms involved in the antinociceptive action of NSAIDs at central and peripheral sites. *Pharmacology and Therapeutics* **107**, 139–154

Burm A (1989) Clinical pharmacokinetics of epidural and spinal anaesthesia. *Clinical Pharmacokinetics* **5**, 283–311

Carroll GL, Narbe R, Kerwin SC *et al.* (2011) Dose range finding study for the efficacy of meloxicam administered prior to sodium urate-induced synovitis in cats. *Veterinary Anaesthesia and Analgesia* **38**, 394–406

Cashman JN (1996) The mechanisms of action of NSAIDs in analgesia. *Drugs* **52**, 13–23

Cashmore RG, Harcourt-Brown TR, Freeman PM, Jeffery ND and Granger N (2009) Clinical diagnosis and treatment of suspected neuropathic pain in three dogs. *Australian Veterinary Journal* **87**, 45–50

Chadwick HS (1985) Toxicity and resuscitation in lidocaine- or bupivacaine-infused cats. *Anesthesiology* **63**, 385–390

Chahar P and Cummings III K (2012) Liposomal bupivacaine: a review of a new bupivacaine formulation. *Journal of Pain Research* **5**, 257–258

Chan MT, Wan AC, Gin T, Leslie K and Myles PS (2011) Chronic postsurgical pain after nitrous oxide anesthesia. *Pain* **152**, 2514–2520

Chew DJ, Buffington CA, Kendall MS, DiBartola SP and Woodworth BE (1998) Amitriptyline treatment for severe recurrent idiopathic cystitis in cats. *Journal of the American Veterinary Medicine Association* **213**, 1282–1286

Clark TP, Chieffo C, Huhn JC *et al.* (2003) The steady-state pharmacokinetics and bioequivalence of carprofen administered orally and subcutaneously in dogs. *Journal of Veterinary Pharmacology and Therapeutics* **26**, 187–192

Clement R, Malinovsky JM, Le Corre P and Dollo G (1999) Cerebrospinal fluid bioavailability and pharmacokinetics of bupivacaine and lidocaine after intrathecal and epidural administrations in rabbits using microdialysis. *Journal of Pharmacology and Experimental Therapeutics* **289**, 1015–1021

Cox B, Durieux ME and Marcus MAE (2003) Toxicity of local anaesthetics. *Best Practice and Research Clinical Anaesthesiology* **17**, 111–136

Cox SR, Lesman SP, Boucher JF *et al.* (2010) The pharmacokinetics of mavacoxib, a long-acting COX-2 inhibitor, in young adult laboratory dogs. *Journal of Veterinary Pharmacology and Therapeutics* **33**, 461–470

Cox SR, Liao S, Payne-Johnson M, Zielinksi RJ and Stegemann MR (2011) Population pharmacokinetics of mavacoxib in osteoarthritic dogs. *Journal of Veterinary Pharmacology and Therapeutics* **34**, 1–11

Craven M, Chandler ML, Steiner JM *et al.* (2007) Acute effects of carprofen and meloxicam on canine gastrointestinal permeability and mucosal absorptive capacity. *Journal of Veterinary Internal Medicine* **21**, 917–923

Crociolli GC, Cassu RN, Barbero RC *et al.* (2015) Gabapentin as an adjuvant for postoperative pain management in dogs undergoing mastectomy. *Journal of Veterinary Medical Science* **77**, 1011–1015

Cronstein BN, Van De Stouwe M, Druska L, Levin RI and Weissman G (1994) Nonsteroidal antiinflammatory agents inhibit stimulated neutrophil adhesion to endothelium: Adenosine dependent and independent mechanisms. *Inflammation* **18**, 323–335

De Gennaro C, Vettorato E and Corletto F (2014) Retrospective clinical evaluation of hypobaric spinal anaesthesia in dogs undergoing pelvic limb orthopaedic surgery. *Journal of Small Animal Practice* **55**, 497–503

Di Salvo A, Bufalari A, De Monte V *et al.* (2014) Intra-articular administration of lidocaine in anaesthetized dogs: pharmacokinetic profile and safety on cardiovascular and nervous systems. *Journal of Veterinary Pharmacology and Therapeutics* **38**, 350–356

Di Salvo A, Chiaradia E, della Rocca G *et al.* (2015) Intra-articular administration of lidocaine plus adrenaline in dogs: pharmacokinetic profile and evaluation of toxicity *in vivo* and *in vitro*. *Veterinary Journal* **208**, 2081–2024

Dowers KL, Uhrig SR, Mama KR, Gaynor JS and Hellyer PW (2006) Effect of short-term sequential administration of nonsteroidal anti-inflammatory drugs on the stomach and proximal portion of the duodenum in healthy dogs. *American Journal of Veterinary Research* **67**, 1794–1801

Dum JE and Herz A (1981) *In vivo* receptor binding of the opiate partial agonist, buprenorphine, correlated with its agonist and antagonistic actions. *British Journal of Pharmacology* **74**, 637–633

Eisenberg E, River Y, Shifrin A and Krivoy N (2007) Antiepileptic drugs in the treatment of neuropathic pain. *Drugs* **67**, 1265–1289

Englesson S (1974) The influence of acid-base changes on central nervous system toxicity of local anaesthetic agents I: an experimental study in cats. *Acta Anaesthesiologica Scandinavica* **18**, 79–87

Feldman HS, Arthur GR and Covino BG (1989) Comparative systemic toxicity of convulsant and supraconvulsant doses of intravenous ropivacaine, bupivacaine, and lidocaine in the conscious dog. *Anesthesia and Analgesia* **69**, 794–801

Feldman HS, Arthur GR, Pitkanen M *et al.* (1991) Treatment of acute systemic toxicity after the rapid intravenous injection of ropivacaine and bupivacaine in the conscious dog. *Anesthesia and Analgesia* **73**, 373–384

Feldman HS, Dvoskin S, Halldin MH, Ask AL and Doucette AM (1997) Comparative local anesthetic efficacy and pharmacokinetics of epidurally administered ropivacaine and bupivacaine in the sheep. *Regional Anesthesia and Pain Medicine* **22**, 451–460

Flecknell PA, Liles JH and Wootton R (1989) Reversal of fentanyl/fluanisone neuroleptanalgesia using mixed agonist/ antagonist opioids. *Laboratory Animals* **23**, 147–155

Frendin J, Boström, IM, Kampa N et al. (2006) Effects of carprofen on renal function during medetomidine-propofol-isoflurane anesthesia in dogs. *American Journal of Veterinary Research* **67**, 1967–1973

Galer BS, Harle J and Rowbotham MC (1996) Response to intravenous lidocaine infusion predicts subsequent response to oral mexiletine: a prospective study. *Journal of Pain and Symptom Management* **12**, 161–167

Gilhooly D, McGarvey B, O'Mahony H and O'Connor TC (2011) Topical lidocaine patch 5% for acute postoperative pain control. *BMJ Case Reports* Feb 8, doi: 10.1136/bcr.06.2010.3074

Giorgi M, Meizler A and Mills PC (2012) Pharmacokinetics of the novel atypical opioid tapentadol after oral and intravenous administration in dogs. *Veterinary Journal* **194**, 309–313

Giorgi M, Saccomanni G, Lebkowska-Wieruszewska B and Kowalski C (2009) Pharmacokinetic evaluation of tramadol and its major metabolites after single oral sustained tablet administration in the dog: a pilot study. *Veterinary Journal* **180**, 253–255

Gowan RA, Baral RM, Lingard AE et al. (2012) A retrospective analysis of the effects of meloxicam on the longevity of aged cats with and without overt chronic kidney disease. *Journal of Feline Medicine and Surgery* **14**, 876–881

Gowan RA, Lingard AE, Johnston L et al. (2011) Retrospective case–control study of the effects of long-term dosing with meloxicam on renal function in aged cats with degenerative joint disease. *Journal of Feline Medicine and Surgery* **13**, 752–761

Graham GG, Davies MJ, Day RO, Mohamudally A and Scott KF (2013) The modern pharmacology of paracetamol: therapeutic actions, mechanism of action, metabolism, toxicity and recent pharmacological findings. *Inflammopharmacology* **21**, 201–232

Grandemange E, Fournel S and Woehrlé F (2013) Efficacy and safety of cimicoxib in the control of perioperative pain in dogs. *Journal of Small Animal Practice* **54**, 304–312

Groban L, Deal DD, Vernon JC, James RL and Butterworth J (2001) Cardiac resuscitation after incremental overdosage with lidocaine, bupivacaine, levobupivacaine, and ropivacaine in anesthetized dogs. *Anesthesia and Analgesia* **92**, 37–43

Guedes AGP, Papich MG, Rude EP and Rider MA (2007) Pharmacokinetics and physiological effects of two intravenous infusion rates of morphine in conscious dogs. *Journal of Veterinary Pharmacology and Therapeutics* **30**, 224–233

Guillot M, Moreau M, Heit M et al. (2013) Characterization of osteoarthritis in cats and meloxicam efficacy using objective chronic pain evaluation tools. *Veterinary Journal* **196**, 360–367

Gunew M, Menrath V and Marshall R (2008) Long-term safety, efficacy and palatability of oral meloxicam at 0.01–0.03mg/ kg for treatment of osteoarthritic pain in cats. *Journal of Feline Medicine and Surgery* **10**, 235–241

Horstman CL, Conzemius MG, Evans R and Gordon WJ (2004) Assessing the efficacy of perioperative oral carprofen after cranial cruciate surgery using noninvasive, objective pressure platform gait analysis. *Veterinary Surgery* **33**, 286–292

Hunt JR, Attenburrow PM, Slingsby LS and Murrell JC (2013) Comparison of premedication with buprenorphine or methadone with meloxicam for postoperative analgesia in dogs undergoing orthopaedic surgery. *Journal of Small Animal Practice* **54**, 418–424

Hutson P, Backonja M and Knurr H (2015) Intravenous lidocaine for neuropathic pain: a retrospective analysis of tolerability and efficacy. *Pain Medicine* **16**, 531–536

Ingvast-Larsson C, Holgersson A, Bondesson U, Lagerstedt AS and Olsson K (2010) Clinical pharmacology of methadone in dogs. *Veterinary Anaesthesia and Analgesia* **37**, 48–56

Jolliffe CT, Leece EA, Adams V and Marlin DJ (2007) Effect of intravenous lidocaine on heart rate, systolic arterial blood pressure and cough responses to endotracheal intubation in propofol-anaesthetized dogs. *Veterinary Anaesthesia and Analgesia* **34**, 322–330

Joshi G, Patou G and Kharitonov V (2015) The safety of liposome bupivacaine following various routes of administration in animals. *Journal of Pain Research* **8**, 781–789

Joudrey SD, Robinson DA, Kearney MT, Papich MG and Da Cunha AF (2015) Plasma concentrations of lidocaine in dogs following lidocaine patch application over an incision compared to intact skin. *Journal of Veterinary Pharmacology and Therapeutics* **38**, 575–580

Kay-Mugford P, Benn SJ, LaMarre J and Conlon P (2000) *In vitro* effects of nonsteroidal anti-inflammatory drugs on cyclooxygenase activity in dogs. *American Journal of Veterinary Research* **61**, 802–810

Kim S-I, Ha K-Y and Oh I-S (2015) Preemptive multimodal analgesia for postoperative pain management after lumbar fusion surgery: a randomized controlled trial. *European Spine Journal* **25**, 1614–1619

Kim TW, Łebkowska-Wieruszewska B, Owen H et al. (2014) Pharmacokinetic profiles of the novel COX-2 selective inhibitor cimicoxib in dogs. *Veterinary Journal* **200**, 77–81

King JN, Rudaz C, Borer L et al. (2010) *In vitro* and *ex vivo* inhibition of canine cyclooxygenase isoforms by robenacoxib: A comparative study. *Research in Veterinary Science* **88**, 497–506

Ko JC, Freeman LJ, Barletta M et al. (2011) Efficacy of oral transmucosal and intravenous administration of buprenorphine before surgery for postoperative analgesia in dogs undergoing ovariohysterectomy. *Journal of the American Veterinary Medical Association* **238**, 318–328

Ko JCH, Maxwell LK, Abbo LA and Weil AB (2008) Pharmacokinetics of lidocaine following the application of 5 lidocaine patches to cats. *Journal of Veterinary Pharmacology and Therapeutics* **31**, 359–367

Ko JCH, Weil AB, Maxwell LK, Kitao T and Haydon T (2007) Plasma concentrations of lidocaine in dogs following lidocaine patch application. *Journal of the American Animal Hospital Association* **43**, 280–283

Kogel B, Terlinden R and Schneider J (2014) Characterisation of tramadol, morphine and tapentadol in an acute pain model in Beagle dogs. *Veterinary Anaesthesia and Analgesia* **41**, 297–304

Koh RB, Isaza N, Huisheng X, Cooke K and Robertson SA (2014) Effects of maropitant, acepromazine and electroacupuncture on vomiting associated with administration of morphine in dogs. *Journal of the American Veterinary Medical Association* **244**, 820–829

Kranke P, Jokinen J, Pace NL et al. (2015) Continuous intravenous perioperative lidocaine infusion for postoperative pain and recovery. *The Cochrane Database of Systematic Reviews* **7**, CD009642

KuKanich B (2010) Pharmacokinetics of acetaminophen, codeine, and the codeine metabolites morphine and codeine-6-glucuronide in healthy Greyhound dogs. *Journal of Veterinary Pharmacology and Therapeutics* **33**, 15–21

KuKanich B (2013) Outpatient oral analgesics in dogs and cats beyond non-steroidal anti-inflammatory drugs: an evidence-based approach. *Veterinary Clinics of North America: Small Animal Practice* **43**, 1109–1125

KuKanich B and Cohen RL (2011) Pharmacokinetics of oral gabapentin in greyhound dogs. *Veterinary Journal* **187**, 133–135

Lascelles BDX, Cripps PJ, Jones A and Waterman Pearson AE (1998) Efficacy and kinetics of carprofen, administered preoperatively or postoperatively, for the prevention of pain in dogs undergoing ovariohysterectomy. *Veterinary Surgery* **27**, 568–582

Lascelles BDX, Gaynor JS, Smith ES et al. (2012) Amantadine in a multimodal analgesic regimen for alleviation of refractory osteoarthritis pain in dogs. *Journal of Veterinary Internal Medicine* **22**, 53–59

Lascelles BDX, Henderson AJ and Hackett IJ (2001) Evaluation of the clinical efficacy of meloxicam in cats with painful locomotor disorders. *Journal of Small Animal Practice* **42**, 587–593

Lascelles BDX and Kirkby Shaw K (2016) An extended release local anaesthetic: potential for future use in veterinary surgical patients? *Veterinary Medicine and Science* **2**, 229–238

Lees P, Pelligand L, Elliott J et al. (2014) Pharmacokinetics, pharmacodynamics, toxicology and therapeutics of mavacoxib in the dog: a review. *Journal of Veterinary Pharmacology and Therapeutics* **38**, 1–14

Lees P, Taylor PM, Landoni FM, Arifah AK and Waters C (2003) Ketoprofen in the cat: pharmacodynamics and chiral pharmacokinetics. *Veterinary Journal* **165**, 21–35

Lenkey N, Karoly R, Kiss JP et al. (2006) The mechanism of activity-dependent sodium channel inhibition by the antidepressants fluoxetine and desipramine. *Molecular Pharmacology* **70**, 2052–2063

Lipscomb VJ, AliAbadi FS, Lees P, Pead MJ and Muir P (2002) Clinical efficacy and pharmacokinetics of carprofen in the treatment of dogs with osteoarthritis. *Veterinary Record* **150**, 684–689

Liu PL, Feldman HS, Giasi R, Patterson MK and Covino BG (1983) Comparative CNS toxicity of lidocaine, etidocaine, bupivacaine, and tetracaine in awake dogs following rapid intravenous administration. *Anesthesia and Analgesia* **62**, 375–379

Lobetti RG and Joubert KE (2000) Effect of administration of nonsteroidal anti-inflammatory drugs before surgery on renal function in clinically normal dogs. *American Journal of Veterinary Research* **61**, 1501–1506

Lorenz ND, Comerford EJ and Iff I (2012) Long-term use of gabapentin for musculoskeletal disease and trauma in three cats. *Journal of Feline Medicine and Surgery* **15**, 507–512

Lucas AN, Firth AM, Anderson GA, Vine JH and Edwards GA (2001) Comparison of the effects of morphine administered by constant-rate intravenous infusion or intermittent intramuscular injection in dogs. *Journal of the American Veterinary Medical Association* **218**, 884–891

Luna S, Basilio AC, Steagall P et al. (2007) Evaluation of adverse effects of long-term oral administration of carprofen, etodolac, flunixin meglumine, ketoprofen, and meloxicam in dogs. *American Journal of Veterinary Research* **68**, 258–264

Madden M, Gurney M and Bright S (2014) Amantadine, an N-Methyl-D-Aspartate antagonist, for treatment of chronic neuropathic pain in a dog. *Veterinary Anaesthesia and Analgesia* **41**, 440–441

Mansa S, Palmer E, Grøndahl C, Lønaas L and Nyman G (2007) Long-term treatment with carprofen of 805 dogs with osteoarthritis. *Veterinary Record* **160**, 427–430

Mathews KA (2005) Analgesia for the pregnant, lactating and neonatal to pediatric cat and dog. *Veterinary Emergency and Critical Care* **15**, 273–284

Mathews KA (2008) Neuropathic pain in dogs and cats: if only they could tell us if they hurt. *Veterinary Clinics of North America: Small Animal Practice* **38**, 1365–1414

Mburu DN, Mbugua SW, Skoglund LA and Lökken P (1988) Effects of paracetamol and acetylsalicylic acid on the post-operative course after experimental orthopaedic surgery in dogs. *Journal of Veterinary Pharmacology and Therapeutics* **11**, 163–170

McKellar QA, Delatour P and Lees P (1994a) Stereospecific pharmacodynamics and pharmacokinetics of carprofen in the dog. *Journal of Veterinary Pharmacology and Therapeutics* **17**, 447–454

McKellar QA, Lees P and Gettinby G (1994b) Pharmacodynamics of tolfenamic acid in dogs. Evaluation of dose response relationships. *European Journal of Pharmacology* **253**, 191–200

McKellar QA, Pearson T, Galbraith EA et al. (1991) Pharmacokinetics and clinical efficacy of a cinchophen and prednisolone combination in the dog. *Journal of Small Animal Practice* **32**, 53–58

Mehta S, Guy S, Lam T, Teasell R and Loh E (2015) Antidepressants are effective in decreasing neuropathic pain after SCI: A meta-analysis. *Topics in Spinal Cord Injury Rehabilitation* **21**, 166–173

Meier T, Wasner G, Faust M et al. (2003) Efficacy of lidocaine patch 5% in the treatment of focal peripheral neuropathic pain syndromes: a randomized, double-blind, placebo-controlled study. *Pain* **106**, 151–158

Messenger KM, Wofford JA and Papich MG (2016) Carprofen pharmacokinetics in plasma and in control and inflamed canine tissue fluid using *in vivo* ultrafiltration. *Journal of Veterinary Pharmacology and Therapeutics* **39**, 32–39

Miranda P, Corvetto MA, Altermatt FR et al. (2016) Levobupivacaine absorption pharmacokinetics with and without epinephrine during TAP block: analysis of doses based on the associated risk of local anaesthetic toxicity. *European Journal of Clinical Pharmacology* **72**, 1–7

Monteiro ER, Figueroa CD, Choma JC, Campagnol D and Bettini CM (2008) Effects of methadone, alone or in combination with acepromazine or xylazine, on sedation and physiologic values in dogs. *Veterinary Anaesthesia and Analgesia* **35**, 519–527

Monteiro-Steagall BP, Steagall PVM and Lascelles BDX (2013) Systematic review of nonsteroidal anti-inflammatory drug-induced adverse effects in dogs. *Journal of Veterinary Internal Medicine* **27**, 1011–1019

Montoya L, Ambros L, Kreil V et al. (2004) A pharmacokinetic comparison of meloxicam and ketoprofen following oral administration to healthy dogs. *Veterinary Research Communications* **28**, 415–428

Moore RA, Derry S, Aldington D, Cole P and Wiffen PJ (2015) Amitriptyline for neuropathic pain in adults. *The Cochrane Database of Systematic Reviews* **7**, CD008242

Moore SA (2016) Managing neuropathic pain in dogs. *Frontiers in Veterinary Science* **3**, 9177–9178

Mullins KB, Thomason JM, Lunsford KV et al. (2012) Effects of carprofen, meloxicam and deracoxib on platelet function in dogs. *Veterinary Anaesthesia and Analgesia* **39**, 206–217

Murrell J, Grandemange E, Woehrle F, Menard J and White K (2014) Clinical efficacy and tolerability of cimicoxib in dogs with osteoarthritis: a multicentre prospective study. *Open Journal of Veterinary Medicine* **4**, 78–90

Murrell JC and Hellebrekers LJ (2005) Medetomidine and dexmedetomidine: a review of cardiovascular effects and antinociceptive properties in the dog. *Veterinary Anaesthesia and Analgesia* **32**, 117–127

Nakahira K, Oshita K, Itoh M *et al.* (2016) Clinical concentrations of local anesthetics bupivacaine and lidocaine differentially inhibit human Kir2.x inward rectifier K+ channels. *Anesthesia and Analgesia* **122**, 1038–1047

Nir R-R, Nahman-Averbuch H, Moont R, Sprecher E and Yarnitsky D (2016) Preoperative preemptive drug administration for acute postoperative pain: A systematic review and meta-analysis. *European Journal of Pain* **20**, 1025–1043

NOAH Compendium (2016) *Pardale-V™ Oral Tablets – Dechra Veterinary Products.* Available at: http://www.noahcompendium.co.uk/?id=-450073

Norkus C, Rankin D and KuKanich B (2015a) Evaluation of the pharmacokinetics of oral amitriptyline and its active metabolite nortriptyline in fed and fasted Greyhound dogs. *Journal of Veterinary Pharmacology and Therapeutics* **38**, 619–622

Norkus C, Rankin D and KuKanich B (2015b) Pharmacokinetics of intravenous and oral amitriptyline and its active metabolite nortriptyline in Greyhound dogs. *Veterinary Anaesthesia and Analgesia* **42**, 580–589

Norkus C, Rankin D, Warner M and KuKanich B (2015c) Pharmacokinetics of oral amantadine in greyhound dogs. *Journal of Veterinary Pharmacology and Therapeutics* **38**, 305–308

O'Brien TQ, Clark-Price SC, Evans EE, Di Fazio R and McMichael MA (2010) Infusion of a lipid emulsion to treat lidocaine intoxication in a cat. *Journal of the American Veterinary Association* **237**, 1455–1458

O'Donohoe PB and Pandit JJ (2012) Physiology and pharmacology of spinal and epidural anaesthesia. *Surgery (Oxford)* **30**, 317–319

Paganelli MA and Popescu GK (2015) Actions of bupivacaine, a widely used local anesthetic, on NMDA receptor responses. *Journal of Neuroscience* **35**, 831–842

Papapetrou P, Kumar AJ, Muppuri R and Chakrabortty S (2015) Intravenous lidocaine infusion to treat chemotherapy-induced peripheral neuropathy. *A & A Case Reports* **5**, 154–155

Parton K, Balmer TV, Boyle J, Whittem T and Machon R (2000) The pharmokinetics and effects of intravenously administered carprofen and salicylate on gastrointestinal mucosa and selected biochemical measurements in healthy cats. *Journal of Veterinary Pharmacology and Therapeutics* **23**, 73–79

Patel N and Sadoughi A (2014) Pharmacology of local anesthetics. In: *Essentials of Pharmacology for Anesthesia, Pain Medicine, and Critical Care,* ed. AD Kaye, AM Kaye and RD Urman, pp. 179–194. Springer, New York

Payne-Johnson M, Becskei C, Chaudhry Y and Stegemann MR (2015) Comparative efficacy and safety of mavacoxib and carprofen in the treatment of canine osteoarthritis. *Veterinary Record* **176**, 284

Pelligand L, King JN, Hormazabal V *et al.* (2014) Differential pharmacokinetics and pharmacokinetic/pharmacodynamic modelling of robenacoxib and ketoprofen in a feline model of inflammation. *Journal of Veterinary Pharmacology and Therapeutics* **37**, 354–366

Peterson NW, Buote NJ and Bergman P (2014) Effect of epidural analgesia with opioids on the prevalence of urinary retention in dogs undergoing surgery for cranial cruciate ligament rupture. *Journal of the American Veterinary Medical Association* **244**, 940–943

Picard J and Meek T (2016) Lipid emulsion for intoxication by local anaesthetic: sunken sink? *Anaesthesia* **71**, 879–882

Pollmeier M, Toulemonde C, Fleishman C and Hanson PD (2006) Clinical evaluation of firocoxib and carprofen for the treatment of dogs with osteoarthritis. *Veterinary Record* **159**, 547–551

Posner LP, Gleed RD, Erb HN and Ludders JW (2007) Post-anesthetic hyperthermia in cats. *Veterinary Anaesthesia and Analgesia* **34**, 40–47

Posner LP, Pavuk AA, Rokshar JL, Carter JE and Levine JF (2010) Effects of opioids and anesthetic drugs on body temperature in cats. *Veterinary Anaesthesia and Analgesia* **37**, 35–43

Przeklasa-Muszyńska A, Kocot-Kępska M, Dobrogowski J, Wiatr M and Mika J (2016) Intravenous lidocaine infusions in a multidirectional model of treatment of neuropathic pain patients. *Pharmacological Reports* **68**, 1–7

Pypendop BH and Ilkiw JE (2008) Pharmacokinetics of tramadol, and its metabolite O-desmethyl-tramadol, in cats. *Journal of Veterinary Pharmacology and Therapeutics* **31**, 52–59

Pypendop BH, Siao KT and Ilkiw JE (2010) Thermal antinociceptive effect of orally administered gabapentin in healthy cats. *American Journal of Veterinary Research* **71**, 1027–1032

Rahimi HR, Shiri M and Razmi A (2012) Antidepressants can treat inflammatory bowel disease through regulation of the nuclear factor-κB/nitric oxide pathway and inhibition of cytokine production: a hypothesis. *World Journal of Gastrointestinal Pharmacology and Therapeutics* **6**, 83–85

Ratajczak-Enselme M, Estebe JP, Rose FX *et al.* (2007) Effect of epinephrine on epidural, intrathecal, and plasma pharmacokinetics of ropivacaine and bupivacaine in sheep. *British Journal of Anaesthesia* **99**, 881–890

Reed F, Burrow R, Poels KLC *et al.* (2011) Evaluation of transdermal fentanyl patch attachment in dogs and analysis of residual fentanyl content following removal. *Veterinary Anaesthesia and Analgesia* **38**, 407–412

Reid P, Pypendop BH and Ilkiw, JE (2010) The effects of intravenous gabapentin administration on the minimum alveolar concentration of isoflurane in cats. *Anesthesia and Analgesia* **111**, 633–637

Reymond N, Speranza C, Gruet P, Seewald W and King JN (2011) Robenacoxib *versus* carprofen for the treatment of canine osteoarthritis: a randomized, noninferiority clinical trial. *Journal of Veterinary Pharmacology and Therapeutics* **35**, 175–183

Rhen T and Cidlowski JA (2005) Antiinflammatory action of glucocorticoids — new mechanisms for old drugs. *The New England Journal of Medicine* **353**, 1–13

Robertson SA, Taylor PM, Lascelles BDX and Dixon MJ (2003) Changes in thermal threshold response in eight cats after administration of buprenorphine, butorphanol and morphine. *Veterinary Record* **153**, 462–465

Romundstad L, Breivik H, Niemi G, Helle A and Stubhaug A (2004) Methylprednisolone intravenously 1 day after surgery has sustained analgesic and opioid-sparing effects. *Acta Anaesthesiologica Scandinavica* **48**, 1223–1231

Rose FO-X, Estebe J-P, Ratajczak M *et al.* (2007) Epidural, intrathecal pharmacokinetics, and intrathecal bioavailability of ropivacaine. *Anesthesia and Analgesia* **105**, 859–867

Rosenberg PH (2016) Current evidence is not in support of lipid rescue therapy in local anaesthetic systemic toxicity. *Acta Anaesthesiologica Scandinavica* **60**, 1029–1032

Rosenberg PH, Veering B and Urmey W (2004) Maximum recommended doses of local anesthetics: A multifactorial concept. *Regional Anesthesia and Pain Medicine* **29**, 564–575

Rusbridge C, Heath S, Gunn-Moore DA et al. (2010) Case series – Feline orofacial pain syndrome (FOPS): a retrospective study of 113 cases. Journal of Feline Medicine and Surgery 12, 498–508

Rusbridge C and Jeffery ND (2008) Pathophysiology and treatment of neuropathic pain associated with syringomyelia. Veterinary Journal 175, 164–172

Ryan WG, Carithers D, Moldave K and Bell M (2010) Field comparison of canine NSAIDs firocoxib and deracoxib. Journal of Applied Research in Veterinary Medicine 8, 114–123

Saber AA, Elgamal MH, Rao AJ, Itawi EA and Martinez RL (2009) Early experience with lidocaine patch for postoperative pain control after laparoscopic ventral hernia repair. International Journal of Surgery 7, 36–38

Salazar V, Dewey CW, Schwark W et al. (2009) Pharmacokinetics of single-dose oral pregabalin administration in normal dogs. Veterinary Anaesthesia and Analgesia 36, 574–580

Sano T, Nishimura R, Kanazawa H et al. (2006) Pharmacokinetics of fentanyl after single intravenous injection and constant rate infusion in dogs. Veterinary Anaesthesia and Analgesia 33, 266–273

Sarotti D, Rabozzi R and Corletto F (2011) Efficacy and side effects of intraoperative analgesia with intrathecal bupivacaine and levobupivacaine: a retrospective study in 82 dogs. Veterinary Anaesthesia and Analgesia 38, 240–251

Sarotti D, Rabozzi R and Franci P (2013) A retrospective study of efficacy and side effects of intrathecal administration of hyperbaric bupivacaine and morphine solution in 39 dogs undergoing hind limb orthopaedic surgery. Veterinary Anaesthesia and Analgesia 40, 220–224

Savides MC, Oehme FW, Nash SL and Leipold HW (1984) The toxicity and biotransformation of single doses of acetaminophen in dogs and cats. Toxicology and Applied Pharmacology 74, 26–34

Schmid VB, Seewald W, Lees P and King JN (2010) In vitro and ex vivo inhibition of COX isoforms by robenacoxib in the cat: a comparative study. Journal of Veterinary Pharmacology and Therapeutics 33, 444–452

Schneider M, Kuchta A, Dron F and Woehrlé F (2015) Disposition of cimicoxib in plasma and milk of whelping bitches and in their puppies. BMC Veterinary Research 11, 178

Scholz A (2002) Mechanisms of (local) anaesthetics on voltage-gated sodium and other ion channels. British Journal of Anaesthesia 89, 52–61

Sessions JK, Reynolds LR and Budsberg SC (2005) In vivo effects of carprofen, deracoxib, and etodolac on prostanoid production in blood, gastric mucosa, and synovial fluid in dogs with chronic osteoarthritis. American Journal of Veterinary Research 66, 812–817

Sherman SL, James C, Stoker AM et al. (2015) In vivo toxicity of local anesthetics and corticosteroids on chondrocyte and synoviocyte viability and metabolism. Cartilage 6, 106–112

Shih AC, Robertson S, Isaza N, Pablo L and Davies W (2008) Comparison between analgesic effects of buprenorphine, carprofen, and buprenorphine with carprofen for canine ovariohysterectomy. Veterinary Anaesthesia and Analgesia 35, 69–79

Siafaka I (n.d.) Epidural and CSF pharmacokinetics of drugs. European Society of Regional Anaesthesia. Available at: http://www.esrahellas.gr/uploads/files/SIAFAKA_Epidural%20and%20CSF%20esra%20hellas.pdf

Siao KT, Pypendop BH and Ilkiw JE (2010) Pharmacokinetics of gabapentin in cats. American Journal of Veterinary Research 71, 817–821

Siao KT, Pypendop BH, Stanley SD and Ilkiw JE (2011) Pharmacokinetics of amantadine in cats. Journal of Veterinary Pharmacology and Therapeutics 34, 599–604

Silber HE, Burgener C, Letellier IM et al. (2010) Population pharmacokinetic analysis of blood and joint synovial fluid concentrations of robenacoxib from healthy dogs and dogs with osteoarthritis. Pharmaceutical Research 27, 2633–2645

Silver K and Lillich J (2016) NSAIDs inhibit cell migration by disrupting the cellular adhesion signaling cascade. The FASEB Journal 30, lb696

Slingsby LS, Sear JW, Taylor PM and Murrell JC (2016) Effect of intramuscular methadone on pharmacokinetic data and thermal and mechanical nociceptive thresholds in the cat. Journal of Feline Medicine and Surgery 18, 875–881

Snow LA, McConnico RS, Morgan TW et al. (2014) Carprofen-induced oxidative stress in mitochondria of the colonic mucosa of the dog. Canadian Journal of Veterinary Research 78, 183–192

Sparkes AH, Heiene R, Lascelles BDX et al. (2010) ISFM and AAFP consensus guidelines. Long-term use of NSAIDs in cats. Journal of Feline Medicine and Surgery 12, 521–538

Stanway GW, Taylor PM and Brodbelt DC (2002) A preliminary investigation comparing pre-operative morphine and buprenorphine for post-operative analgesia and sedation in cats. Veterinary Anaesthesia and Analgesia 29, 29–35

Steagall PV, Carnicelli P, Taylor PM et al. (2006) Effects of subcutaneous methadone, morphine, buprenorphine or saline on thermal and pressure thresholds in cats. Journal of Veterinary Pharmacology and Therapeutics 29, 531–537

Steagall PV and Monteiro-Steagall BP (2013) Multimodal analgesia for perioperative pain in three cats. Journal of Feline Medicine and Surgery 15, 737–743

Steagall PVM, Pelligand L, Giordano T et al. (2013) Pharmacokinetic and pharmacodynamic modelling of intravenous, intramuscular and subcutaneous buprenorphine in conscious cats. Veterinary Anaesthesia and Analgesia 40, 83–95

Stiglitz DK, Amaratunge LN, Konstantanos AH and Lindholm DE (2010) Intraoperative nitrous oxide as a preventive analgesic. Anaesthesia and Intensive Care 38, 890–893

Surdyk KK, Brown CA and Brown SA (2013) Evaluation of glomerular filtration rate in cats with reduced renal mass and administered meloxicam and acetylsalicylic acid. American Journal of Veterinary Research 74, 648–651

Surdyk KK, Sloan DL and Brown SA (2012) Renal effects of carprofen and etodolac in euvolemic and volume-depleted dogs. American Journal of Veterinary Research 73, 1485–1490

Taylor CP, Gee NS, Su TZ et al. (1998) A summary of mechanistic hypotheses of gabapentin pharmacology. Epilepsy Research 29, 233–249

Taylor PM, Steagall PVM, Dixon MJ, Ferreira TH and Luna SP (2007) Carprofen and buprenorphine prevent hyperalgesia in a model of inflammatory pain in cats. Research in Veterinary Science 83, 369–375

Tucker GT (1986) Pharmacokinetics of local anaesthetics. British Journal of Anaesthesia 58, 717–731

Tucker GT and Mather LE (1979) Clinical pharmacokinetics of local anaesthetics. Clinical Pharmacokinetics 4, 241–278

Ulrich CM, Bigler J and Potter JD (2006) Non-steroidal anti-inflammatory drugs for cancer prevention: promise, perils and pharmacogenetics. Nature Reviews Cancer 6, 130–140

Valtolina C, Robben JH, Uilenreef J et al. (2009) Clinical evaluation of the efficacy and safety of a constant rate infusion of dexmedetomidine for postoperative pain management in dogs. Veterinary Anaesthesia and Analgesia 36, 369–383

Valverde A, Dyson DH and McDonell WN (1989) Epidural morphine reduces halothane MAC in the dog. Canadian Journal of Anaesthesia 36, 629–632

Vane JR and Botting RM (1997) Mechanism of aspirin-like drugs. *Seminars in Arthritis and Rheumatism* **26**, 2–10

Vanegas H, Vazquez E and Tortorici V (2010) NSAIDs, opioids, cannabinoids and the control of pain by the central nervous system. *Pharmaceuticals* **3**, 1335–1347

Vettorato E and Corletto F (2011) Gabapentin as part of multi-modal analgesia in two cats suffering multiple injuries. *Veterinary Anaesthesia and Analgesia* **38**, 518–520

Vilar JM, Morales M, Santana A *et al.* (2013) Long-term valuation of oral mavacoxib in osteoarthrosic dogs using force platform analysis. *Pakistan Veterinary Journal* **33**, 229–233

Viscusi ER, Sinatra R, Onel E and Ramamoorthy SL (2014) The safety of liposome bupivacaine, a novel local analgesic formulation. *The Clinical Journal of Pain* **30**, 102

Wagner AE, Mich PM, Uhrig SR and Hellyer PW (2010) Clinical evaluation of perioperative administration of gabapentin as an adjunct for postoperative analgesia in dogs undergoing amputation of a forelimb. *Journal of the American Veterinary Medical Association* **236**, 751–756

Wagner AE, Walton JA, Hellyer PW, Gaynor JS and Mama KR (2002) Use of low doses of ketamine administered by constant rate infusion as an adjunct for postoperative analgesia in dogs. *Journal of the American Veterinary Medical Association* **221**, 72–75

Waldron NH, Jones CA, Gan TJ, Allen TK and Habib AS (2013) Impact of perioperative dexamethasone on postoperative analgesia and side-effects: systematic review and meta-analysis. *British Journal of Anaesthesia* **110**, 191–200

Walton MB, Cowderoy EC, Wustefeld-Janssens B, Lascelles BD and Innes JF (2014) Mavacoxib and meloxicam for canine osteoarthritis: a randomised clinical comparator trial. *Veterinary Record* **175**, 280

Weil AB, Ko J and Inoue T (2007) The use of lidocaine patches. *Compendium on Continuing Education for the Practicing Veterinarian* **29**, 208–210

Weiland L, Croubels S, Baert K *et al.* (2006) Pharmacokinetics of a lidocaine patch 5% in dogs. *Transboundary and Emerging Diseases* **53**, 34–39

Weinberg G, Ripper R, Feinstein DL and Hoffman W (2003) Lipid emulsion infusion rescues dogs from bupivacaine-induced cardiac toxicity. *Regional Anesthesia and Pain Medicine* **28**, 198–202

Westropp JL and Buffington C (2004) Feline idiopathic cystitis: current understanding of pathophysiology and management. *Veterinary Clinics of North America: Small Animal Practice* **34**, 1043–1055

Wilson DV, Evans AT and Mauer WA (2007) Pre-anesthetic meperidine: associated vomiting and gastroesophageal reflux during the subsequent anesthetic in dogs. *Veterinary Anaesthesia and Analgesia* **34**, 15–22

Wilson JE, Chandrasekharan NV, Westover KD, Eager KB and Simmons DL (2004) Determination of expression of cyclooxygenase-1 and -2 isozymes in canine tissues and their differential sensitivity to nonsteroidal anti-inflammatory drugs. *American Journal of Veterinary Research* **65**, 810–818

Wooten JG, Blikslager AT, Ryan KA *et al.* (2008) Cyclooxygenase expression and prostanoid production in pyloric and duodenal mucosae in dogs after administration of nonsteroidal anti-inflammatory drugs. *American Journal of Veterinary Research* **69**, 457–464

Zychowska M, Rojewska E, Makuch W, Przewlocka B and Mika J (2015) The influence of microglia activation on the efficacy of amitriptyline, doxepin, milnacipran, venlafaxine and fluoxetine in a rat model of neuropathic pain. *European Journal of Pharmacology* **15**, 115–123

Physical methods used to alleviate pain: nursing considerations

Fiona Scarlett

Veterinary nurses look after day patients for elective procedures, as well as sick and longer-stay patients, all with varying demands. The importance of nursing care is highlighted when dealing with painful patients. The emphasis of this chapter, which describes physical methods of alleviating pain, will be split between inpatients and outpatients. While some topics discussed in this chapter may not have an obvious association with the alleviation of pain, the focus will be on suffering and the emotional component that is involved in pain modulation. It is easy to focus on the day-to-day patients and deliberate on the acute pain associated with procedures such as subcutaneous mass removal, castration, and digit amputation. Most veterinary clinics have protocols for premedication and analgesic medications prescribed at discharge, but it may be important to go beyond this rudimentary level of care. Pain is a complex syndrome that has a multitude of factors impacting on the extent of suffering of the patient. Pain assessment in non-verbal patients is challenging and requires the use of behavioural and physiological indicators, which has largely been addressed in Chapter 2.

Veterinary nursing staff play a fundamental role in effective pain management; they are the integral link between veterinary surgeon (veterinarian), owner and patient. Under the guidance of a veterinary surgeon and in accordance with the Royal College of Veterinary Surgeons (RCVS) Schedule 3, a skilled and experienced veterinary nurse is uniquely positioned to have a key role in patient pain management and comfort. Veterinary nurses often spend more time with patients and are therefore excellently placed to detect subtle changes in behaviour. Nurses often liaise closely with clients, thus can identify further nuances related to the patient and its behaviour. Aside from time observing patient behaviour, nurses spend a lot of time collecting objective data, such as vital signs, demeanour, response to handling and exercise levels of the patient. This data collection allows for the development of nursing care plans. Nurses are involved in most interventions in hospitalized patients. Under RCVS Schedule 3 guidance, veterinary nurses can administer pain medication and a multitude of additional therapeutic approaches to relieve pain and suffering. Nurses may uncover other factors contributing to discomfort, such as uncomfortable body

BSAVA Guide to Pain Management in Small Animal Practice. Edited by Ian Self. ©BSAVA 2019

positions, slipped or soiled dressings, or the need to urinate. A veterinary nurse is typically responsible for documenting any interventions, and the patient's response to these interventions, in medical records. Nurses then ensure the intervention plan and patient's unique needs are communicated to all members of the team.

Inpatient focus

Many patients admitted for day procedures, such as imaging, dentals, and mass removals, will have concurrent disease. This disease may be diagnosed and clinically obvious or subclinical. Degenerative joint disease is a very common concurrent disease of veterinary patients. First, it is important to consider appropriate kennel size and adequate bedding for the comfort of these patients. An arthritic large-breed dog in a medium-sized kennel with only newspaper bedding is not appropriate. Longer duration recumbent patient care will be covered in more detail below, but an anaesthetized patient is essentially a recumbent patient. Although some procedures are short, the total anaesthesia and recovery time should be the emphasis for care. Particular discomfort is caused by remaining in a single position for prolonged periods, by the limbs being tied in various positions for improved surgical access, or by having the hips 'frog legged' during dorsal recumbency. This discomfort will contribute to a less settled anaesthetic state and, furthermore, the patient will have additional postoperative discomfort in areas other than that associated with the procedure just undertaken. Comfort and padding are important to prevent pain from positioning during anaesthesia (Figure 6.1); a wide variety of aids are available through both veterinary and human medical suppliers. Vacuum positioning cushions allow a variety of patient positions to be achieved while also providing superior comfort and insulation compared with solid cradles. A huge variety of foam shapes, operating table accessories such as padded arm retainers (Figure 6.2), and anaesthetic tubing holders exist, which aid in

Position	Ideas
Sternal	• Padding in the groin area to lift the pelvis in better alignment with the spine • Padding under the elbows or in the axilla to reduce force through the elbow • Padding under the chin/neck being careful not to occlude jugular vessels
Dorsal	• Vacuum positioning cushions • Sandbags either side of the thorax or abdomen depending on surgical access • Cradles with padding and the use of foam wedges to minimize rotation • Padding under each thigh (lateral side) to reduce the 'spread' of pelvis
Lateral	• Vacuum positioning cushions • Use of padded retainers to help secure limbs out of surgical fields • Padding between stifles

6.1 Alternative ideas to achieve routine patient positioning for procedures.

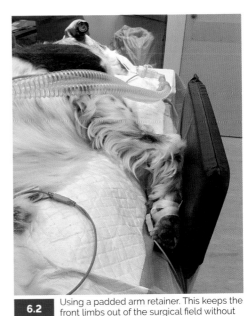

6.2 Using a padded arm retainer. This keeps the front limbs out of the surgical field without the need for tying.

comfort, ease of patient positioning and reduced drag from anaesthetic equipment.

Prolonged care of recumbent patients presents a multitude of challenges, not least, the additional pressure it places on veterinary staff to provide the high level of care required for these patients. Several pathologies can lead to prolonged recumbency; for example, neurological, neuromuscular or musculoskeletal conditions.

Prolonged recumbency is an unnatural state for any species to maintain. Extended immobility leads to physiological changes in the muscles, joints and bones. Muscles atrophy, bones demineralize and joints contract. Lungs develop dependent airway closure and atelectasis. Pulmonary secretions pool and stagnate, leading to infections. Integument pressure damage can occur over bony prominences where local soft tissue is compressed against a surface. Excessive moisture from urinary or faecal incontinence or wound drainage can also damage the integument. Pathology of the cardiorespiratory system due to prolonged recumbency can easily be missed without appropriate monitoring. Other organ systems affected by recumbency are the endocrine system, the gastrointestinal system, the immune system, and fluid and electrolyte balance.

Human intensive care units have dedicated staff trained in a multitude of physical therapies to aid recumbent patients. These physical therapists incorporate treatments such as passive range of motion, active range of motion, active-assisted range of motion, active-resisted range of motion, and exercise. In veterinary medicine, this responsibility for physical therapies usually resides with the veterinary nurse. Details of these therapies are addressed elsewhere in this book, and further practical continuing education in this area is valuable. For example, staff training by a qualified veterinary physiotherapist in techniques appropriate for recumbent patients with various conditions will enhance patient care and outcomes.

Supported standing in recumbent patients should be encouraged if no contraindications exist, for instance spinal instability or an unstable fracture. Standing exercises provide many benefits to a recumbent patient; they restore the body to its natural orientation, allow for proprioceptive development, and promote 'normalization' of neuronal firing. Standing exercises provide a degree of pulmonary rehabilitation, mental stimulation, permit expenditure of energy, and may encourage toileting behaviour. If manual thoracic physiotherapy such as coupage is required, it is essential that the patient is upright to allow for postural drainage and coughing. Specialized hoists, standing frames, slings, harnesses (Figure 6.3) and manual supports are physical aids that can be used to allow patients to stand upright. Some harnesses (e.g. the Pet Support Suit™ by Animal Suspension Technology, USA) can be worn for prolonged periods, making it easier to move these patients as often as necessary.

Bedding and padding

Two major types of support surfaces exist for comfort and pressure relief: static and dynamic. Static surfaces are more common and include air, foam, and water mattress overlays. Dynamic surfaces for more advanced pressure reduction (e.g. alternating air overlay, low air-loss beds and air-fluidized beds) are commonly used in human medical care to reduce the incidence of bed sores; however, these are uncommon in the veterinary practice. Foam mattresses of varying materials are readily available for the veterinary patient. Given the abundant evidence proving the positive effect of appropriate padded bedding in the care of recumbent human patients, mattresses for all veterinary inpatients should be standard. Additional methods of padding may further aid in pressure relief. Improvise with pillows, towels, blankets (Figure 6.4) or use more specialized equipment such as foam shapes and gel protectors. Carers should be proactive in padding areas that are naturally bony and can be in direct contact with surfaces during recumbency, for example, the stifles and hocks.

Moisture accumulation in bedding can be avoided by using padding that wicks away moisture, by creating a regular faecal and urinary voiding schedule, by using highly

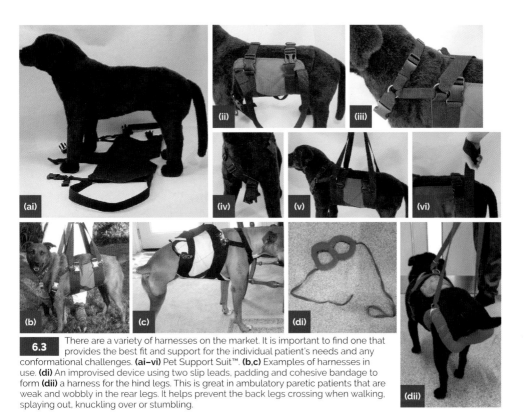

6.3 There are a variety of harnesses on the market. It is important to find one that provides the best fit and support for the individual patient's needs and any conformational challenges. **(ai–vi)** Pet Support Suit™. **(b,c)** Examples of harnesses in use. **(di)** An improvised device using two slip leads, padding and cohesive bandage to form **(dii)** a harness for the hind legs. This is great in ambulatory paretic patients that are weak and wobbly in the rear legs. It helps prevent the back legs crossing when walking, splaying out, knuckling over or stumbling.

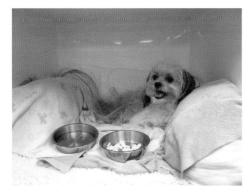

6.4 A kennel padded out using a mattress and pillows for the recumbent patient to be able to lean against and remain upright.

absorbent dressings to capture excessive exudate from wounds, and by wiping away saliva (Figure 6.5), food and water that may collect around Elizabethan collars or other movement-restricting devices.

Any friction or shearing of integument across a surface will increase the likelihood of skin breakdown. This is especially relevant when considering both moving patients and the type of bedding provided. Interestingly, the use of doughnut-type cushions and devices is not recommended. They may increase pressure where the doughnut ring sits, potentially causing further skin breakdown. Additionally, the doughnut may become displaced and increase risk to areas of otherwise unaffected skin.

89

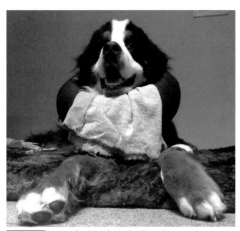

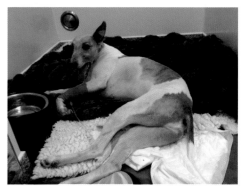

6.6 Sighthounds with little body fat are particularly susceptible to urine scalding and skin irritations when recumbent.

6.5 Use of a Comfy Collar™ and a towel to absorb drool from the patient.

A useful resource for further information regarding preventing and treating pressure sores is the guidelines document available from the National Pressure Ulcer Advisory Panel. These guidelines are available from their website (www.npuap.org) and provide the most up-to-date recommendations in human medicine.

Turning

Frequent turning is common practice in recumbent patients. In human medical care, recumbent patients are turned every 2 to 4 hours. This frequency of turning developed from historical nursing shortages: the time it took for the nurses to rotate all patients on the wards was 2 hours (Bansal *et al.*, 2005). Turning frequency should be increased for patients with respiratory compromise or if the integument had lost integrity with signs of ulceration and infection. Decubitus ulcers, also known as bed sores and pressure sores, result from impaired blood supply and tissue malnutrition caused by prolonged pressure over skin, soft tissue, muscle, and bone. Patients with very little body fat are at a higher risk (Figure 6.6). The cornerstone of decubitus ulcer therapy is to reduce or eliminate pressure, through the provision of support surfaces, turning, padding, positioning, and, if possible, mobilization of the patient (Bansal *et al.*, 2005).

Low-stress handling techniques, such as those taught by the late veterinary behaviourist Dr Sophia Yin (https://lowstresshandling.com/), are increasingly embraced by veterinary staff to improve patient welfare and comfort. However, many practices and individuals remain unaware of the handling techniques and behaviour theory that this practice highlights. Many veterinary surgeons, veterinary nurses and support staff receive very little training on subtle canine and feline body language and proper handling of cats, for example. The practices of pinning patients down and scruffing cats are outdated and should be superseded with far more effective and safe practices.

Toileting

Patients receiving intravenous fluids and/or diuretics, and any polydipsic patient, should have more frequently scheduled toileting opportunities. Any patient that can be taken outside to toilet should have this as a primary option. Not only does going outside increase patient activity levels but it also provides patients with stimulation and social interaction.

Indwelling urinary catheters are often used to assist with the management of recumbent veterinary patients. For inpatients with critical illness, neurogenic bladder dysfunction, paraparesis or tetraparesis, close monitoring of fluids in and out is required. Indwelling urinary catheters assist ease of patient care, assessing fluid balance and decreasing risk of urine-related dermatitis, but they also hold potential for significant risk such as the development of urinary tract infections. Smarick *et al.* (2004) found that antimicrobial administration can be associated with the development of antimicrobial-resistant bacterial infections in dogs undergoing prolonged catheterization. Aseptic catheter placement and maintenance every 8 hours, or whenever the urinary catheter becomes visibly soiled, is recommended. The practice of clipping hair to help with incontinent veterinary patients is often adopted. This involves clipping hair away from the perineum and dorsal surface of the proximal tail. The tail can be wrapped to minimize contamination of fur and reduce the need for regular bathing. Care should be taken as clipper blades can cause skin disturbance and, in the worst cases, may contribute to irritation, erythema and development of dermatitis.

Veterinary nurses should be taught proper techniques for manual bladder expression by their supervising veterinary surgeons. Effective manual bladder expression technique takes practice and varies from patient to patient. Another essential technique for veterinary nurses to master is the basic use of an ultrasound machine to assess bladder size. Giving veterinary nurses the confidence to incorporate this skill is invaluable for accurate assessment of patients and decreases potential complications arising from patient handling and poor technique.

Feeding and nutrition

Bodyweight and body condition scoring are familiar to veterinary nurses. Proper nutritional requirements and meeting caloric needs in hospitalized patients can be challenging. The World Small Animal Veterinary Association's (WSAVA) Global Nutrition Guidelines are a great resource for both veterinary staff and owners to assist in providing appropriate nutrition.

Cats often pose the biggest challenges in the face of inappetence. Many animals will have factors that significantly influence food intake, such as psychological state, learned behaviours, circadian rhythm and the external environment. Cats tend to form fixed food preferences and are influenced by the timing and location of meals, the type of bowl or dish the food is offered in, and social stimuli such as the presence or absence of other household members and pets (Michel, 2001). All species are susceptible to learned food aversions, which may be associated with nausea, pain, malady, with the act of eating or even the sight or scent of food. Food aversions are especially relevant to hospitalized patients. Hospitalized patients that excessively swallow, gulp or drool at the sight or smell of food, who turn their heads away from the food, spit it out when it is put in their mouths, or try to escape from offered food, should be left alone. Equally, providing a buffet banquet of all food choices is incorrect methodology; this is an unnatural approach to feeding behaviour in veterinary patients. Nausea, like pain, has a sensory and affective component. Nausea is considered a highly noteworthy cause of suffering in humans. Overt signs of nausea and discomfort should be addressed first. See Figure 6.7 for suggestions for feeding an inpatient that is showing signs of food aversion.

Some patients will require more efficient means to increase nutritional intake. Serious complications are linked with poor nutrition, and cats are particularly prone to the effects of early malnutrition. Veterinary nurses must be

- Offer food in a novel setting
- Have someone different do the feeding
- Make mealtimes as comfortable and as stress-free as possible
- Try to offer food in a quiet setting
- Try to schedule feedings at a different time from other treatments such as pilling
- Avoid pushing food on the patient
- Stroke and talk to the patient
- Try feeding using different dishes/bowl types, e.g. wide shallow bowls or flat plates for cats
- Chilled food from the fridge can be warmed
- Be careful when warming food as this can be counterproductive in some patients with food aversions
- Get the owner involved. They can cook or bring something in and spend time with their pet to try and encourage eating

6.7   Ideas to stimulate feeding.

proactive and advocate early intervention for these patients. Enteral feeding via feeding tubes, such as oesophagostomy tubes, is associated with minimal complications.

Visceral pain disorders are observed commonly in veterinary patients. Visceral pain can range in intensity. Common conditions seen are irritable bowel syndrome, pancreatitis and interstitial cystitis. Visceral pain signals travel through both spinal and vagal routes, and sensitization of peripheral nerves can induce central sensitization at both spinal and supraspinal levels. We often use dietary changes when managing conditions such as feline idiopathic cystitis, for example, low-fat high-fibre regimes, sometimes combined with behavioural modifications. In acute flares, these patients may be admitted for supportive care and analgesia. Treatment options for cats with feline idiopathic cystitis or patients with pancreatitis are often unsatisfactory due to various factors that affect the perception and maintenance of this type of pain.

There has been a recent interest in examining the role of gut microbiota in regulating visceral pain in humans. Gut microbiota are commonly associated with maintenance of intestinal homoeostasis, peristalsis, intestinal mucosal integrity, protection against pathogens and priming of the immune response. A review by O'Mahony et al. (2017) discusses several mechanisms by which the microbiota influence brain function and that this microbiome likely works in concert with reciprocal signalling from the brain. A growing body of literature links central nervous system (CNS) diseases to the mechanism of communication between the gut microbiota and the CNS. Furthermore, a study done by Braniste et al. (2014) showed that the blood–brain barrier integrity in the frontal cortex, hippocampus, and striatum is influenced by gut microbiota. Enhanced pain signalling has been shown in adult mice when they had disturbed gut microbiota. Human and animal models have demonstrated that stress, either chronic or in early life, is a key factor potentiating visceral pain responses and some of the associated co-morbidities. Early life antibiotic

administration has been shown to induce long-lasting effects on visceral pain responses. As the mechanisms by which gut microbiota influence or reduce visceral hypersensitivity are further understood, great potential benefits for veterinary patients will arise.

Feeding techniques for pets are constantly evolving. Various techniques should be utilized more readily in veterinary practice for inpatient enrichment. Studies in dogs investigating different food receptacles and puzzle feeders demonstrate increased time spent on both feeding behaviour and activity. Furthermore, the frequency of barking behaviour was reduced (Schipper et al., 2008). In cats, Dantes et al. (2016) reviewed the use and introduction of puzzle feeders. Another option for cats is the NoBowl Feeding System™. Devised by a US veterinary surgeon, it allows a meal to be split between five NoBowls, which are then hidden around the house. It allows for natural feeding behaviour by encouraging cats to hunt, find, pounce and manipulate the device to dispense small meals.

Further considerations

The placement of a peripheral venous cannula is standard care for many inpatients. These cannulae are often placed by veterinary surgeons, nurses or nurses in training to administer medications and infusions. Cannula-associated phlebitis results in pain, erythema, swelling, and both increased morbidity and cost in veterinary patients. Quality of cannula material, site, placement and maintenance technique, duration of insertion and type of infusions have been identified as factors influencing the occurrence of phlebitis. Palese et al. (2016) found a robust link between nursing care and level of nursing experience in rates of phlebitis in human care. Peripheral venous cannulation is an unpleasant experience; it can be time-consuming, exacerbate patient stress and have associated increases in costs to both clinics and clients. Instigating a cannulation policy is sensible, such as a 'two stick' rule to avoid incidences of multiple attempts, in multiple limbs, by one individual. Certain patient groups are more susceptible to phlebitis, for example, immunosuppressed patients, neutropenic patients, malnourished patients and patients with circulatory impairments. Extra caution with sterility and technique should be applied in these higher risk patient populations.

Clear guidelines do not exist in the veterinary patient for replacement of long-term peripheral venous cannulae. A 2015 Cochrane review suggests that, in humans, removal should only take place when clinically necessary. The report found that there was no evidence to support changing catheters every 72–96 hours and suggested that clinicians consider changing to a policy whereby catheters are changed only if clinically indicated (Webster *et al.*, 2015).

To minimize peripheral cannula-related complications:

- Place under strict aseptic technique, including a generous area of clipped hair in veterinary patients
- In emergency cases, it is worth replacing a peripheral cannula that was pre-placed urgently when asepsis was compromised
- Insertion site should be inspected at each changeover of staff, including complete removal of bandaging and observation of the entry point of the cannula
- The cannula should be removed if signs of inflammation, infiltration or blockage occur.

Recumbent patients are a high-risk patient group for compromised eye integrity and thus are dependent on regular eye care. These patients are susceptible to corneal dehydration, abrasions and infection because of impairment of primary eye protective measures, and the effects of certain medications. In human intensive care units, eye care is performed every 2 hours to prevent corneal abrasions, dehydration and infection; this interval is similarly recommended by veterinary ophthalmologists. Eye care consists of gentle cleaning of the area around both eyes and application of appropriate lubrication to the cornea.

Frequency of oral care has been reported at 2, 3 and 12 hour intervals in human intensive care patients. Oral care at 2- and 4-hour

intervals improved oral hygiene in human patients. While traditional tooth brushing is not common practice in veterinary inpatients, oral health should be attended to. This is particularly important in inappetant or tube-fed patients.

Aural hygiene is also imperative as recumbent animals can be predisposed to ear infections and irritation of the pinnae. They may be unable to display behaviours that would give evidence of this, such as head shaking or scratching. Any patient with skin folds should have regular examinations and cleansing of these areas as required.

Stress and sleep

Hospital environments are stressful for veterinary patients, and hospitalization has been shown to increase psychological stress in humans. Typical problems that are encountered in hospitalized veterinary patients are:

- Struggling during handling
- Difficulty in treating
- Anxious patients being aggressive or unpredictable
- Frustrated dogs barking and whining continually, or chewing through dressings and giving sets
- Stress-related anorexia
- Urinary and faecal retention.

Stress is a cognitive perception of uncontrollability and unpredictability that is expressed in physiological and behavioural responses (Geva *et al.*, 2014). Individuals experience this phenomenon in different degrees. In veterinary patients, there are individuals that are strongly influenced by stress and others that are more resilient; this variation in resilience to stress is mirrored in humans. There are studies that link stress and pain modulation in people, with findings relating stress to a reduction in pain inhibition, and pain intensification (Geva *et al.*, 2014). Exposing animals to prolonged stress without the ability to adjust to their immediate environment has negative consequences. Stress makes the patient harder to care for and contributes to adverse associations. These negative associations are linked to the clinic and individual animal carer. Veterinary patients' senses are far more acute than the senses of humans. The hospital environment is an unnatural setting, which may have strong aversive smells, stark hospital cages, wards that create abnormal social groups, intermixing of species, noise, lighting, and evoked sleep deprivation, all affecting a patient that may already have negative physical feelings, such as hunger, pain and nausea (Hewson, 2014a).

Brachycephalic breeds need particular attention when hospitalized. Any form of stress or excitement can cause severe respiratory distress in this category of patient. They have an impaired ability to thermoregulate and therefore have a propensity to overheat. Basic science supports the value of using an oscillating fan to provide air movement and flows within the environment, and a 'wind chill' effect to help cool and calm the patient. Fans need to be directed at the patient or in very close proximity to have a beneficial effect (Figure 6.8).

Sleep deprivation is often massively overlooked in the care strategy of critically ill patients (Figure 6.9). Frequent interruption of sleep is a significant problem and a noted stressor in human intensive care settings. Sleep is a basic physiological need. The average canine spends approximately 50% of the day sleeping, 30% lying around awake, and just 20% being active. These percentages vary dependent on breed, in particular the inherent use for which the animal was bred (e.g. Labradors are a highly active retrieving breed), and age.

Sleep deprivation in people has been associated with behavioural changes such as becoming short-tempered, irritable, over-reactive, and an inability to cope effectively with situations or society. This mental stress induces a catabolic state and negatively affects the immune system and healing process, thus reducing good patient outcomes.

Feline patients can be particularly prone to the adverse effects of stress. A recent review by Amat *et al.* (2016) observed that highly stressed cats are five times more likely to develop upper respiratory tract infections

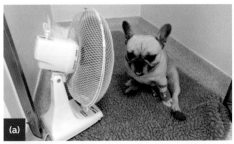

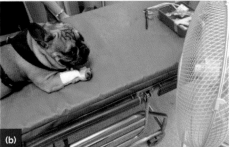

6.8 **(a)** Brachycephalic breed being cooled by a fan. **(b)** Brachycephalic breed stressed and dyspnoeic after a car journey. A fan is used to cool and destress the patient prior to examination. Note the airway management kit on standby.

Cause	Examples
Environmental noise	• Phones ringing • Talking • Beepers • Overhead speakers • Equipment sounds (e.g. suction, drip pumps)
Lighting	• Overhead lights • Spotlights
General discomfort	• Monitoring attached • Dressings • Elizabethan collars • Intravenous lines
Oxygen	• Drying of nasal passages
Room temperature	• Too hot or cold, poor air quality
Pain	• Pathology, surgery, injury
Psychological stressors	• Physical and social

6.9 Causes of sleep deprivation.

compared with cats with lower stress levels. Stress has been associated with gastrointestinal signs such as diarrhoea and vomiting. Stress can alter the integrity of the intestinal mucosa, predispose cats to feline interstitial cystitis and reactivate dormant feline herpesvirus. Atopic dermatitis, acral licks and perpetuation of pruritus are affected by stress. Extreme or chronic stress can lead to compulsive behaviours such as feline hyperaesthesia syndrome (FHS), psychogenic alopecia and pica (Amat *et al.*, 2016).

Core territory is of particular importance in feline patients but too often cannot be incorporated in the hospital setting. Cats also need to be able to perch, to hide, and be elevated, to feel safe and to reduce anxiety, and these very helpful provisions need not be expensive. The cat's carrier, if appropriate (Figure 6.10), or a cardboard box is an ideal 'hiding place'. Cats prefer to use edges for facial marking, so this should be an important consideration when investing in 'furniture' for their environment. Keeping cats separate from dogs has been shown to reduce stress levels and has led to the development of feline-specific waiting areas, wards and intensive care units at many veterinary hospitals.

Cats and dogs have a high degree of olfactory acuity. The use of odours for psychological well being is well documented in humans and some captive animals. Recent studies have examined the effects of certain scents in both cats and dogs in the rescue shelter setting. In dogs, lavender resulted in more behaviours suggestive of relaxation with less time spent moving and more time resting, as well as reduction in barking behaviours. In another example, cats interact significantly more with catnip than with lavender, the scent from a domestic rabbit or a control; 50–75% of cats exhibit a positive response to catnip. An extensive review by Frank *et al.* (2010) of the use of synthetic pheromone therapy found that, while synthetic pheromone application is worthwhile in some scenarios, there is no evidence of efficacy in veterinary hospital wards. Some animals use their own pheromones to establish an area in which they feel control and reassurance. Often, kennels are cleaned daily using strong-smelling disinfectants and new bedding is put in, and this may hugely influence behaviour and anxiety in some inpatients. Anxiety is suffering, and carers must acknowledge it as a negative outcome and address this as part of the patient experience. If good practices of infection prevention and control exist and any evident soiling is removed in a timely manner, the need for daily cleaning and disinfection is reduced for some patients, thus reducing their anxiety levels.

Mental or physical distraction is an essential technique to incorporate in both inpatient care and for outpatients where owners need assistance. Literature supports the use of music and music therapy. Well *et al.* (2002) demonstrated that dogs display behaviours suggestive of relaxation in response to classical music. Pop music and talk radio did not have the same effect. In a study by Snowden *et al.* (2015), cats expressed a preference for species-appropriate music over music composed for humans. This is not surprising as many species are sensitive to different frequency ranges and tempos. Auditory communication varies between species, so while auditory enrichment can be useful, music needs to be selected carefully. It is insufficient to just turn on the radio or play standard classical music.

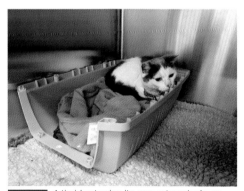

6.10 A timid cat using its own cat carrier base as a secure space. Blankets inside are from the cat's home environment so will have familiar pheromones.

Outpatient focus

Veterinary nursing clinics have become more common in many hospitals throughout Britain. Veterinary nurses have long been the intermediary between clients and veterinary surgeons. Their roles in education, provision of care and utilization of a myriad of clinical skills makes veterinary nurses key team members, especially when considering painful patients. Most nurses are already familiar with postoperative check-ups and addressing commonly related concerns such as:

- Is the patient eating regularly?
- Are any side effects to the medications dispensed apparent?
- Has the patient been interfering with the wound?
- Can the wound be palpated without adverse reaction?
- Has the wound healed as expected?
- Can the patient go outside/exercise off leash?

Geriatric and arthritis nursing clinics

The nurse consultation involves assessing the patient's comfort level and how well both patient and client are coping at home. Geriatric and arthritis clinics have a commonality in that during this stage in a patient's life cycle the top priority is to minimize suffering. Patient suffering may arise in response to an illness or disease. Suffering can encompass many contributing states such as pain, anxiety, stress and starvation. Some of these states arise from a dysfunctional care delivery system or may vary based on differences in how clinics provide care. Ultimately, these states are avoidable. Some animals suffer more by imposed lifestyle restrictions than by the suffering caused by the pain induced by regular lifestyle activities; for example, a patient may mentally suffer more by not playing with the ball or going out for walks than they would suffer physically if they performed the activities.

Pain has a strong emotional component. Chronic pain in humans is frequently associated with disorders such as anxiety and depression. This aspect is not well researched in veterinary patients. However, understanding of pain pathology and processing in mammalian species supports the presence of emotional states in some veterinary patients that are unaddressed. Assessment and examination of chronic pain cases are discussed in Chapter 4.

For chronic pain patients, the support provided by a nurse clinic can be instrumental in successful management. Any chronic condition involves a period of both client education and adjustment. Clients may not understand the condition, how it affects their animal, how it affects themselves, and the continuing management required. Nurses can competently advise clients on topics such as diet, nutraceuticals, exercise, modifications around the home, medication dosing and side effects, and pain recognition and assessment. Of importance are both owner awareness of the support network available to them and provision of an interdisciplinary, holistic approach to chronic pain management. Owners need to understand that most chronic conditions are incurable and that a long-term commitment to management is required. The aim of long-term management of arthritic cases is to slow down the progression of this degenerative disease. Good management of an arthritic patient will both reduce patient suffering and produce improvements in mobility. In the geriatric patient with cognitive dysfunction, it can be challenging to distinguish pain from other signs of cognitive decline. Maintaining organ function when concurrent disease is present may influence drug choices. Owners may need advice and reassurance that they will recognize the correct time for euthanasia of their pet. Quality of life (QoL) assessments are critical in assessing both geriatric and arthritic patients. A validated measure of health-related QoL and pain in animals is available through NewMetrica and the University of Glasgow (see Appendix 1). These QoL assessments support veterinary staff and owners by providing a meaningful shift in veterinary care and animal welfare.

A very simple mnemonic, ABCDE (courtesy of Professor Stuart Carmichael), can be used to guide treatment and recommendations for geriatric or chronically painful patients; see also Chapters 4 and 7g.

- A – analgesia.
- B – bodyweight and body score.
- C – comfort, compliance, common sense, complications, core territory.
- D – disease modifications.
- E – exercise, environment enrichment.

Each of these categories are outlined in more detail below.

Analgesia

Analgesia tends to form the cornerstone of treatment in chronic pain cases. Educating owners about all the options available, and informing them that it may take some time to find the right balance for their pet, is important.

- Pharmaceutical therapies (see Chapter 5).
- Physical therapies, for example acupuncture (Figure 6.11; see also Chapter 6b), transcutaneous electrical nerve stimulation (TENS), physiotherapy, hydrotherapy and laser therapy.
- Interventions, such as platelet rich plasma injections and stem cell therapy.

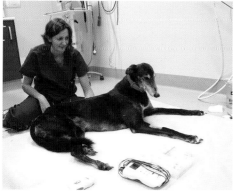

6.11 Author performing acupuncture in an elderly Greyhound. A thick mattress is used for comfort. The patient is calm, unrestrained and does not need sedation. Veterinary nurses can perform acupuncture under the direction of a trained veterinary surgeon.

Nausea and side effects should be discussed during the consultation. Salivating, lip licking, eating more grass, yawning, stretching, pica, and coprophagia may all be signs of nausea. Cats experiencing nausea tend to become anorexic whereas dogs often keep eating. Owners must also look out for side effects of analgesic therapies. Combinations of drugs may be prescribed and the pharmacokinetics/pharmacodynamics may be unknown. Some drugs are psychoactive so will influence behaviour, anxiety and disinhibition.

While veterinary surgeons are responsible for prescribing drugs, veterinary nurses can explain the reason for prescription and correct use of the drugs, side effects, licensing and further information where human drugs are used and repurposed.

Analgesia checklist

- Start simple but prepare the owner for the possibility of multiple interventions.
- Listen to owner concerns about medication types (they may have personal experience or friend/family who experienced negative effects).
- Listen for signs of misunderstanding – 'aren't we just masking the pain?'
- Offer physical interventions with positive associations – gentle touch, gentle massage (flat hand), gentle stretching.
- Establish clear targets of treatment.

PRACTICAL TIP

Pain is a stressor and causes all the same physiological changes as chronic stress. This is important to communicate to owners as most will understand the detrimental effects of stress

Bodyweight and body score

When deciding if a patient is under- or overweight it is important to also consider fat and muscle distribution. Adipose tissue is well established as an endocrine gland that produces adipokines. Adipokines possess pro- and anti-inflammatory properties that play a vital function in systemic metabolism and immune function. Obesity promotes a pro-inflammatory state that contributes to a chronic low-grade state of systemic inflammation. Adipokines also influence metabolic conditions linked with obesity. This pro-inflammatory state will contribute directly to any coexisting pain.

Veterinary nurses can teach owners how to body condition score and direct them to helpful resources such as videos available on the WSAVA nutritional toolkit website. Resources are also available to teach owners about human caloric equivalents. The Association for Pet Obesity Prevention has some great resources, for example, the Pet-Human Weight Translator, and other weight loss tools for cats and dogs that can be printed and passed on to owners. If medication is only administered with cheese or a hot dog, the calories of these foods need to be factored into calorie counting. Lower calorie alternatives or other methods of medication administration should be discussed. Delivering food in different ways (Figure 6.12) will increase patient interest. 'Just feed less' is not a workable solution if food is an important resource for that pet or the owner. Methods to incorporate this need to be considered.

Comfort

This can encompass a myriad of solutions that may improve welfare and well being, some of the more obvious being all the areas where the pet enjoys resting and sleeping. For some pets this will also involve thinking about access to the sleeping area, e.g. steps to the back of the sofa. There will be perhaps less obvious areas to deal with such as how the pet travels in the car; if they have exposed nail beds from scuffing their feet, can they manage a walk; and also more owner-centred considerations such as how able they are to lift a dog into the car or make changes around the home.

- Beds: best for patient, not what matches décor or owner's aesthetic preferences.
- Flooring: slippery floors may be problematic; use rugs, runners and consider nail grips such as Dr Buzby™ nail grips.
- Car rides: ask owners what the patient does specifically while in the car and when the

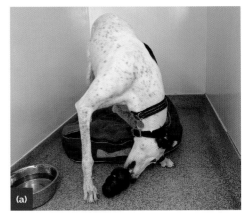

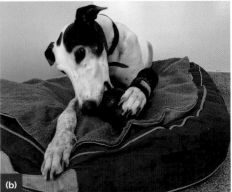

6.12 **(a,b)** A toy (Kong™) used as a method of feeding a Greyhound in hospital. This method of feeding encourages natural feeding behaviours, increases the time taken for the patient to eat and provides a great distraction.

car is travelling. Are they pacing, salivating, panting excessively, falling over, jamming themselves into a corner? A big open-spaced boot is not always helpful for dogs struggling against a moving car.
- Scuffed nails: down to the quick can be very uncomfortable; nail covers such as Soft Paws™ are available.
- Mobility aids: these may help owners take their pet out more easily or frequently and can be used in combination with conventional walks. Aids such as wheels, harnesses, buggies and ramps warrant consideration.

Compliance
Veterinary staff must take the time to explore owner and patient motivations, and understand how involved the owner can be and realistically how much time they have to put towards additional measures.

- Positive interventions help.
- Give owners tasks to complete.

Common sense
It is important to help maintain and strengthen the human–animal bond. In some instances, this will involve coming up with solutions to scenarios that are important to the client and the pet, for example, ways to allow the patient to be with the owner such as on sofas.

Complications
The need for close monitoring in these patients is paramount. Co-morbidities and/or polypharmacy will require frequent assessment for potential side effects and organ function. Complications may exist from the outset or develop along the way with the owner, for example, if they have limited resources or are going through a personal crisis of their own.

- Ongoing monitoring for side effects (e.g. blood tests).
- Explain complications to owners.
- Owner-related complications may occur at any time.

Core territory (cats)
Core territory is extremely important to cats and is smaller in size than a cat's home range. It consists of the area where the cat feels secure enough to eat, sleep, play, groom and avoid conflict with other household pets. Cats like the use of vertical space for resting and security. Providing shelves or cat trees are easy ways to increase vertical space, but remember to provide access to these areas, particularly for older or less mobile cats.

- Provide access to heights and hiding places.
- An arthritic cat may struggle to use vertical scratching posts; horizontal or sloped scratching posts may be more accessible.

- Provide access to food and water, which should ideally be a room apart.
- Think about access and accessibility of toilet areas; walls of litter boxes may be too high for the patient to comfortably traverse.
- Increase play opportunities by rotating toys.
- Grooming should be performed with a soft brush.

Use of video to assess mobility and core territory can be invaluable. Cats in a consult room are not easy to assess and will often move unnaturally, for example, they often have a very low body carriage or may just 'freeze'.

Disease modification
Veterinary nurses should educate clients about ways of slowing the progression and worsening of the disease.

- Try to limit repeated concussion of affected joints, as may occur with jumping in and out of vehicles or bounding in anticipation of a walk.
- Improve muscle strength with appropriate, regular exercise.
- Discuss direct joint interventions, including surgical options.
- Explore the use of nutraceuticals.
- Provide appropriate analgesia.

Exercise
Optimization of exercise training is key in prevention and treatment for many chronic conditions. It needs to be engaging and sustained and realistically balanced with the owner's schedule.

- The right type, the right amount.
- Structured.
- Aim to progress.
- Keep it interesting; different walks, different parks, different entrances, visit a café or pet store.
- Consider the substrate; concrete *versus* sand *versus* uneven surfaces.
- Consider how the patient behaves at home and possible physical impacts, for example jumping up at the window every time a bus goes past.

- Consider whether the dog pulls on the lead; trigger points, lipomas/masses that may get compressed with halter/collars.
- What exercise makes them worse? What exercise makes them better?
- Outdoor cats spend 60–80% of their waking hours seeking their prey. This predatory search is a cat's natural exercise, as well as mental stimulation.

Exercise restriction is not always the answer; often, restriction will worsen chronic conditions. Patients need to keep moving. They need to be kept interested and stimulated.

Environmental enrichment

All captive animals need environmental enrichment and this includes family pets. The idea is to influence the animal's environment to increase physical activity and normal species-typical behaviour that will satisfy their physical and psychological needs.

Enrichments must be dynamic and sensible for the intended species; for example, the same Kong™ toy, at the same time, with the same filling every day provides limited enrichment. If you restrict a resource (e.g. food, exercise, play) then it needs to be replaced with something else where possible, otherwise this could contribute to increased suffering. These resources are requirements that an animal needs to survive; patients will suffer if they do not receive these resources.

Techniques used to improve an environment include:

- Food-based enrichment
- Sensory enrichment (sight, smell, touch, taste and hearing)
- Novel objects
- Social enrichment
- Positive training techniques.

PRACTICAL TIP

Suggestions such as keeping a diary to record owner-perceived pain levels, activity levels, and sleep quality, will assist review periods, titration of medication and further interventions such as physiotherapy, hydrotherapy, and acupuncture

---

References and further reading

Amat M, Camps T and Manteca X (2016) Stress in owned cats: behavioural changes and welfare implications. *Journal of Feline Medicine and Surgery* **18**, 577–586

Bansal C, Scott R, Stewart D and Cockerell CJ (2005) Decubitus ulcers: A review of the literature. *International Journal of Dermatology* **44**, 805–810

Braniste V, Al-Asmakh M, Kowal C et al. (2014) The gut microbiota influences blood-brain barrier permeability in mice. *Science Translational Medicine* **6**, 263ra158

Coyer FM, Wheeler MK, Wetzig SM and Couchman BA (2007) Nursing care of the mechanically ventilated patient: What does the evidence say? *Intensive and Critical Care Nursing* **23**, 71–80

Dantas LM, Delgado MM, Johnson I and Buffington CT (2016) Food puzzles for cats: Feeding for physical and emotional wellbeing. *Journal of Feline Medicine and Surgery* **18**, 723–732

Ellis SLH and Wells DL (2010) The influence of olfactory stimulation on the behaviour of cats housed in a rescue shelter. *Applied Animal Behaviour Science* **123**, 56–62

Frank D, Beauchamp G and Palestrini C (2010) Systematic review of the use of pheromones for treatment of undesirable behavior in cats and dogs. *Journal of the American Veterinary Medical Association* **236**, 1308–1316

Geva N, Pruessner J and Defrin R (2014) Acute psychosocial stress reduces pain modulation capabilities in healthy men. *Pain* **155**, 2418–2425

Graham L, Wells DL and Hepper PG (2005) The influence of olfactory stimulation on the behaviour of dogs housed in a rescue shelter. *Applied Animal Behaviour Science* **91**, 143–153

Hewson C (2014b) Evidence-based approaches to reducing in-patient stress – Part 1: Why animals' sensory capacities make hospitalization stressful to them. *Veterinary Nursing Journal* **29**, 130–132

Hewson C (2014a) Evidence-based approaches to reducing in-patient stress — Part 3: How to reduce in-patient stress. *Veterinary Nursing Journal* **29**, 234–236

Honkus VL (2003) Sleep deprivation in critical care units. *Critical Care Nursing Quarterly* **26**, 179–189

Li M-J, Liu L-Y, Chen L et al. (2017) Chronic stress exacerbates neuropathic pain via the integration of stress-affect-related information with nociceptive information in the central nucleus of the amygdala. *Pain* **158**, 717–739

Mancuso P (2016) The role of adipokines in chronic inflammation. *Immuno Targets and Therapy* **5**, 47–56

Michel K (2001) Management of anorexia in the cat. *Journal of Feline Medicine and Surgery* **3**, 3–8

NPUAP (2014) *NEW 2014 Prevention and Treatment of Pressure Ulcers: Clinical Practice Guideline* [online]. The National Pressure Ulcer Advisory Panel. Available at: http://www.npuap.org/resources/educational-and-clinical-resources/prevention-and-treatment-of-pressure-ulcers-clinical-practice-guideline/

O'Mahony SM, Dinan TG and Cryan JF (2017) The gut microbiota as a key regulator of visceral pain. *Pain* **158**, S19–S28

Palese A, Ambrosi E, Fabris F et al. (2016) Nursing care as a predictor of phlebitis related to insertion of a peripheral venous cannula in emergency departments: findings from a prospective study. *Journal of Hospital Infection* **92**, 280–286

Schipper LL, Vinke CM, Schilder MBH and Spruijt BM (2008) The effect of feeding enrichment toys on the behaviour of kennelled dogs (*Canis familiaris*). *Applied Animal Behaviour Science* **114**, 182–195

Smarick SD, Haskins SC, Aldrich J et al. (2004) Incidence of catheter-associated urinary tract infection among dogs in a small animal intensive care unit. Journal of the American Veterinary Medical Association **224**, 1936–1940

Snowdon CT, Teie D and Savage M (2015) Cats prefer species-appropriate music. Applied Animal Behaviour Science **166**, 106–111

Webster J, Osborne S, Rickard CM and New K (2015) Clinically-indicated replacement versus routine replacement of peripheral venous catheters. Cochrane Database of Systematic Reviews **17**

Wells DL, Graham L and Hepper PG (2002) The influence of auditory stimulation on the behaviour of dogs housed in a rescue shelter. Animal Welfare **11**, 385–393

Some useful websites

Association for Pet Obesity Prevention:
http://petobesityprevention.org/

Fear free certification program:
https://fearfreepets.com

Fenzi Dog Sports Academy Cooperative Canine Care program:
https://fenzidogsportsacademy.com/index.php/courses/2392

Hill's Pet Nutrition – What Human Food Does to Your Pet:
http://www.hillspet.com/en/us/pet-care/nutrition-feeding/human-food-treat-translator

Low Stress Handling® – Dr Sophia Yin:
https://drsophiayin.com/low-stress-handling/

NewMetrica Quality of Life measurement:
http://www.newmetrica.com

WSAVA Nutritional Toolkit:
http://www.wsava.org/nutrition-toolkit

Stockists

The following list includes stockists of products and product types mentioned in the text. Please note, this list is not exhaustive.

Aneticaid:
http://www.aneticaid.co.uk
Stockist of theatre equipment including arm retainer pads and anaesthetic tube holders.

Comfy Collars:
https://www.comfycollars.co.uk

Cosy Dogs Harnesses:
https://www.cosydogs.com/harnesses-shop/cosy-dogs-harnesses.html

Doc and Phoebe Cat Co.:
https://docandphoebe.com/
Manufacturer of The NoBowl Feeding System™.

KONG toys:
https://www.kongcompany.com/en-uk

Kruuse:
https://www.kruuse.com/en-GB.aspx
Stockists of BUSTER thermal vac support sets.

Medipaw Protective Pet Wound Management:
http://medivetproducts.com
Protective pet clothing.

OrthoPets:
http://www.orthopets.co.uk
Stockist of Help'EmUp Harness and Dr Buzyby's ToeGrips.

Pet Support Suit:
http://petsupportsuit.com

Ruffwear:
http://www.ruffwear.co.uk

Soft Paws Nail Caps:
http://www.softpaws.co.uk

Chapter 6b

Physical methods used to alleviate pain: complementary therapies

Samantha Lindley

Acupoint abbreviations used in this chapter:

BL – Bladder
CV – Conception vessel
GB – Gallbladder
GV – Governing vessel
LI – Large intestine
PC – Pericardium
SP – Spleen
ST – Stomach

■ Acupuncture
■ Physiotherapy
■ Hydrotherapy
■ Chiropractic
■ Osteopathy
■ Bowen therapy
■ Pressure point massage/therapeutic massage

6.13 Physical therapies commonly used in veterinary pain management.

The use of physical therapies in veterinary pain management is increasingly popular with clients (Figure 6.13). This is partly because they have a sense that such approaches must be safe; partly because they feel that such treatments allow them to have some active involvement in their pet's care; and partly because they assume (not always correctly) that such approaches will avoid or limit pharmacological analgesia.

Quality research on the specific efficacy of an intervention is inherently more difficult for physical therapies than for pharmacological treatments because blinding of the subject and owner (and therapist) is not straightforward. As soon as physical contact occurs between therapist and animal, changes occur in the animal that may have non-specific effects on the pain. Positive social interactions cause a reduction in blood pressure and release of neurotransmitters that improve mood, but are also associated with pain relief (Uvnas-Moberg et al., 1993; Odendaal, 2002).

Notwithstanding the difficulties of a veterinary, clinically oriented evidence base, some physical therapies do have a convincing body of (animal) experimental and human clinical studies.

Acupuncture

Acupuncture, although perhaps not immediately thought of as a physical therapy, must be considered as such because physical interactions occur during examination and treatment of the patient. However, despite the potential for non-specific effects, there are plenty of experimental (animal) and clinical (human) studies to demonstrate specific efficacy of the needle insertion (i.e. over and above placebo and non-specific effects) (Filshie *et al.*, 2016).

For the purposes of this chapter, acupuncture is defined as: 'the insertion of a solid needle into the body for the purpose of therapy and pain relief'.

Summary of the mechanisms

Acupuncture stimulates afferent nerves, competes with other inputs at the dorsal horn of the spinal cord, and triggers effects on the brain, which include, but are not limited to: deactivation of the limbic system; facilitation of descending inhibitory pain pathways; stimulation of the hypothalamus; and release of beta endorphins from the periaqueductal gray (PAG).

Local effects

An acupuncture needle is a solid, non-traumatic needle that is inserted through the skin. Where it goes thereafter depends on what the acupuncturist is trying to achieve. From a Western perspective, the therapist is not necessarily aiming for a very specific anatomical location with a specific name (i.e. an acupuncture point such as LI 4), although these are used, but they will have a specific structure in mind. Such structures include: myofascial trigger points (MTrPs – tiny ischaemic areas within the end plate zones of muscles, which give rise to potentially intense pain, referral of pain, muscle weakness and muscle shortening (Figure 6.14) – MTrPs are not inflammatory and are not equivalent to muscle spasm), tendon insertions, joint margins, the most prominent part or the raphae of muscles, ligaments, tender areas of fascia, and periosteum.

When treating pain, the aim of the acupuncturist is to place the needle *as close as possible to the source of pain without making it worse*.

Acupuncture points

Terms such as ST and PC refer to specific point or 'meridians'. The meridian name is given first, followed by a number. In Western acupuncture, these notations are simply shorthand for a (reasonably) specific anatomical area in which needles are commonly placed. For example: ST36 is a point in the cranial tibial muscle just lateral to the tibial crest in the most prominent part of the muscle, oriented from the cranial to the caudal aspect of the limb.

The high threshold stimulus of needle insertion stimulates afferent nerves. These nerves, despite their name, release most of their neurotransmitters at their prodromal (peripheral) end. These include substance P (SP), calcitonin gene-related peptide (CGRP), vasoactive intestinal peptide (VIP), and nerve growth factor (NGF), amongst others. These are healing factors, released normally in response to damage and trauma. Adenosine is also released and achieves analgesia locally.

Segmental effects

The afferent nerves stimulated are alpha-delta fibres (in skin) and type II/III fibres (in muscle). These nerves signal so-called 'fast pain', which indicates actual or potential tissue damage and limits such damage by its rapid transmission to the central nervous system, resulting in the withdrawal of the affected part of the body from the threat. The transmission of fast pain is mediated in the dorsal horn by the activation of enkephalinergic interneurons in the substantia gelatinosa of the dorsal horn. These interneurons release enkephalins and block the onward transmission of so-called 'slow pain' from the C fibres (type IV fibres in muscle) – this is the 'competition' aspect of an acupuncture stimulus.

The 'fast pain' signal is then transmitted to the brain where it stimulates the release of beta endorphins from the PAG, which circulate humerally, and 5-hydroxytryptamine (5-HT) and noradrenaline from the locus coeruleus, which facilitate the descending inhibitory pain pathways.

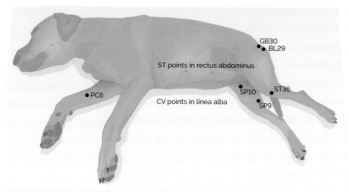

6.14

General location of needling points.

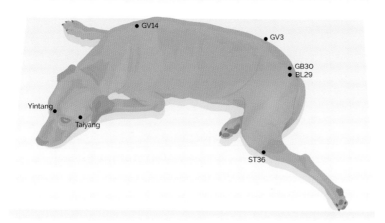

This whole effect occurs most potently at the spinal segment stimulated by the acupuncture needle. This is segmental acupuncture and justifies the approach of needling as close as possible to the source of pain.

Heterosegmental effects

The release of 5-HT and noradrenaline and consequent facilitation of the descending inhibitory pain pathways occurs throughout the spinal cord (although it is most potent at the segment stimulated).

General effects

One of the primary effects of dry needling (or manual acupuncture) is to deactivate the limbic system. The limbic system is the major area of the brain associated with emotion and is overactive in (especially) chronic pain, when suffering is significant. Functional magnetic resonance imaging (MRI) studies by Hui *et al.* (2000) have demonstrated that acupuncture deactivates the limbic system and thus reduces the emotional component of pain, i.e. it reduces suffering. This is pertinent when considering the 'outcome measures' used for assessing the effects of acupuncture.

The general effects of circulating endorphins and other neurotransmitters in the cerebrospinal fluid (CSF) and blood contribute to mood and arousal states in the patient.

Long-term relief of pain

Acupuncture may result in a cumulative response to signs such as pain or dysfunction. In terms of pain, this is mediated at least in part by the upregulation of messenger RNA for preproenkephalin, i.e. more precursors of endorphins are produced. This means that the body responds to new or returning pain sensation by rapidly producing more pain relief.

Essentially, acupuncture 'fools' the brain into thinking that the body has been damaged, so that it triggers very potent pain-relieving mechanisms that are then directed to the area that most needs the pain relief.

This sounds impressive and, although these effects have been reliably demonstrated, the potency of acupuncture depends on the inherent ability of the patient to respond to the stimulus and the ability of the acupuncturist to deliver an effective 'dose' for the individual and for the condition under treatment.

Legal status of veterinary acupuncture

Acupuncture is an act of veterinary surgery. However, veterinary nurses may perform acupuncture under Schedule 3 if directed to do so by a veterinary surgeon (veterinarian) trained in acupuncture and who directs the depth and position of needling.

Physiotherapy

Physiotherapy is defined as a range of physical therapies used to prevent and treat injuries, restore function, and maximize physical potential. It includes any of the manipulative therapies such as osteopathy and chiropractic, but, although acupuncture is a physical therapy, acupuncture is not included within the scope of veterinary physiotherapy, as it is an act of veterinary surgery, as noted above.

Access to a veterinary physiotherapist is not universal and, even if it were, it is not necessarily appropriate for all conditions and all patients. What will be described here are the simple techniques that can be employed and demonstrated by the veterinary team to help

owners to help improve their pet's mobility, muscle strength and balance.

Techniques that fall under the umbrella of 'physiotherapy' include any skill (except acupuncture) in which the physiotherapist is included, e.g. hydrotherapy, laser therapy, massage, pressure point massage and manipulations. However, each of these may also be offered by practitioners who specialize in one technique only (e.g. hydrotherapists and chiropractors).

Hydrotherapy

Hydrotherapy uses the inherent properties of water to facilitate rehabilitation of patients who may find land-based exercises too difficult or painful. Where a hydrotherapy facility is available to the practice it will obviously be used, but there are some patients that do not accept formal hydrotherapy and some owners may not have the time or resources to use it.

In these cases, so-called do it yourself (DIY) hydrotherapy may be employed, but owners need advice on minimizing risk and optimizing benefits. Hydrotherapy is not a panacea, it can be hard work for the patient, and can result in a worsening of pain if used improperly.

Hydrotherapy services available include:

- Pools/tanks: swimming in pools generally expends greater effort than walking on an underwater treadmill, so it is not suitable for older or frail animals or those with cardiovascular disease. Moreover, swimming in a pool, while allowing greater joint flexion than land-based exercise, does not contribute to joint extension
- Underwater treadmills: allow better joint flexion and extension than land-based exercise; can contribute to an improvement in proprioception; and reduce loading and concussion on the joints (Figure 6.15)
- 'DIY' hydrotherapy: this can mimic some of the effects of pools and water walking, depending on how the owner controls the patient. The main risks with such an approach are the access to and exit from the water – diving in and scrabbling out is likely to be detrimental and so owners must source shallow beach type areas for their

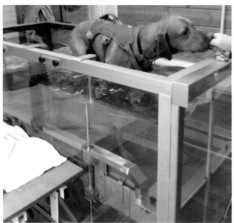

6.15 Underwater treadmills help to achieve better flexion and extension of joints than a pool.

dog and control the way they approach the water. They must also prevent the dog from becoming too cold. Advantages include: dogs that are anxious about formal hydrotherapy can benefit and even enjoy the therapy; it is free; and it may be more frequently accessed than the formal version.

Potential benefits of all hydrotherapy forms include: a theoretical decrease in pain perception; increase in blood circulation; increase in sodium excretion by the kidneys; and reduction of oedema.

Massage and touch therapies

Touch, if the patient enjoys it, is useful in the treatment of pain because it reduces blood pressure (and pain is a stressor that can increase blood pressure) and releases mood neurotransmitters that include endorphins, serotonin, noradrenaline, dopamine, oxytocin, and prolactin. These are variously related to analgesia, mood, arousal states, and bonding (Figure 6.16).

The safest approach to massage is to use a flat hand approach. Owners often want to use their fingers to try to tackle the 'knots' they can feel (trigger points) in the way they may enjoy a therapeutic massage for themselves. This may be helpful, but it may also cause a worsening of

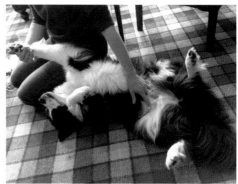

6.16 Touch can release neurotransmitters associated with pain relief.

PRACTICAL TIPS

For old, frail animals and animals with spinal problems only use an underwater treadmill or gentle DIY hydrotherapy.

Key points of DIY hydrotherapy:

- Access to and exit from the water are the most important aspects of safety. Gentle slopes should be found, preferably flat beach areas with a smooth surface
- The dog should be well dried and kept warm after the session
- Starting gently with the water up to hock and carpus, get the dog used to walking back and forth along a short stretch of water (5 m). Work up to having the water at the level of the greater trochanter over four sessions, once or twice weekly. Then repeat twice or three times weekly, gradually increasing the number of 'lengths' from two to six over a month. Teach the owner to monitor heart rate and to be aware of signs of excessive tiring
- Check that the pain is not getting worse after 3 weeks.

pain, especially in dogs that patiently put up with anything their owner does to them. Use the palm of the hand in contact with the skin; move the hand and the skin together over the underlying muscles (Figure 6.17). Use the animal's body language and facial expressions to determine whether the touch is too firm or if they would enjoy greater pressure. Ideally, this massage should be done before and after exercise.

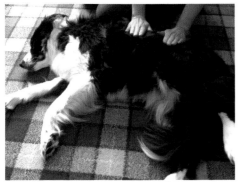

6.17 Flat hand massage is the safest form of massage to teach an owner.

Use of physical therapies in veterinary pain management

Acute pain

Generally speaking, acupuncture will be the main physical therapy used in acute pain presentations, as an adjunct to pharmacological analgesia. Physiotherapy and hydrotherapy are indicated postoperatively in intervertebral disc disease and orthopaedic conditions (depending on the procedure used). Hydrotherapy can be started almost as soon as the wound is healed, but the ideal timescale varies for different orthopaedic conditions.

Acute neurological pain – intervertebral disc disease

Clearly, the primary importance for intervertebral disc disease (IVDD) is making the correct assessment. Contrary to some reports

Acupuncture may be added where pharmacological analgesia does not appear to be reducing signs of distress and discomfort. The addition of acupuncture will sometimes give sufficient relaxation and endogenous pain relief to allow the medical analgesia to work. Needles can be placed near the source of pain if appropriate; segmentally; peri-segmentally; or in non-painful general points such as ST36, GV14, GV3, and Yintang (Figure 6.18). Physiotherapy and hydrotherapy should be used in conjunction with professional advice in acute neurological and orthopaedic pain.

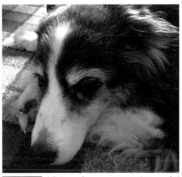

6.18 Yintang is an acupuncture point between the eyes (the Chinese name is only used here because the point is an extra one to the normal numbering system).

(e.g. Joaquim *et al.*, 2010), acupuncture is not an alternative to decompressive surgery, where such surgery is indicated, but it does appear to be a useful adjunct at different stages of the disease.

At first presentation, without delaying assessment or surgery, acupuncture should be performed at the suspected site of disc prolapse into the epaxial muscles. If electroacupuncture is available and appropriate this should be used (Figure 6.19).

- Outcomes: pain relief; relaxation; decrease of anxiety and secondary muscle spasm.
- Conservative management: acupuncture should be used twice weekly initially (to

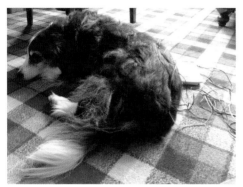

6.19 Electroacupuncture is the most potent form of stimulation with acupuncture needles.

'ramp up' the cumulative effects) in the relevant epaxial muscles, using electroacupuncture if tolerated.

- Post-surgically: acupuncture can be applied initially at the segments either side of the surgical site into the epaxial muscles or paraspinally into multifidus muscles.
- Once the wound has healed: the affected segments can be treated directly.

It should be noted that acupuncture will optimize wound healing (see Chronic dermatological pain, below) but, unless wound healing is poor, the surgical site is avoided initially because it is likely to be bruised and hyperalgesic.

Acute orthopaedic pain

Acupuncture can be used for adjunctive pain relief in patients with acute orthopaedic pain. Probably the most useful indication is for cruciate disease prior to assessment for surgery. Acupuncture around (not into) the knee joint into ST36, BL40, SP9 and SP10 and into the hip girdle (GB30, BL29) for an acute presentation should be performed (Figure 6.20). If the disease has been present for some time before the acute presentation then secondary trigger points will be identified in the contralateral pelvic limb and the epaxial muscles (possibly also the contralateral thoracic limb). The sooner acupuncture is started, the better the prospects for effective rehabilitation post-surgically or if conservative treatment is chosen.

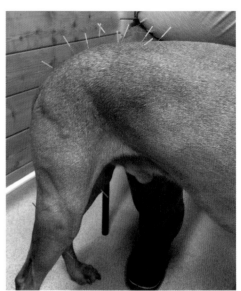

6.20 Acupuncture around the stifle and hip girdle muscles for cruciate and other stifle pain.

Acute gastrointestinal pain

While the main thrust of treatment is fluid support and resolution of the main signs of disease, pain and nausea should not be ignored and may be treated adjunctively with acupuncture. There is experimental (dogs, rats, mice) evidence that acupuncture can also normalize function, reduce gastric acid, and stimulate dopamine release from the adrenals, which may have an impact in acute septic conditions (Sato *et al.*, 1993; Torres-Rosas *et al.*, 2014).

Very painful visceral disease (such as pancreatitis) can also create myofascial pain in epaxial and abdominal muscles supplied by the same spinal nerves as the affected viscera. These trigger points will contribute to the pain of the acute disease and also maintain pain and signs in between acute episodes of disease.

Treat segmentally into the paraspinal (multifidus) muscles in the appropriate segments. For stomach, pancreatic and kidney disease, needle the caudal thoracic and cranial lumbar segments; for small intestinal disease use the cranial lumbar segments; for large intestinal, uterine and bladder disease, use the caudal lumbar and sacral segments. Abdominal points such as abdominal CV points in linea alba or, for safety and probably better efficacy, the ST points in rectus abdominus in the pain referral zones (cranial for stomach and pancreas; middle for small intestine; caudal for large intestine, uterus and bladder) can also be used if safely accessible. Add ST36 and PC6, if accessible, for antiemesis, gastric acid reduction and dopamine release (Figure 6.21).

Acute bladder pain

Acupuncture can be used adjunctively for the management of pain associated with acute cystitis and to reduce straining around the time of treatment of urethral obstruction. Needle paraspinally L1–L4 in the dog and L2–L5 in the cat, with needles down to the sacrum at S1–S3 for both species for any painful or functional condition of the bladder (Figure 6.22). If accessible and tolerated, use electroacupuncture for acute presentations, particularly obstructions (as well as rectal prolapse). For speed, needle S1–S3

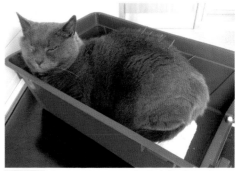

6.22 Acupuncture paraspinally in L2–L5 and over the sacrum for pain and functional bladder problems in the cat.

over the sacrum only (bilaterally two to four needles, through the multifidus muscle and down to the level of the sacrum to be sure of reaching the correct segments).

Acute ocular and aural pain

Acupuncture may be a helpful adjunct for the treatment of pain associated with acute otitis externa, conjunctivitis, glaucoma, and corneal ulceration. Needles should be placed as close as possible to the eye and ear. This is often tolerated remarkably well: Yintang and Taiyang are obvious choices, with the temporal muscles generally being easy to access close to the eye and around the base of the ear (Figure 6.23). For recurrent conditions look also at the dorsal neck muscles, masseter and sternomastoid/cleidomastoid muscles for trigger points that may be contributing to the pain.

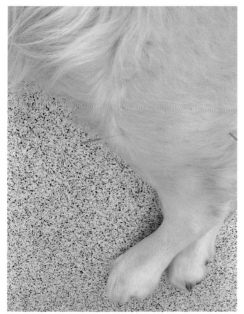

6.21 ST36 is a point in the cranial tibial muscle just lateral to the tibial crest.

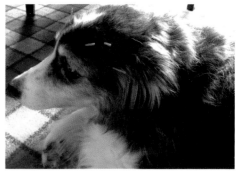

6.23 Acupuncture in the temporal muscles around the eye is often well tolerated.

Chronic pain

Acupuncture, physiotherapy and hydrotherapy are more usually thought of as treatments for chronic, rather than acute, pain. This is because such conditions traditionally cause owners to seek out non-pharmacological interventions. The evidence for acupuncture in veterinary clinical conditions is sparse (note: not negative, just very underpowered, poor quality studies with many confounding factors). Funding for large-scale research into human clinical conditions has provided evidence to the level of systematic review to show that acupuncture works (beyond sham) for chronic lower back pain, allergic rhinitis, migraine and tension headache and osteoarthritis in the knee, as well as postoperative and post-chemotherapeutic nausea and vomiting.

For the conditions discussed below the reader can assume that formal physiotherapy and hydrotherapy are preferred where available, affordable and tolerated by the patient.

Physiotherapy

For any neurological or orthopaedic condition where there is obvious muscle wastage and weakness the simple physical approaches are:

- Hindlimbs:
  - Sit to stand: from a 'square' sitting position, encourage the dog to stand with a word, hand gesture or treat. Repeat three times, three times daily initially (Figure 6.24). This will work the thigh muscles, but only if the dog starts from a proper sitting position. Most dogs will sit 'squarely' if there is a suggestion of a reward ('muscle memory' from puppy training, even if they do not sit properly of their own accord). If they cannot sit squarely because one leg is abducted, start with them sitting against a wall
- All limbs:
  - Steps: using two or three shallow steps, put the dog on the lead and slowly walk them up and down the steps, such that they use each leg individually. If they are allowed to go at their own pace they will likely hop up the steps and avoid using the affected limb. Going down slowly is as important as going up. Repeat three times, twice daily
  - Slopes: use a gentle slope initially and walk the dog up and down it slowly on a lead so that it uses each leg separately. Repeat twice, once or twice a day. Increase frequency after 1 month if there is no worsening of pain.

Stretching

Stretches can help to reduce pain and stiffness in the muscles and help mobilize joints.

- Hindlimbs:
  - When the animal is lying on its side or back at rest, stroke the flank or belly so that the dog voluntarily extends the hindlimb or limbs. When this happens, apply gentle pressure against the cranial thigh muscles to maintain that stretch for 3 seconds, then release gently and repeat. Do the set three times, three times daily for each limb (Figure 6.25).

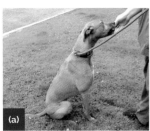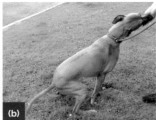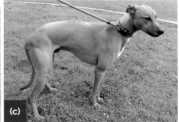

6.24 (a–c) Sit to stand exercises use and strengthen the hindlimb muscles.

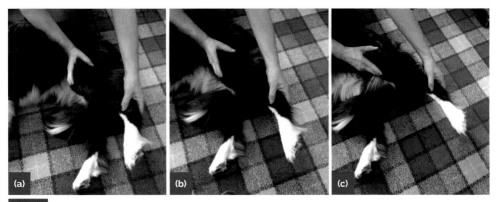

6.25 **(a–c)** Sequential steps for stretching the hindlimbs.

■ Forelimbs:
  • Some dogs can be taught to do a play bow and hold it (Figure 6.26), and this will stretch the triceps and infraspinatus muscles (common sources of pain in forelimb dysfunction and disease).
  • With a hand under the carpus for support, push gently on the point of the elbow so that elbow and forelimb extend. Hold for 3 seconds, release and repeat. Do the set three times, three times daily for each limb (Figure 6.27). If the dog resists and jerks the limb do not persist.

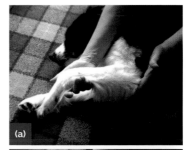

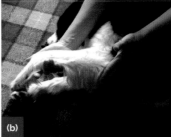

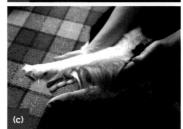

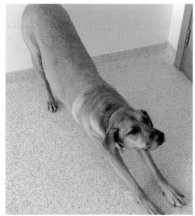

6.26 Some dogs can be taught to perform a 'play bow' or stretch and hold the position to stretch the front legs.

6.27 **(a–c)** Sequential steps for stretching the forelimbs.

- Spine:
  - Use weaving poles to encourage lateral movement of the spine and spinal muscles. Start with poles a body-width apart (Figure 6.28).

For balance and to encourage the limbs to be lifted and joints to be flexed use Cavaletti poles (Figure 6.29) a body-width apart, starting with them on the ground and progressively raising them as the dog gets used to stepping over them.

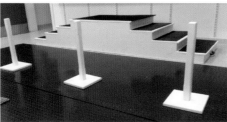

| 6.28 | Weaving poles to encourage lateral spine flexibility. |

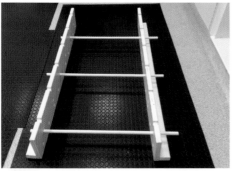

| 6.29 | Cavaletti poles to encourage lifting the legs, balance and proprioception. |

Chronic neurological pain

The expected effects of acupuncture are pain relief with consequent improvement in mobility, and return to function. Physiotherapy and hydrotherapy will be used for pain relief, to improve or maintain muscle strength and mass, and to improve proprioception.

> **WARNING**
>
> Care should be taken with any physical therapy when there is evidence of central sensitization. If light touch or gentle pressure is interpreted by the patient as pain, the therapy will be unpleasant and, almost certainly, less effective or detrimental

Physical therapies will not directly have therapeutic effects on neuropathic conditions, for example for compression of, and direct impingement on, nervous tissue. However, for some so-called 'dynamic' lesions, where the posture of the animal determines how much compression or impingement occurs, the physical therapies appear to have a part to play.

- IVDD: apply acupuncture as for the acute presentation, but also examine and treat secondary muscular pain in the epaxial and limb muscles.
- Foraminal stenosis: treat the secondary muscle pain found on examination to try to prevent the cycle of physical hunching and further nerve impingement. Treatment will inevitably have to be frequent and long-term.

> **WARNING**
>
> - Reduce the pain first with acupuncture and other analgesia before starting these exercises.
> - More is NOT better, so start slowly and infrequently.
> - Check that the exercises are not making the pain worse.
> - If the pain is worse, check what the owner is doing.
> - Avoid swimming especially where there are cervical lesions but also in any condition where lordosis of the spine is obviously associated with a worsening of signs.
> - Care with underwater treadmills when the animal's stride is lengthened to the point where hip extension also causes pelvic tilting when lordosis exacerbates pain.

- Spondylosis/spondylitis: acupuncture can be used for the secondary muscular pain in the epaxial muscles, but also in the sublumbar muscles, pectoral muscles and limbs if affected.
- Chiari malformation/syringomyelia: acupuncture may improve the secondary muscle pain around the neck and should be added to the treatment regime where there is: a) palpable muscle pain; and b) signs of discomfort and suffering in between attacks of yelping/screaming and phantom scratching. It will not usually reduce the screaming and scratching, nor would it be expected to, given the cause of these signs.

Chronic orthopaedic pain – arthritis

Sources of arthritic pain include: joint inflammation; bone on bone impingement; fragments or fissures within the joint; ligament and tendon pain; secondary muscle pain; and potential central sensitization. Acupuncture may reduce the nociceptive input from the joint, reduce secondary muscle and soft tissue pain, and reduce central sensitization. Treat as close to the joint as possible without entering the joint–joint margins can be needled if safely identified; trigger the points in the adjacent muscles and those affected by postural shift, especially the epaxials. If the affected joint is too painful to needle, target areas above and below the joint and 'mirror points' on the contralateral limb. Treatments can often be limited to monthly or 6-weekly once the pain is controlled. Electroacupuncture should be used as the animal gets older and the treatment appears less effective (because there is more input with which to compete).

Chronic dermatological pain – self-trauma and wound healing

There is good evidence for the use of acupuncture in wound healing (Jansen *et al.*, 1989). Place needles as close as possible to the edge of the wound in healthy skin to the depth of the tissue damage and 2.5 cm apart (Figure 6.30). Acupuncture appears to be helpful for acral lick dermatitis: treat as for open wounds, but also add ST36, LI11 and GV14 and GV3.

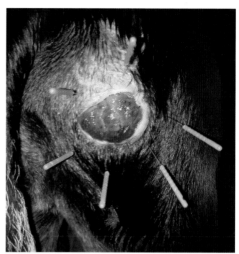

6.30 Wound healing is promoted by acupuncture.
(Courtesy of Vicky Emmott)

Chronic gastrointestinal pain

Acupuncture can modify function and reduce pain in the viscera. A secondary consideration is the potential for 'viscerosomatic' pain, where painful visceral stimuli cause trigger points in the body wall (Figure 6.31). These trigger points may then maintain or exacerbate the signs of

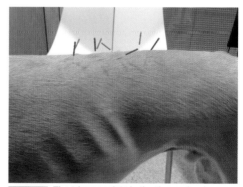

6.31 The trigger points in the thoracolumbar epaxial muscles of this lurcher appeared to maintain daily 'classical' signs of pancreatitis (lip licking, 'praying', excessive yawning, 'swan' posture) in the absence of a positive canine pancreatic lipase immunoreactivity (cPLI) test. Treatment of these points appeared to resolve the signs completely.

the original disease. Treat segmentally as for acute pain. Examine the epaxial muscles, abdominal oblique muscles and rectus abdominus muscles in the segmental referral zone for trigger points and treat. Add ST36 (and PC6 if accessible) for effects on appetite, gastric acid secretion and nausea.

Chronic bladder pain

Treat chronic bladder pain as for acute pain, but also look for segmentally relevant trigger points in the caudal rectus abdominus muscle and lumbar epaxial muscles.

Chronic otitis externa

There is some evidence that acupuncture may reduce the severity and frequency of chronic otitis externa (Sanchez-Araujo and Puchi, 2011). Treat at the time of presentation and/or weekly/ biweekly around the base of the ear and dorsal neck muscles, checking the sternomastoid and cranial trapezius muscles for trigger points.

Ocular pain (dry eye)

For palliation and optimization of remaining tear production, place needles around the eye (see 'Acute ocular and aural pain', above).

Oral pain

For dental pain, stomatitis and facial pain, needle along the muzzle, in masseter, Yintang, and the temporal muscles. It should be noted that for some of these conditions, the appearance of the disease may not alter, but the owner may report improved mood, appetite

and attitude. Where conventional treatment has failed and palliation of chronic suffering is required, the outcome measure of the animal's suffering should be included.

References and further reading

Filshie J, White A and Cummings M (2016) *Medical Acupuncture: A Western Scientific Approach 2nd edn*. Elsevier, London

Hui KKS, Liu J, Makris N *et al.* (2000) Acupuncture modulates the limbic system and subcortical gray structures of the human brain: Evidence from fMRI studies in normal studies. *Human Brain Mapping* **9**, 13–25

Jansen G, Lundeberg T, Kjartsson J *et al.* (1989) Acupuncture and sensory neuropeptides increase cutaneous blood flow in rats. *Neuroscience Letters* **97**, 305–309

Joaquim JGF, Luna SPL, Brondani JT *et al.* (2010) Comparison of decompressive surgery, electroacupuncture, and decompressive surgery followed by electroacupuncture for the treatment of dogs with intervertebral disk disease with long-standing severe neurologic deficits. *Journal of the American Veterinary Medical Association* **236**, 1225–1229

Lindley S and Watson P (2010) *BSAVA Manual of Canine and Feline Rehabilitation, Palliative and Supportive Care*. BSAVA Publications, Gloucester

Odendaal J (2002) *Pets and Our Mental Health: the Why, the What and the How*. Vantage Press, New York

Sanchez-Araujo M and Puchi A (2011) Acupuncture prevents relapses of recurrent otitis in dogs: a 1 year follow up of a randomized controlled trial. *Acupuncture in Medicine* **29**, 21–26

Sato A, Sato Y, Suzuki A *et al.* (1993) Neural mechanisms of the reflex inhibition and excitation of gastric motility elicited by acupuncture-like stimulation in anaesthetized rats. *Neuroscience Research* **18**, 53–62

Torres-Rosas R, Yehia G and Pena G (2014) Dopamine mediates vagal modulation of the immune system by electroacupuncture. *Nature Medicine* **20**, 291–295

Uvnas-Moberg K, Bruzelius G, Alister P *et al.* (1993) The antinociceptive effect on non-noxious sensory stimulation is mediated partly through oxytocinergic mechanisms. *Acta Physiologica Scandinavia* **149**, 199–204

Chapter 7a

Trauma and emergency pain

Dominic Barfield

In emergency situations there are many factors that the veterinary team need to consider and manage. It should be paramount to alleviate pain by the most reliable and safe method. Physical examination parameters and pain scores are often unreliable in the acute setting to evaluate pain in our patients; therefore, analgesia should always be given if in any doubt. A fast-acting, potent, titratable drug would be ideal, making full mu agonist opioids the preferred choice. As with the administration of any drug, the five rights (patient, drug, dose, route, time) apply and in addition, veterinary surgeons (veterinarians) might be limited by the availability of specific drugs and vascular access in the patient. For reliable delivery, the intravenous route is preferable, and intraosseous is better than intramuscular. Fentanyl has a faster onset of action and is more potent (50 times) than morphine or methadone. Although pethidine has a fast onset of action it should only be administered intramuscularly.

The benefit of opioids being titratable cannot be overlooked. That being said, it is important to start at the lower end of the dose range (*starting dose*), **do not** be tempted to give more as the patient looks worse, and always wait for the peak time of effect to be reached; if the animal is still in pain give half of the starting dose again. If using fentanyl, make the bolus equal the background (e.g. if 1 µg/kg is given as a bolus, then start 1 µg/kg/hr continuous rate infusion (CRI). Increase the bolus and background by 30–50% after the peak time of effect if the patient is still in pain.

It is important to remember that mu opioids can be antagonized by naloxone although other methods of providing analgesia must be considered if naloxone is used. The cardiorespiratory side effects of mu agonists are highly unlikely to be significant at clinical doses in veterinary species.

When do you start an additional analgesic?

This should be considered if the pain has not been adequately controlled after two rational increases in opioid dose. The next analgesic to add would be either ketamine or lidocaine (in dogs only). Ketamine is good for peritoneal pain and at low doses augments opioid analgesia as opioid sensitivity is mediated through *N*-methyl-D-aspartate (NMDA) receptors.

Ketamine should be given as a loading dose (bolus) of 250 µg/kg followed by a CRI of 2–10 µg/kg/min. Lidocaine requires a slow intravenous loading dose of 1 mg/kg, followed by a CRI of 20–60 µg/kg/min.

What drugs to avoid

Non-steroidal anti-inflammatory drugs (NSAIDs) should be avoided initially in every emergency patient due to their prostaglandin-mediated side effects (renal and gastric blood flow). NSAIDs can be added in later once blood pressure is stabilized and hydration and blood volume status addressed. Alpha-2 agonists, while having analgesic effects, have profound dose-dependent effects on cardiac output and should not be used. Butorphanol has a rapid onset of action but has only mild analgesic effects and should be avoided. Buprenorphine might have similar analgesic effects in cats to full mu opioids; however, it takes 40–50 minutes for full effect to be reached, which is not appropriate in an emergency.

References and further reading

Epstein ME, Rodan I, Griffenhagen G et al. (2015a) 2015 AAHA/AAFP pain management guidelines for dogs and cats. Journal of Feline Medicine and Surgery **17**, 251–272

Epstein ME, Rodan I, Griffenhagen G et al. (2015b) 2015 AAHA/AAFP pain management guidelines for dogs and cats. Journal of the American Animal Hospital Association **51**, 67–84

Robertson S (2016) Anaesthetic management for Caesarean sections in dogs and cats. In Practice **38**, 327–339

Case example 1: Gastric dilatation–volvulus

HISTORY AND PRESENTATION

Gastric dilatation–volvulus (GDV) mostly affects large- to giant-breed, deep-chested dogs. Patients present with acute signs, with some association with exercise and eating.

CLINICAL SIGNS

These vary from agitation to collapse, depending upon cardiovascular stability. There are often signs of hypovolaemic and obstructive shock, tachycardia and tachypnoea.

SIGNS OF PAIN

These originate from abdominal distention (stretch), which can cause considerable pain.

TREATMENT

A full mu opioid is ideal (morphine, methadone or fentanyl), administered intravenously. Due to a high proportion of dogs having postoperative arrhythmias, the use of lidocaine can also be considered. If an escalation of analgesia is required then lidocaine would be a good first choice.

Case example 2: Caesarean section

HISTORY AND PRESENTATION

There are many fetal and maternal causes leading to the requirement for a Caesarean section. Brachycephalic breeds are over-represented and these are often elective procedures. Number of fetuses should be known prior to surgery, which requires radiographs to be taken.

CLINICAL SIGNS

These include agitation; other signs can be related to hypocalcaemia and hypoglycaemia.

SIGNS OF PAIN

These can be related to contractions, abnormal fetal presentation in the birth canal, and fetopelvic disproportion. There might not be any obvious signs of pain with uterine inertia.

TREATMENT

Antiemetics are often given as patients are at risk of aspiration. Premedication should ideally include an opioid; methadone might be the most appropriate, buprenorphine can be used postoperatively. Although methadone can cause fetal bradycardia, it can be antagonized. If there is concern about narcotic effects on the neonates then opioids can be given to the bitch/queen after delivery and prior to recovery. A local anaesthetic line block can be considered and/or an epidural, depending on time and technical ability, and being cognisant of the side effects (hypotension intraoperatively, motor deficits postoperatively). The epidural dose can be reduced to one-third of that used in non-parturient patients (volumetric 1:1 lidocaine:bupivacaine has been suggested to extend the duration of analgesia; however, this is controversial and might lead to an unpredictable blockade). NSAIDs are likely to be beneficial without compromising the neonates, as only small levels reach the milk.

Case example 3: Septic abdomen

HISTORY AND PRESENTATION

In dogs this is often secondary to foreign body ingestion, or the use of NSAIDs. However, it can occur secondary to trauma, neoplasia and biliary tract leakage, amongst other causes. Patients present with variable signs depending on cause, from lethargy and inappetance to marked vomiting and collapse.

CLINICAL SIGNS

These are often related to cardiovascular compromise and reflect appropriate or excessive inflammatory response and sepsis. Patients are often neurologically obtunded, which could be related to the inflammation or metabolic effects of sepsis (e.g. hypoglycaemia).

SIGNS OF PAIN

These can vary from mild to marked abdominal pain from the peritonitis itself; there may be a tense or guarded abdomen on palpation with groaning. If the patient is neurologically impaired it would likely mask obvious signs of pain and discomfort.

→ **CASE EXAMPLE 3 CONTINUED**

TREATMENT

Initial analgesia with mu agonist opioids would be ideal, though cautious use is required if the patient requires vasopressors to maintain adequate mean arterial blood pressure (≥65 mmHg). Patients often require multimodal analgesia including ketamine and lidocaine both as CRIs. These can be given as separate infusions or mixed together in the same bag, which is more convenient though has much less flexibility to titrate the right dose of the analgesics to the patient.

If concerned about the cardiovascular stability of the patient (e.g. sepsis), then start at the lower end of the dose.

Case example 4: Road traffic accident

PRESENTATION AND HISTORY

Both dogs and cats, usually young, can be victims of a road traffic accident. Dogs are often witnessed to have been hit by a car; with cats it is usually presumed when they return home.

CLINICAL SIGNS

Respiratory signs are common secondary to pulmonary contusions. Orthopaedic and soft tissue injuries can be significant.

SIGNS OF PAIN

Signs of pain are often focal and relate to the main site of injury. The main focus is on the obvious musculoskeletal injuries, though head injuries, for example, can include ocular, dental, neurological and dermatological (burns) pain. If the patient has nerve damage, this can be misleading in their pain assessment. Signs attributable to an acute abdomen can be seen with traumatic injuries to the abdomen, from injury to the gastrointestinal tract, urogenital system, or abdominal musculature (abdominal wall rupture).

TREATMENT

Mu agonist opioids would be the first line of treatment; the intramuscular route could be considered if there is any difficulty in obtaining intravenous access. Additional pain medications, such as NSAIDs, can be considered once the patient is deemed cardiovascularly stable, with adequate sustained blood pressure. The variation in analgesia provided is likely to reflect the individual patient's response, the severity of their injuries and pre-emptive analgesia, for example, for fracture stabilization. It is always better to start with a drug that can be titrated to effect than to start with drug that cannot be escalated. It is not uncommon for these patients, depending on the time of their injury relative to presentation, to become more painful after initial assessment as their endogenous endorphins wear off.

Chapter 7b

Thoracic pain

Ana Marques

Thoracotomy is associated with severe acute postoperative pain. It can adversely affect coughing and deep breathing, resulting in respiratory complications such as hypoxia, atelectasis, chest infection, and respiratory failure that may delay recovery or, if severe, be life-threatening (Kavanagh et al., 1994; Pavlidou et al., 2009).

Acute pain control is important to prevent splinting and stretching of the surgical incisions as a result of breathing, and to help provide effective pre-emptive analgesia. Pain is relayed via the intercostal and phrenic nerves and leads to an inflammatory cascade, which decreases the pain threshold and sensitizes the affected peripheral nerves. Continued stimulation can result in central sensitization and higher incidence of chronic pain (Sabanathan et al., 1993; Katz et al., 1996).

A multitude of strategies for pain control and the timing of analgesia administration have been widely discussed. Experimental and clinical studies have shown that neuronal afferent blockade applied before injury can reduce postoperative pain, providing a rationale for pre-emptive analgesia (Woolf and Chong, 1993).

Opioids are commonly used as a first line of analgesia and delivered as an intravenous bolus. In humans, opioids can cause central respiratory depression and contribute to postoperative hypoventilation. In animals, these side effects are rarely observed at clinical doses; however, monitoring is advisable. Intravenous constant rate infusions (CRI) can minimize dose-dependent adverse effects by avoiding peaks in serum concentrations. Changes in dosage are also easily accomplished and have a predictable onset when infusion pumps are used.

The use of regional analgesia can minimize the pain associated with rib spreading, which is considered one of the most important factors involved in post-thoracotomy pain (Fibla et al., 2009). It has the potential advantage of providing analgesia without central respiratory depression or sedation, allowing improved ventilation and easier evaluation (Pascoe and Dyson, 1993; Conzemius et al., 1994). Local anaesthetics, such as bupivacaine and lidocaine, can be delivered in the form of intercostal nerve blocks, as a single injection across a range of dermatomes or through placement of sterile catheters (paravertebral catheter, thoracostomy drain and wound soaker catheter) (Helms et al., 2011; Franci et al., 2012; Wildgaard et al., 2012). Thoracostomy drains allow delivery of local anaesthetics intrapleurally and can provide adequate regional analgesia. Wound soaker catheters are flexible indwelling catheters that are placed in the surgical site and can deliver boluses or a continuous infusion of local anaesthetics. They provide local pain relief and can reduce systemic opioid administration in the postoperative period (Radlinsky *et al.*, 2005).

The use of lumbosacral epidural morphine provides analgesia for upper abdominal and thoracic procedures (Campoy, 2004; Freitas *et al.*, 2011) with localized and more intense effects when compared with systemic administration (Hansen, 2001). Administration near to the site of action also allows a reduction of the total dose and provides pain relief for about 24 hours in dogs following thoracotomy (Popilskis *et al.*, 1993; Carregaro *et al.*, 2014).

The use of non-opioid analgesics has been explored in an effort to enhance postoperative analgesia. Numerous classes of drugs including gabanoids, *N*-methyl-D-aspartate (NMDA)-receptor antagonists, and non-steroidal anti-inflammatory drugs (NSAIDs) have been used in the treatment of postoperative pain after thoracic surgery.

Video-assisted thoracoscopic surgery (VATS) has been developed to minimize surgical trauma and postoperative pain. In contrast to a standard thoracotomy, VATS causes less acute pain due to smaller incisions, less muscular trauma and avoidance of rib retraction or resection (Walsh *et al.*, 1999; Kaplowitz and Papadakos, 2102). The ideal anaesthetic regimen for VATS is currently unknown, but it likely involves the use of regional analgesia in conjunction with opioid and non-opioid analgesics (Wildgaard *et al.*, 2102; Komatsu *et al.*, 2014).

References and further reading

Abelson AL, McCobb EC, Shaw S *et al.* (2009) Use of wound soaker catheters for the administration of local anesthetic for post-operative analgesia: 56 cases. *Veterinary Anaesthesia and Analgesia* **36**, 597–602

Bernard F, Kudnig ST and Monnet E (2006) Hemodynamic effects of interpleural lidocaine and bupivacaine combination in anesthetized dogs with and without an open pericardium. *Veterinary Surgery* **35**, 252–258

Campoy L (2004) Epidural and spinal anaesthesia in the dog. *In Practice* **26**, 262–269

Carregaro AB, Freitas GC, Lopes C *et al.* (2014) Evaluation of analgesic and physiologic effects of epidural morphine administered at a thoracic or lumbar level in dogs undergoing thoracotomy. *Veterinary Anaesthesia and Analgesia* **41**, 205–211

Conzemius MG, Brockman DJ, King LG *et al.* (1994) Analgesia in dogs after intercostal thoracotomy: a clinical trial comparing intravenous buprenorphine and interpleural bupivacaine. *Veterinary Surgery* **23**, 291–298

DeRossi R, Frazilio FO, Jardim PH *et al.* (2011) Evaluation of thoracic epidural analgesia induced by lidocaine, ketamine, or both administered via a lumbosacral approach in dogs. *American Journal of Veterinary Research* **72**, 1580–1585

Fibla JJ, Molins L, Mier JM *et al.* (2009) A prospective study of analgesic quality after a thoracotomy: paravertebral block with ropivacaine before and after rib spreading. *European Journal of Cardio-Thoracic Surgery* **36**, 901–905

Franci P, Leece EA and Corletto F (2012) Thoracic epidural catheter placement using a paramedian approach with cephalad angulation in three dogs. *Veterinary Surgery* **41**, 884–889

Freitas GC, Carregaro AB, Gehrcke MI *et al.* (2011) Epidural analgesia with morphine or buprenorphine in ponies with lipopolysaccharide (LPS)-induced carpal synovitis. *Canadian Journal of Veterinary Research* **75**, 141–146

Hansen B (2001) Epidural catheter analgesia in dogs and cats: technique and review of 182 cases (1991–1999). *Journal of Veterinary Emergency and Critical Care* **11**, 95–103

Hansen B, Lascelles BD, Thomson A *et al.* (2013) Variability of performance of wound infusion catheters. *Veterinary Anaesthesia and Analgesia* **40**, 308–315

Helms O, Mariano J, Hentz JG *et al.* (2011) Intra-operative paravertebral block for postoperative analgesia in thoracotomy patients: A randomized, double-blind, placebo-controlled study. *European Journal of Cardio-Thoracic Surgery* **40**, 902–906

Kaplowitz J and Papadakos PJ (2012) Acute pain management for video-assisted thoracoscopic surgery: an update. *Journal of Cardiothoracic and Vascular Anesthesia* **26**, 312–321

Katz J, Jackson M, Kavanagh BP *et al.* (1996) Acute pain after thoracic surgery predicts long-term post-thoracotomy pain. *The Clinical Journal of Pain* **12**, 50–55

Kavanagh BP, Katz J and Sandler AN (1994) Pain control after thoracic surgery. *Anesthesiology* **81**, 737–759

Komatsu T, Kino A, Inoue M *et al.* (2014) Paravertebral block for video-assisted thoracoscopic surgery: analgesic effectiveness and role in fast-track surgery. *International Journal of Surgery* **12**, 936–939

Pascoe PJ and Dyson DH (1993) Analgesia after lateral thoracotomy in dogs. Epidural morphine *versus* intercostal bupivacaine. *Veterinary Surgery* **22**, 141–147

Pavlidou K, Papazoglou L, Savvas I *et al.* (2009) Analgesia for small animal thoracic surgery. *Compendium of Continuing Education for the Practicing Veterinarian* **31**, 432–436

Popilskis S, Kohn DF, Laurent L *et al.* (1993) Efficacy of epidural morphine *versus* intravenous morphine for post-thoracotomy pain in dogs. *Veterinary Anaesthesia and Analgesia* **20**, 21–25

Radlinsky MG, Mason DE, Roush JK *et al.* (2005) Use of a continuous, local infusion of bupivacaine for postoperative analgesia in dogs undergoing total ear canal ablation. *Journal of the American Veterinary Medical Association* **227**, 414–419

Robinson R, Chang YM, Seymour CJ *et al.* (2014) Predictors of outcome in dogs undergoing thoracic surgery (2002–2011). *Veterinary Anaesthesia and Analgesia* **41**, 259–268

Sabanathan S, Richardson J and Mearns A (1993) Management of pain in thoracic surgery. *British Journal of Hospital Medicine* **50**, 114–120

Tillson DM (2015) Thoracic surgery; important considerations and practical steps. *Veterinary Clinics of North America: Small Animal Practice* **45**, 489–506

Walsh PJ, Remedios AM, Ferguson JF *et al.* (1999) Thoracoscopic *versus* open partial pericardectomy in dogs: comparison of postoperative pain and morbidity. *Veterinary Surgery* **28**, 472–479

Wildgaard K, Petersen RH, Hansen HJ *et al.* (2012) Multimodal analgesic treatment in video-assisted thoracic surgery lobectomy using an intraoperative intercostal catheter. *European Journal of Cardio-Thoracic Surgery* **41**, 1072–1077

Woolf CJ and Chong MS (1993) Preemptive analgesia-treating postoperative pain by preventing the establishment of central sensitization. *Anesthesia and Analgesia* **77**, 362–379

Case example 1: Pneumothorax

HISTORY AND PRESENTATION

An 8-year-old male neutered Labrador Retriever presented with a 9-day history of increased respiratory effort, tachypnoea and lethargy. The owner reported no history of trauma and that the dog had been quieter than normal for the last couple of months.

CLINICAL SIGNS

Clinical signs included pink and moist mucous membranes, a capillary refill time of less than 2 seconds, a heart rate of 92 bpm, palpable and synchronous femoral pulses, panting, increased expiratory effort, and a temperature of 37°C. Thoracic auscultation showed loud inspiratory and expiratory noises but no crackles or wheezes. Peripheral lymph nodes and abdominal palpation were unremarkable. No signs of pain were present.

INVESTIGATIONS AND TREATMENT

Thoracic radiographs revealed a pneumothorax. Thoracentesis retrieved 500 ml of air. Routine haematology and biochemistry were unremarkable. Computed tomography (CT) showed a bilateral pneumothorax and pneumomediastinum. At the periphery of the mid ventral portions of the right middle and right cranial lung lobes there were multiple thin-walled, gas-filled structures, the largest of which was at least 5.6 cm long, which also contained a fine network of thin soft tissue dense stranding. The CT findings were consistent with a pneumothorax and pneumomediastinum secondary to rupture of pulmonary bullae. The animal was anaesthetized and prepared for surgery.

Case 1 anaesthesia protocol

- **Premedication:** acepromazine 0.01 mg/kg i.v. + methadone 0.2 mg/kg i.v.
- **Induction:** propofol 12 ml i.v.
- **Endotracheal tube size:** 9.5 mm
- **Breathing system:** circle ventilator
- **Fluid therapy:** 2–5 ml/kg/h

A median sternotomy was performed. Bullae were identified on the right middle, right cranial and left caudal lung lobes. No obvious leaks were identified at surgery but two of the bullae (right middle and left caudal) appeared to have healing scars in their central portions. Stapled partial lobectomy of the left caudal lung lobe and hilar lobectomy of the right middle lung lobe were performed and a thoracic drain placed. The thoracic cavity was flooded and no further leaks were identified. Routine closure and placement of a wound soaker catheter was achieved with appropriate intra-thoracic pressure being reached.

PERIOPERATIVE MANAGEMENT

A bolus of fentanyl (1 μg/kg i.v.) was given at the beginning of surgery followed by a continuous rate infusion (CRI) of fentanyl (2.5–5 μg/kg/h) throughout the procedure. The fentanyl CRI was stopped at end of the procedure and a bolus of morphine ➜

→ CASE EXAMPLE 1 CONTINUED

(0.25 mg/kg i.v.) was administered 4.5 hours after premedication. A splash block on the sternotomy wound was performed via the wound soaker catheter with bupivacaine 0.25% (1 mg/kg).

POSTOPERATIVE MANAGEMENT

Pain assessment was regularly performed and guided by the use of the Glasgow Composite Measure Short Form Pain Scale. Intravenous boluses of morphine (0.2 mg/kg) were continued every 4 hours for the first 48 hours followed by buprenorphine (20 μg/kg) every 8 hours, for 3 days. Splash blocks, via the wound soaker catheter, with bupivacaine 0.25% (1 mg/kg) were performed every 6 hours for 48 hours. At this stage the catheter was removed. The dog was discharged 5 days postoperatively on a course of meloxicam (0.1 mg/kg orally once daily) and 400 mg paracetamol/9 mg codeine phosphate (half tablet, twice daily).

TIPS FROM THE AUTHOR – PLACEMENT OF A WOUND SOAKER CATHETER

Wound soaker catheters are also known as diffusion catheters and are available in several lengths.

- Choose a length of catheter that encompasses the length of the wound.
- The catheter should be buried in the deepest layer of the closure, just ventral to the sternum (on top of) in a median sternotomy and medial to the latissimus dorsi muscle in an intercostal thoracotomy (Figure 7.1ab).
- The catheter should exit the wound dorsally and all micropores must be situated under the skin.
- An in-line bacterial filter (arrow towards the wound) should be attached to the open end of the catheter followed by a needle-free valve to prevent contamination (Figure 7.1c).

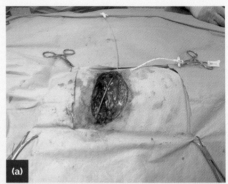

(a)

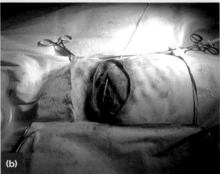

(b)

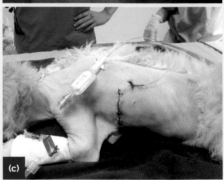

(c)

7.1 Intercostal thoracotomy wound. **(a)** The wound soaker catheter has been placed along the length of the wound, just dorsal to the circumcostal sutures. A minimal profile thoracostomy drain (white) has also been placed. **(b)** The latissimus dorsi muscle is apposed laterally to the wound soaker catheter. **(c)** The wound has been completely closed. Note the in-line bacterial filter attached to the open end of the catheter → followed by a needle-free valve.

→ **CASE EXAMPLE 1 CONTINUED**

- Postoperatively, bupivacaine may be given as an intermittent bolus every 6 hours at a dose of 0.5–2 mg/kg in dogs (Hansen *et al.*, 2013).

- The maximum recommended time that a catheter should be left in place is 3 days (McCobb, protocol written for Mila International).

Case example 2: Pleural effusion

HISTORY AND PRESENTATION

A 3-year-old female entire Whippet, presented with a 4-month history of episodes of tachypnoea and laboured breathing at rest.

CLINICAL SIGNS

Clinical signs included pink and moist mucous membranes, a capillary refill time of less than 2 seconds, a heart rate of 170 bpm, palpable and synchronous femoral pulses, a respiratory rate of 50 breaths per minute, increased expiratory effort and a temperature of 38.6°C. Thoracic auscultation showed muffled lung sounds. Peripheral lymph nodes and abdominal palpation were unremarkable. No signs of pain were present.

INVESTIGATIONS AND TREATMENT

A conscious lateral thoracic radiograph revealed marked pleural effusion. Thoracic ultrasonography confirmed marked bilateral pleural effusion. Thoracic drainage retrieved 600 ml of a lightly red, turbid fluid. Cytological and biochemical evaluation of the fluid were consistent with a chylous effusion. Bacteriological analysis yielded no growth. Echocardiography and computed tomographic imaging showed no cause for the effusion and were consistent with a presumptive diagnosis of idiopathic chylothorax. Medical management was initiated. No improvement was observed in the following weeks and surgical intervention was elected. The animal was anaesthetized and prepared for surgery.

Case 2 anaesthesia protocol

Premedication: fentanyl 5 μg/kg i.v. + midazolam 0.15 mg/kg i.v.
Induction: alfaxalone 1 ml i.v.
Endotracheal tube size: 7.5 mm
Breathing system: circle ventilator
Fluid therapy: 5–10 ml/kg/h

Surgical management comprised thoracic duct ligation and subtotal pericardiectomy via a thoracoscopic approach and cisterna chyli ablation via a right paracostal approach. Bilateral pleural ports were also placed.

PERIOPERATIVE MANAGEMENT

A bolus of methadone (0.2 mg/kg i.v.) was given and a fentanyl continuous rate infusion (CRI) (3 μg/kg/h) started before the beginning of surgery. An intercostal nerve block was performed before port placement with bupivacaine 0.25% (2 mg/kg). A lumbosacral epidural block with morphine (0.15 mg/kg) was performed before recovery and a bolus of methadone (0.3 mg/kg) was repeated 4 hours after the first dose. Meloxicam (0.2 mg/kg i.v.) was given at recovery.

POSTOPERATIVE MANAGEMENT

Pain assessment was regularly performed and guided by the use of the Glasgow Composite Measure Short Form Pain Scale. The fentanyl CRI (4 μg/kg/h) was continued for 6 hours and methadone

→ CASE EXAMPLE 2 CONTINUED

boluses were administered every 4 hours (0.2 mg/kg i.v.) for 48 hours followed by buprenorphine (20 µg/kg i.v.) every 8 hours for 72 hours. Meloxicam (0.1 mg/kg orally) was continued every 24 hours and the animal was discharged on this medication.

TIPS FROM THE AUTHOR

When performing intercostal nerve blocks make sure to block three consecutive intercostal nerves cranial and caudal to the incision. For this purpose, inject bupivacaine caudal to each rib and near the intervertebral foramen (Figure 7.2). Before injecting, aspirate to make sure you are not in a vessel. The author prefers to apply intercostal nerve blocks before the incision is made rather then prior to closure of the thoracotomy wound.

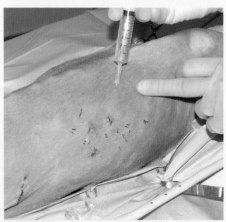

7.2 Intercostal nerve blocks performed prior to port placement in a dog with recurrent chylothorax. Note the needle caudal to the rib and in a dorsal location. Pen-marked numbers indicate respective ribs.

Case example 3: Thoracic trauma

HISTORY AND PRESENTATION

A 1-year-old male neutered Cavapoo presented with severe thoracic wounds after being bitten by a Bullmastiff.

CLINICAL SIGNS

On clinical examination the dog was in lateral recumbency but alert and responsive. Clinical signs included pink and moist mucous membranes, a capillary refill time of less than 2 seconds, a heart rate of 128 bpm, palpable and synchronous femoral pulses, a respiratory rate of 40 breaths per minute, with mildly increased effort but no paradoxical movement. Subcutaneous emphysema was present over the thoracic region bilaterally. Rectal temperature was 38.1°C.

SIGNS OF PAIN

The dog cried when touched on the torso and was reluctant to stand.

INVESTIGATIONS AND INITIAL MANAGEMENT

A bolus of methadone was given (0.3 mg/kg i.v.). The affected areas were clipped and the wounds cleaned and covered. Thoracic radiographs showed a moderate pneumothorax in the right hemithorax, a possible intercostal tear at the left seventh intercostal space, collapse of the right lung lobes and fracture of the fourth rib at the level of the costochondral junction on the right. A morphine (0.1 mg/kg/h) continuous rate infusion (CRI) and lidocaine CRI (40 µg/kg/min) were initiated and the animal was stabilized overnight. →

→ CASE EXAMPLE 3 CONTINUED

PERIOPERATIVE MANAGEMENT

Following overnight stabilization, the animal was anaesthetized. A fentanyl CRI (3 µg/kg/h) and ketamine CRI (2 µg/kg/min) were started before surgery. Bupivacaine 0.25% (2 mg/kg) intercostal nerve blocks were performed. Exploration and resection of the affected areas over both hemithoraces was performed. The thoracic cavity was lavaged and all wounds apposed. A minimal profile thoracostomy drain was placed in the right hemithorax and an oesophagostomy tube was left in place.

Case 3 anaesthesia protocol

Premedication: methadone 0.1 mg/kg i.v.
Induction: propofol 2.2 ml i.v.
Endotracheal tube size: 6.5 mm
Breathing system: circle ventilator
Fluid therapy: 5–10 ml/kg/h

POSTOPERATIVE MANAGEMENT

Pain assessment was regularly performed and guided by the use of the Glasgow Composite Measure Short Form Pain Scale. A morphine CRI (0.1 mg/kg/h) and ketamine CRI (2 µg/kg/min) were administered for the first 24 hours and bupivacaine 0.25% (1 mg/kg q6h) was instilled through the thoracostomy tube. After this period, feeding via the oesophagostomy tube was initiated and the ketamine CRI stopped. The morphine CRI was continued for another 48 hours followed by buprenorphine (20 µg/kg) for another 72 hours. The dog was sent home on meloxicam (0.1 mg/kg orally once daily) and 400 mg paracetamol/9 mg codeine phosphate (half tablet, twice daily).

TIPS FROM THE AUTHOR

The author uses minimal profile thoracostomy drains from Mila International. The drains are placed using a modified Seldinger wire technique (Figure 7.3). The drains are ideally placed before closure of the thoracotomy wound so that correct placement can be confirmed by visual inspection. When placed in a closed chest, radiographic confirmation is necessary. When instilling bupivacaine via the thoracostomy tube, make sure the animal is positioned in lateral recumbency with the incision site down or in dorsal recumbency to allow the local anaesthetic to pool near the incision site and close to the intercostal nerves.

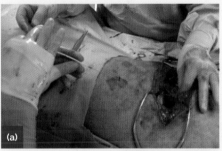

(a)

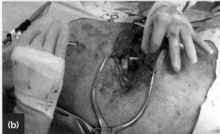

(b)

7.3 Placement of a minimal profile thoracostomy drain during an intercostal thoracotomy using a modified Seldinger wire technique. **(a)** The catheter is tunnelled subcutaneously and introduced into the thoracic cavity over a stylet, away from the surgical incision. The J-wire is threaded through the catheter and advanced cranioventrally. **(b)** The catheter is removed over the guide wire and the minimal profile drain advanced into the thoracic cavity over the guide wire. The guide wire is then removed and the thoracostomy tube is secured in place.

Chapter 7c

Abdominal pain

Caroline Kisielewicz

Pain of viscera in the abdominal or pelvic cavities results from the activation of nociceptors within the organs. Stimuli that can result in visceral pain include distension of hollow organs, traction on the mesentery, ischaemia and endogenous inflammatory mediators. As a result of the various stimuli that can be involved in inducing visceral pain, it is possible that this pain can occur without significant visceral injury or obvious pathology. There is also a poor correlation between the degree of visceral pathology and the intensity of pain in some cases; for example, intestinal ulceration or perforation can occur with minimal or no pain. Certain viscera, such as the liver and kidneys, appear relatively insensitive to stimulation; however, their capsules do have nociceptors that are sensitive to inflammatory mediators and distension.

Visceral pain is typically diffuse and poorly localized, partly due to sparse visceral afferent innervation relative to somatic innervation. Visceral pain can be referred and perceived in a somatic area. Clinically, abdominal pain can be confused with spinal or back pain and *vice versa*, likely as a result of referred pain. Referred pain occurs particularly when the process in the viscus inducing the pain is intense and long-lasting or recurs frequently.

Multiple physiological mechanisms are involved with the development of referred pain, which are beyond the scope of this chapter.

There are several abdominal conditions, such as pancreatitis and peritonitis, which cause abdominal pain in dogs and cats. This assessment is based on extrapolation from humans, where it is recognized that these conditions are painful, as well as clinical assessment of the affected animal. Abdominal pain is underdiagnosed in animals for a number of reasons including difficulties in communication with the patient, not recognizing clinical signs associated with pain, variation in individual tolerances to pain, and severity of the disease. Inadequate management of pain can have a major negative impact on the recovery of animals and their welfare. It is recognized in humans that abdominal pain can result from any of over 2500 conditions. Abdominal visceral pain can result from neoplastic infiltration, infection, inflammation, rupture or perforation, obstruction, torsion and ischaemia or infarction of any of the abdominal or pelvic organs as well as metabolic or endocrine disease.

Abdominal visceral pain is associated with strong emotional and autonomic responses and so can occur in conjunction with other clinical

BSAVA Guide to Pain Management in Small Animal Practice. Edited by Ian Self. ©BSAVA 2019

signs, depending on the underlying disease. Figure 7.4 depicts a list of clinical signs that can be associated with abdominal pain. The importance of nurses and technicians in assessing and monitoring pain behaviours in animals and their response to analgesia should not be underestimated. The author takes the view that each individual animal with abdominal disease might have pain, whether or not it can be fully appreciated, and subsequently provides analgesia in most cases. Figure 7.5 lists different treatment options available for abdominal pain.

Summary

There are many different causes of abdominal pain in dogs and cats. With any single condition, the intensity of pain can vary in individuals depending on many factors such as tolerance, concurrent conditions and medications. There are no set analgesia protocols available for specific abdominal conditions to manage pain due to these variations.

References and further reading

Catanzaro A, Di Salvo A, Steagall PV *et al.* (2016) Preliminary study on attitudes, opinions and knowledge of Italian veterinarians with regards to abdominal visceral pain in dogs. *Veterinary Anaesthesia and Analgesia* **43**, 361–370

Coleman DL and Slingsby LS (2007) Attitudes of veterinary nurses to the assessment of pain and the use of pain scales. *Veterinary Record* **160**, 541–544

Hunt JR, Knowles TG, Lascelles BD and Murrell JC (2015) Prescription of perioperative analgesics by UK small animal veterinary surgeons in 2013. *Veterinary Record* **176**, 493

Lamont LA (2008) Multimodal pain management in veterinary medicine: the physiologic basis of pharmacologic therapies. *Veterinary Clinics of North America: Small Animal Practice* **38**, 1173–1186

Mansfield C and Beths T (2015) Management of acute pancreatitis in dogs: a critical appraisal with focus on feeding and analgesia. *Journal of Small Animal Practice* **56**, 27–39

Shilo M and Pascoe PJ (2014) Anatomy, physiology, and pathophysiology of pain. In: *Pain Management in Veterinary Practice*, ed. CM Egger, L Love and T Doherty, pp. 9–28. Wiley Blackwell, West Sussex

Type of clinical signs	Specific examples
Changes in posture, gait or movement	Hunched, reluctant to move, prayer position/lordosis
Physiological changes	Pallor, tachypnoea, tachycardia, changes in blood pressure, increase in body temperature, sweating, trembling, nausea, vomiting, decrease in appetite, diarrhoea or constipation
Abdominal tenderness	Reaction to palpation of the abdomen
Changes in behaviour	Lethargy, restlessness, aggression, vocalization

7.4 Clinical signs that can manifest as a result of abdominal pain.

Analgesia

- Epidural catheter with local anaesthesia or opioid
- Coeliac plexus ganglion block
- Opioid (morphine, fentanyl) continuous rate infusion ± lidocaine (use cautiously in cats) ± ketamine
- Regular opioid injections (methadone, buprenorphine)
- Alpha-2 agonist continuous rate infusion
- Paracetamol (10 mg/kg) intravenous or oral (dogs only)
- Non-steroidal anti-inflammatory drugs (in appropriate situations only)
- Steroids (in appropriate situations only)

Additional treatment

- Identify and treat underlying disease
- Antiemetics
- Antacids, prokinetics, antispasmodics
- Nutrition
- Nursing care

7.5 List of options available for treating abdominal pain in dogs and cats.

Case example 1: Pancreatitis

Pancreatitis involves inflammatory cell infiltration of the exocrine pancreas but also includes necrotizing and chronic manifestations where inflammation is minimal. Pancreatitis is divided into acute and chronic forms based on the presence or absence of histopathological lesions such as fibrosis and/or atrophy.

HISTORY AND PRESENTATION

Although typically affecting middle-aged to older dogs and cats, animals of any age could be affected. Certain dog breeds, such as Miniature Schnauzers, terriers, Cocker Spaniels, Cavalier King Charles Spaniels, Border Collies and Boxers, are more commonly affected but there is no known breed predisposition in cats. Pancreatitis is commonly idiopathic although several potential risk factors have been identified in dogs, such as hypertriglyceridaemia, drug reactions, prior surgery, dietary factors, infections and endocrine disease.

CLINICAL SIGNS AND SIGNS OF PAIN

Clinical signs vary from mild non-specific signs such as anorexia and lethargy, with or without gastrointestinal signs, in chronic subclinical pancreatitis to cardiovascular shock, disseminated intravascular coagulation and death in severe acute pancreatitis. Clinical signs tend to be more subtle in cats, particularly those with chronic disease. Pain results from inflammation of the pancreas as well as the resulting local peritonitis. Pancreatitis manifests as cranial abdominal pain. The abdomen is typically tender on palpation and dogs may display the 'prayer position' (Figure 7.6).

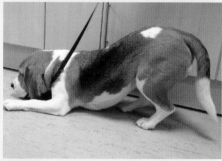

7.6 In between bouts of vomiting, this Beagle was repeatedly demonstrating the 'prayer position', which continued despite administration of intermittent doses of methadone.

TREATMENT

Medical management is supportive. The main focus should be analgesia; untreated pain delays recovery. Cats do not openly show signs of pain in most cases; however, it should not be concluded that they feel less pain than dogs or humans. Acute pancreatitis can be managed with continuous rate infusions of opioids, lidocaine (dogs only) and ketamine, epidural opioids or local anaesthetics, regular opioid injections and intravenous paracetamol (dogs only) (see Chapter 5). Chronic, subclinical cases can be managed with oral opioids, paracetamol and, possibly, non-steroidal anti-inflammatory drugs (NSAIDs). Fluid therapy is imperative in moderate to severe cases to correct hypovolaemia and dehydration as well as manage acid–base and electrolyte imbalances. Additional management includes providing nutrition, antiemetics, antacids and vitamin B12, etc.

Case example 2: Pyelonephritis

Pyelonephritis results from infection of the renal pelvis and can progress to acute kidney injury in both dogs and cats. It typically arises from ascending infection from the lower urinary tract; however, a haematogenous origin is possible. Bacterial endocarditis, discospondylitis and pyometra are recognized predisposing conditions for pyelonephritis. Pain can result from inflammation but also following stretching of the renal capsule when renomegaly develops (Figure 7.7).

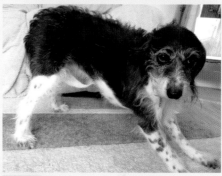

7.7 This female dog was repeatedly stretching while in the home environment prior to presentation, having shown increased drinking and urination in the previous days.

HISTORY AND PRESENTATION

Dogs and cats with systemically compromised immunity (hyper-adrenocorticism, diabetes mellitus), chronic kidney disease or vesico-ureteral reflux are more predisposed to developing pyelonephritis. In acute disease, animals present with severe systemic illness alongside uraemia and possibly sepsis, whereas chronic disease can be insidious with slowly progressive azotaemia and renal failure.

CLINICAL SIGNS AND SIGNS OF PAIN

Abdominal or renal pain, sometimes misinterpreted as back pain, is identified in acute cases. Dogs can occasionally demonstrate the 'prayer position' with renal pain. Palpation of the kidneys, particularly if enlarged, can elicit a pain response. Animals can present as cases of pyrexia of unknown origin. In chronic cases, the clinical signs can be subtle and non-specific.

TREATMENT

Once diagnosed, initial treatment with intravenous antibiotics and fluid therapy is imperative. Analgesia should be administered especially during the intensive management phase in acute presentations. Options could include opioids, lidocaine infusions and paracetamol intravenously. Some would avoid ketamine as this is 100% renally excreted. The use of non-steroidal anti inflammatory drugs is generally avoided because of the potential for worsening renal function. Opioids administered by the epidural route have generally not been used due to the risk of urine retention. However, recent studies have questioned the importance of this. Antibiotics should continue for at least 6–8 weeks with regular urine culture monitoring.

Case example 3: Oesophagitis

Gastrointestinal pain is often underestimated, particularly pain involving the oesophagus. Oesophagitis is under-recognized as there are no pathognomonic signs and diagnosis in the veterinary field requires endoscopic visualization of an erythematous, oedematous and ulcerated oesophageal mucosa.

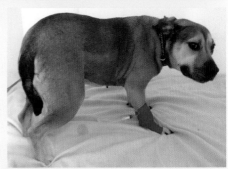

7.8 This dog shows a tucked-up tail, slight hunching of the back and appears unsettled and uncomfortable following abdominal surgery. The anorexia in this case could be due to abdominal pain; however, the dog had gastrointestinal reflux during anaesthesia prompting the concern for concurrent oesophagitis.

HISTORY AND PRESENTATION

It commonly results from gastro-oesophageal reflux but also from local damage of the oesophageal barrier when ingesting irritant materials and possibly from local neoplasia. Reflux can develop with prolonged fasting, intra-abdominal surgery, certain drugs, anatomical abnormalities including hiatal hernia, upper airway obstruction, disorders of gastric emptying and chronic vomiting.

CLINICAL SIGNS AND SIGNS OF PAIN

Clinical signs are often non-specific and influenced by underlying conditions. Signs that have been associated with oesophagitis include regurgitation, ptyalism, odynophagia, anorexia, extending head and neck with swallowing, repeated swallowing, retching, gagging, coughing and vocalizing after eating (especially cats). Affected animals can simply show signs of discomfort, restlessness and non-localizable pain (Figure 7.8).

TREATMENT

Oesophagitis is self-perpetuating; therefore, it is imperative to treat it aggressively. The pain resulting from oesophagitis is often underappreciated; analgesia should be considered a priority, particularly in severe cases. Analgesia could include opioids, lidocaine (dogs only), ketamine and paracetamol (dogs only). Supportive treatment includes the use of cytoprotective agents (sucralfate), antacids (omeprazole 1 mg/kg q12h) and prokinetics (metoclopramide and cisapride; these can increase lower oesophageal sphincter tone, increase gastric motility and possibly oesophageal motility in cats). Oral provision of food may need to be withheld temporarily in some cases with nutrition provided through other routes. Longer term, low-fat diets are recommended, and late night feeding should be avoided. Successful treatment requires identification and management of any underlying conditions where possible.

Chapter 7d

Neuropathic pain

Annette Wessmann

Neuropathic pain is defined as pain arising as a direct consequence of a lesion or disease affecting the somatosensory system and therefore occurs as a consequence of a true insult on the central or peripheral nervous system (Grubb, 2010). Pain of non-neural origin would not be termed neuropathic, even though the persistence of any pain can cause plasticity and changes in the nervous system (this would be termed neurogenic pain). The sensations caused by neuropathic pain may include spontaneous pain, paraesthesia (abnormal sensation that is not unpleasant such as tingling, prickling), dysaesthesia (unpleasant, usually burning sensation), allodynia (pain produced by a stimulus that is not usually painful such as light touch), or hyperalgesia or hyperpathia (exaggerated pain response produced by a normally painful stimulus).

Chronic neuropathic pain develops mostly due to an alteration of the sensory processing caused by an abnormal peripheral input and abnormal central processing. It can be challenging to diagnose and to treat, and it is thought to cause greater impairment of the patient's quality of life compared with other pain syndromes (Grubb, 2010). The history is particularly important, as the pain can be intermittent or not obvious such as in central pain (pain experienced in the area of the body subserved by the lesion originating from a primary lesion of the CNS). The affected animal may show obvious or subtle changes such as intermittent scratching or attacking an area of the body, frequent looking at the same area, hiding and reluctance to go for walks, yelping for no apparent reason, yelping when petted, or exaggerated response to stimuli that would normally cause only mild discomfort (Mathews, 2008).

Author's perspective

Assessment and treatment of neuropathic pain (adapted from O'Connor and Dworkin, 2009).

Step 1 – Assessment

1. Take a detailed history and clarify the signs of pain the patient is showing.
2. Assess pain on examination and establish a diagnosis of neuropathic pain.
3. If possible, identify the cause of the neuropathic pain.

▶

Author's perspective *continued*

4. Identify and treat relevant co-morbidities if indicated (e.g. renal, hepatic, cardiac or musculoskeletal disease). Treatment may need to be adjusted accordingly.
5. Discuss treatment plan and expectations with the client.

Step 2 – Treatment

Mild to moderate neuropathic pain may respond to non-steroidal anti-inflammatory drugs (NSAIDs) alone or in a combination with gabapentin. Chronic or severe neuropathic pain often requires multimodal analgesia.

- Initiate therapy of the disease causing neuropathic pain if applicable.
- **Pharmacological treatment for neuropathic pain: oral medication**
  - **Anti-inflammatory drugs:**
    - Non-steroidal anti-inflammatory drugs. Cyclo-oxygenase inhibition caused by NSAIDs treats associated inflammatory components and has been shown to help alleviate neuropathic pain
    - Corticosteroid therapy. May be preferred depending on the underlying disease process. Corticosteroids have an anti-inflammatory effect as well as an effect on sympathetically mediated pain by decreased substance P expression.
  - **Calcium-channel blockers:**
    - Gabapentin. There is a wide dose range for gabapentin; it should be given to effect. Reported to take up to 2 weeks for full effect, although the author commonly notices a response within a few days. Tapering of the dose is important to avoid possible rebound pain. Dogs: start at 10 mg/kg q8–12h, then increase incrementally up to 60 mg/kg orally, divided q8–12h. Cats: 5–10 mg/kg orally q8–12h
    - Pregabalin. Appears to be more effective in some dogs.
  - **Opioids.** Opioid receptors in the descending pathway may be reduced or inactivated in neuropathic pain; therefore, their efficacy is frequently inadequate when used alone. May be used for treatment of acute pain or breakthrough pain. Sedative effect commonly limits neurological assessment and thus, if possible, opioids should be avoided prior to assessment. Urinary retention is reported as a side effect of long-term opioid use.
    - Fentanyl transdermal (patch or solution). Used only in exceptional circumstances due to long duration of action.
  - *N*-methyl-D-aspartate receptor (NMDA) antagonists:
    - Amantadine. Can help to break a chronic pain cycle. May be beneficial in severe traumatic brain injury.
  - **Tricyclic antidepressants:**
    - Amitriptyline. Blocks the reuptake of catecholamines, thereby enhancing adrenergic transmission. Serves as an NMDA receptor antagonist.
- **Pharmacological treatment for neuropathic pain: injectable medication**
  - **Methadone.** Possibly better for treating neuropathic pain than tramadol. In addition to its opioid analgesic properties it is also an NMDA receptor antagonist and serotonin reuptake inhibitor (SRI).
  - **Ketamine continuous rate infusion (CRI).** Ketamine does not directly dilate cerebral vessels. It did not have an adverse effect on cerebral haemodynamics in patients with head trauma (Mathews, 2008). Ketamine may reduce an increasing intracranial pressure (ICP) in patients with an already increased ICP if combined with a benzodiazepine. Its analgesic effect is via NMDA receptor antagonism. ▶

Author's perspective *continued*

- **Fentanyl CRI.** Fentanyl has a shorter half-life compared with morphine and thus might be a better choice in patients with CNS pain as it can be withdrawn more easily to assess the patient. It seems to have fewer side effects than morphine at higher dosages (especially in cats). However, high doses causing side effects such as cortical depression should be avoided as they can mask increasing intracranial pressure assessment.
- **Medetomidine or dexmedetomidine CRI.** Potent alpha-2 agonists. Can be used individually or combined with other medications such as fentanyl.
- **Lidocaine CRI.** Usually given in combination with methadone or ketamine. Systemic application of lidocaine blocks the ectopic afferent neural activity within the dorsal horn.
- ■ **Non-pharmacological treatment** options such as acupuncture, physiotherapy and other aspects of rehabilitation can be an effective analgesic modality (see Chapter 6).

Step 3 – Follow-up
- ■ Reassess pain and health-related quality of life frequently.
- ■ Check if dispensed medication, dosage and side effect profile is appropriate or requires adjustment.

Common causes of neuropathic pain

Common diseases that cause neuropathic pain include intervertebral disc disease (compressive and non-compressive extrusion, protrusion), degenerative lumbosacral stenosis, meningoencephalitis of unknown origin, steroid-responsive meningitis arteritis (SRMA), infectious diseases such as discospondylitis or vertebral osteomyelitis, trauma to the nervous system, malformation, syringomyelia, neoplasia compressing or infiltrating the nervous system, and vascular causes such as fibrocartilagenous embolic myopathy.

References and further reading

Grubb T (2010) Chronic neuropathic pain in veterinary patients. *Topics in Companion Animal Medicine* **25**, 45–52

Loughin CA (2016) Chiari-like malformation. *Veterinary Clinics of North America: Small Animal Practice* **46**, 231–242

Mathews KA (2008) Neuropathic pain in dogs and cats: if only they could tell us if they hurt. *Veterinary Clinics of North America: Small Animal Practice* **38**, 1365–1414

O'Connor AB and Dworkin RH (2009) Treatment of neuropathic pain: an overview of recent guidelines. *American Journal of Medicine* **122**, S22–S32

Case example 1: Chiari-like malformation and syringomyelia

This disease is characterized by a mismatch between the caudal fossa volume and its contents (the cerebellum and caudal brain stem) leading to an obstruction of the normal cerebrospinal fluid (CSF) flow through the foramen magnum resulting in syringomyelia (fluid-filled cavitation) and dilatation of the central canal within the spinal cord.

HISTORY AND PRESENTATION

Occurs most commonly in young to middle-aged Cavalier King Charles Spaniels, presenting with allodynia or dysaesthesia. They may scratch at usually one side of the neck at rest and while walking and often without making skin contact, yelp for no reason or on light touch, dislike being touched or groomed, with a worsening of signs when a collar is used; they may be less energetic and sleep more than usual, with the head in an elevated position. Signs can be intermittent.

CLINICAL SIGNS AND SIGNS OF PAIN

The dog may exhibit a large variety of signs from normal to severely abnormal. Abnormal mentation may only be evident from the history. Gait can be normal, ataxic, paretic or lame. Cervical pain is often only evident on palpation and not on movement of the neck. Postural reactions may be normal or abnormal. Cranial nerve examination is unremarkable.

TREATMENT

Medical management focuses on analgesia and reduction of CSF production but is not proven to prevent disease progression.

- Anti-inflammatory drugs combined with analgesic action
  - Non-steroidal anti-inflammatory drugs as first choice, or anti-inflammatory dose of corticosteroids (less preferred).
- Analgesia
  - Gabapentin. In some dogs pregabalin appears to be more effective.
  - Other types of analgesia such as amantadine or amitriptyline can be added if necessary.
- Drugs that may have an effect on CSF production and CSF pulse pressure, but for which a clear conclusion of efficacy has not yet been made:
  - Omeprazole. Newer studies suggest that omeprazole may not have the desired effect
  - Furosemide. Decreases intracranial pressure by diuresis and reduced blood volume, but it may not have the desired effect on CSF pressure
  - Corticosteroids. May decrease CSF pulse pressure.
- Use a harness instead of a neck collar.

Case example 2: Steroid-responsive meningitis arteritis (SRMA)

An inflammatory, and suspected immune-mediated, disease occurring most commonly in young (usually less than 2 years old) medium- to large-breed dogs (particularly Beagles, Boxers and Bernese Mountain dogs) characterized by vasculitis of the meningeal arteries, non-suppurative inflammation in the CSF and subclinical coronary arteritis.

HISTORY AND PRESENTATION

Waxing and waning, unchanged or worsening signs of cervical hyperaesthesia, pyrexia and lethargy.

CLINICAL SIGNS AND SIGNS OF PAIN

Pyrexia on physical examination. Rigid neck carriage, neck pain and lethargy are commonly the only neurological deficits.

TREATMENT

Medical management focuses on treatment of the underlying cause. Analgesia is added as necessary.

- Immunosuppressive doses of prednisolone in a tapering fashion over 6–12 months.
- Analgesia. Affected dogs usually respond quickly to the appropriate therapy and are pain-free within a few days. Dogs can be very painful and may require hospitalization with opioid (e.g. methadone) therapy. At home, analgesia may include paracetamol or gabapentin in addition to immunosuppressive therapy.
- Use a harness instead of a neck collar.

Case example 3: Intervertebral disc herniation

INTERVERTEBRAL DISC EXTRUSION (HANSEN TYPE I):

Nucleus pulposus extrusion causing spinal cord or nerve root compression. Associated with disc degeneration.

History and presentation

Mostly chondrodystrophic breeds with usually acute or acute progressive presentation; commonly moderate to severe focal spinal pain.

Clinical signs and signs of pain

Dogs commonly have focal spinal pain, obvious gait abnormalities or are recumbent with urinary incontinence. Para/tetrapareses or para/tetraplegia is common.

Treatment

The acute injury and spinal pain are usually treated. Analgesia should be given to effect including non-steroidal anti-inflammatory drugs (NSAIDs) ± gabapentin, and, if success-ful, should not be required after a few weeks of management. Conservative management includes restricted/controlled exercise, which may include cautious physiotherapy for 4–6 weeks and can be elected if dogs are ambulatory (see Chapter 6b). Decompressive spinal surgery should be discussed and considered if the dog is recumbent or if pain is unmanaged with medical therapy.

→ CASE EXAMPLE 3 CONTINUED

INTERVERTEBRAL DISC PROTRUSION (HANSEN TYPE II)

Anulus fibrosus hypertrophy causing spinal cord or nerve root compression (e.g. degenerative lumbosacral stenosis (cauda equina syndrome)); associated with disc degeneration.

History and presentation

Mostly non-chondrodystrophic breeds, with a usually chronic progressive presentation and reluctance to exercise; can present with acute deterioration. Commonly there is no reported or mild spinal pain.

Clinical signs and signs of pain

Commonly no or mild spinal pain, or pain on tail elevation, in cases of degenerative lumbosacral stenosis. The dog is usually ambulatory with a mild gait abnormality (ataxia or paresis). Some dogs have a chronic history of neuropathic pain, particularly dogs with lumbosacral stenosis.

Treatment

Dogs commonly present with chronic neuropathic pain. NSAIDs and gabapentin should be combined and the response monitored. If pain is severe, other medications such as amantadine, amitriptyline or tramadol can be added to effect (one at a time). Sedation is the limiting factor. A muscle relaxant such as diazepam (0.5 mg/kg orally q8h) or methocarbamol (20–45 mg/kg orally q8h) may be useful if muscle spasms are apparent. In the author's experience, some conservatively managed dogs with Hansen type II disc disease respond better in the long term to prednisolone (0.5 mg/kg orally q24h) compared with NSAID therapy. Conservative management includes restricted/controlled exercise and cautious physiotherapy for 4–6 weeks or longer. Decompressive spinal surgery might be considered depending on the severity.

ACUTE NON-COMPRESSIVE NUCLEUS PULPOSUS EXTRUSION (ANNPE)

Acute nucleus pulposus extrusion into the spinal canal causing spinal cord contusion without spinal cord compression. Often affects normal discs.

History and presentation

Acute non-compressive presentation. Commonly occurs during exercise. Similar in its presentation to fibrocartilaginous embolism (FCE). However, patients with FCE commonly show no pain a few hours after the incident, whereas patients with ANNPE are commonly mildly painful for a few days.

Clinical signs and signs of pain

Commonly mild focal spinal pain. Asymmetrical or symmetrical clinical signs affecting either both hindlimbs (thoracolumbar lesion) or all limbs (cervical lesion), ambulatory or recumbent with possible urinary incontinence. ANNPE is not considered likely if clinical signs continue to deteriorate for more than 24 hours, in which case other differential diagnoses must be considered.

Treatment

Pain is usually mild and is usually present only for a few days. NSAID treatment has been reported to be beneficial. Gabapentin can be added if still painful. It is a non-surgical condition. Management includes a controlled exercise regime and physiotherapy for 4–6 weeks. The physiotherapy protocol can be expanded once a lack of spinal cord compression is confirmed.

Chapter 7e

Dental pain

Cecilia Gorrel

Even in the presence of oral/dental disease it is rare for the dog or cat to stop eating. Usually, they will change their food preferences (e.g. an animal will only eat soft food) or change the way they chew (e.g. chew selectively on one side). A common feedback from clients after their pet has undergone a remedial dental procedure is that the animal is brighter in general, often showing more interest in exercise and games than prior to treatment. One can speculate that this frequently reported change in behaviour after treatment is attributable to the removal of chronic discomfort and pain.

It seems reasonable to assume that, like humans, dogs and cats experience discomfort and pain when afflicted by oral diseases and after receiving treatment. In following this line of reasoning, overtreatment with analgesics may occur, but the adverse consequences of this are minimal compared with the distress of withholding pain relief.

Indications for analgesia

Common conditions that are known to cause discomfort and/or pain in people, and are thus likely to cause similar sensations in an affected animal, include:

- Complications of periodontitis, e.g. lateral periodontal abscess, toxic mucous membrane ulcers, gingivostomatitis
- Pulp and periapical disease, e.g. acute pulpitis, periapical abscess, osteomyelitis
- Traumatic injuries, including soft tissue lacerations and jaw fracture.

Dental procedures that we know are likely to cause postoperative pain in humans, and are therefore likely to cause similar sensations in animals, include:

- Periodontal therapy, e.g. deep subgingival curettage
- Extraction, especially when extraction sockets are left to heal by granulation.

It is important to distinguish between pre-emptive analgesia and alleviation of postoperative pain. In other words, pre-emptive analgesia may block sensitization, but it does not eliminate postoperative pain; additional measures are still required to ensure a comfortable recovery.

The basic analgesic routine

The optimum form of pain therapy is continuous preventive analgesia, constantly preventing the establishment of sensitization. The administration of opioids or local anaesthetic drugs blocks central sensitization and non-steroidal anti-inflammatory drugs (NSAIDs) reduce the severity of the peripheral inflammatory response. The combined use of an opioid and an NSAID is more effective than using either drug alone. Local anaesthetics can produce complete pain relief by blocking all sensory input from the affected area.

A basic analgesic routine, which can be modified as required, is as follows:

■ Include an opioid (such as buprenorphine) in the premedication
■ Administer additional opioids as required intraoperatively
■ Consider using local anaesthetic preoperatively/intraoperatively/postoperatively
■ Give opioids and/or NSAIDs postoperatively
■ Administer NSAIDs during recovery.

The author routinely includes an opioid in the patient's premedication. The animal is then anaesthetized and a meticulous oral examination is performed, including dental radiographs. Based on the findings, a list of problems and a treatment plan is drawn up. The individual analgesic regime will then be decided based on type and severity of disease and the type of remedial procedure that will be performed. As shown below, the basic analgesic routine is flexible and can be modified to suit the individual animal.

Gingivitis or early periodontitis

Gingivitis only or early periodontitis affecting only a few teeth where treatment will consist of supragingival scaling and polishing, minor subgingival debridement and either no extractions or just a few teeth that require extraction. In such cases, the inclusion of an opioid in the premedication is generally sufficient and no further analgesics or NSAIDs at the end of the procdure are required.

Moderate to severe periodontitis

Moderate to severe periodontitis where remedial therapy will involve extensive subgingival curettage and multiple tooth extractions. Use opioids as required intraoperatively ± local anaesthesia intraoperatively. Postoperative pain relief would be opioids and/or NSAIDs. Local anaesthesia could also be used to provide postoperative analgesia. In addition, a 3–5 day course of NSAIDs may facilitate recovery.

Trauma

Traumatic injuries with dental and/or skeletal fracture where treatment involves tooth extraction ± jaw fracture repair. The analgesic regime will be similar to that used for moderate to severe periodontitis.

Gingivostomatitis

For cases of chronic feline gingivostomatitis, where treatment involves extraction of most teeth, consider adding intra- and postoperative local anaesthesia to the basic regime. An added advantage of using local anaesthesia with vasoconstrictors intraoperatively is a reduction in haemorrhage, which allows for better visualization and easier surgery.

Maxillectomy/mandibulectomy procedures

In patients undergoing maxillectomy/mandibulectomy procedures, consider adding intra- and postoperative local anaesthesia to the basic regime.

Local anaesthesia

Local anaesthesia can be used to provide intra- and postoperative analgesia. In contrast with human patients, dogs and cats are not amenable to local anaesthetic injection if conscious, so the techniques are used when the animal is anaesthetized. When given prior to the start of a procedure, the use of local anaesthetic drugs may reduce the requirement for general anaesthetic drugs during surgery. When given at the end of a procedure, prior to recovery from anaesthesia, they will provide postoperative analgesia.

Useful techniques in the oral cavity include infiltration anaesthesia and regional nerve blocks. Infiltration anaesthesia is where a small amount of anaesthetic agent is deposited locally to diffuse into the tissue and exert its effect. Regional anaesthesia is where the anaesthetic agent is deposited as close to the nerve as possible and its effect is thus to block all sensation distally.

Infiltration techniques are easier to perform and safer to use than regional blocks, yet they are often not described in veterinary textbooks. The main risk with regional blocks is damage to the nerve as the anaesthetic agent is placed. Iatrogenic nerve damage (when the needle scratches or perforates the nerve) causes pain and it can take weeks to months before the tissue regenerates and the patient is pain free. In rare instances, there is permanent nerve damage. In veterinary dentistry, the described techniques for regional blocks involve placing a needle well into a foramen/canal. Moreover, this is performed on an anaesthetized animal where there will be no sensory feedback to alert the veterinary surgeon (veterinarian) that the nerve is being damaged. In the author's opinion, regional blocks should be performed with great caution and only be used in areas where infiltration anaesthesia is not possible, i.e. mandibular premolars and molars.

All clinically used local anaesthetics stop or slow conduction of impulses. Sensation disappears in the following order: pain, cold, warmth, touch, joint, and deep pressure. For local anaesthesia in the oral cavity, lidocaine, mepivacaine, bupivacaine and ropivacaine are all suitable. The local anaesthetic drug chosen for postoperative pain relief should ideally have a long duration of action, and therefore bupivacaine (onset 15 minutes, duration 4–6 hours) is the drug of choice. Lidocaine can be used during surgery for more immediate effect. In inflamed or infected tissue, local anaesthetic *may be* virtually ineffective due to the acidic pH interfering with dissociation of anaesthetic base.

In human dentistry and oral surgery, vasoconstrictors (adrenaline, L-noradrenaline) are routinely used in combination with the local anaesthetic. The main reason is to delay systemic absorption of the local anaesthetic, thus reducing the toxicity and increasing the margin of safety. Local anaesthetics produce analgesia when given in small doses intravenously, but are potent proconvulsants and can induce marked myocardial depression and cardiac dysrythmias when administered systemically. The addition of vasoconstrictors, by reducing systemic absorption of the local anaesthetic, will also increase intensity and prolong anaesthetic activity. However, they may increase the risk of cardiac arrhythmias and ventricular fibrillation. In veterinary dentistry and oral surgery, local anaesthetics are generally used without the addition of vasoconstrictors. The author uses local anaesthetics with added vasoconstrictor to ensure that the anaesthetic agent remains locally active for a prolonged period. As already mentioned, it also reduces bleeding and thus allows for better visualization and facilitates many techniques, especially extraction.

The use of a dental local anaesthetic syringe and needle (Figure 7.9) is strongly recommended. Safe maximum doses are 4 mg/kg lidocaine and 1–2 mg/kg bupivacaine. This is calculated for each animal. In general, 0.25–1 ml of local anaesthetic agent is deposited per site. Always aspirate for blood before injecting.

Technique for infiltration anaesthesia

The technique involves depositing a small amount of local anaesthetic (bleb technique) into the gingiva and alveolar periosteum in the region of the apex of the tooth that needs to be desensitized (Figure 7.10). The anaesthetic agent diffuses into the tissue to have local effect on the nerve. The infiltrates are deposited buccally and palatally/lingually as required. This technique can be used to provide desensitization of all teeth in the upper jaw. In fact, regional blocks are not necessary in the upper jaw. Infiltration can also be used

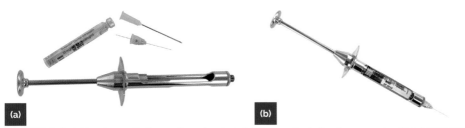

7.9 A dental local anaesthetic needle and syringe. **(a)** The empty device, the ampoule with local anaesthetic agent and the needle. An 18 G needle is also depicted to demonstrate how fine the dental needle is. **(b)** The device assembled and ready for use.

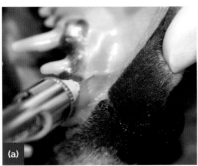

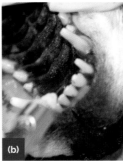

7.10 Technique for infiltration anaesthesia. A small amount of local anaesthetic is deposited into the gingiva and alveolar periosteum in the region of the tooth that needs to be desensitized. The anaesthetic agent diffuses into the tissue to have local effect on the nerve. **(a)** The location for buccal desensitization of an upper incisor is shown on a cadaver. **(b)** It is often necessary to place anaesthetic agent palatally as well. The location for palatal desensitization of an upper incisor is shown on a cadaver.

to desensitize incisors and rostral premolars in the lower jaw. It is only for the caudal premolars and molars in the mandible that a regional block is required.

Technique for regional blocks

Regional anaesthesia is where the anaesthetic agent is deposited as close to the nerve as possible and its effect is thus to block all sensation distally. Techniques that have been described for dental procedures in animals are the infraorbital, the mandibular and the mental blocks.

In the author's opinion, the only regional block that is required for veterinary dentistry is the mandibular block, which is described in Figure 7.11.

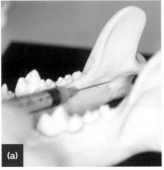

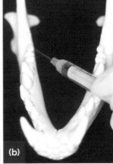

7.11 The intraoral approach to the mandibular block involves palpating the mandibular foramen intraorally and directing the needle to that area using an oral approach. **(a)** The easiest way is to slide the needle along the medial aspect of the ventral mandible, with the syringe held parallel to the hemi-mandible to be blocked. **(b)** When the point of the needle is close to the foramen, move the syringe barrel over to the premolar region of the contralateral side to give better access to the area around the foramen. The needle should be close to the bone of the ventral mandible to avoid inadvertently blocking the lingual nerve. The calculated dose is deposited.

Summary

Preventive and postoperative analgesia using opioids and/or NSAIDs should be used in all animals.

Local anaesthesia can be a useful part of the analgesic regime. Infiltration techniques can be used to desensitize all teeth in the upper jaw as well as incisors and rostral premolars in the lower jaw. It is only for the caudal premolars and molars in the mandible that a regional block is required.

References and further reading

Gorrel C (2013) Anaesthesia and analgesia. In: *Veterinary Dentistry for the General Practitioner 2nd Edn*, ed. C Gorrel, pp. 15–29. Saunders Elsevier, Philadelphia

Chapter 7f

Ophthalmic pain

Carl Bradbrook

Recognition and effective treatment of ophthalmic pain may present the clinician with a challenge due to difficulties in patient assessment. This may result from a combination of factors including a lack of validated ocular pain scales, altered patient temperament due to the presenting condition, and difficulty in assessing the periorbital area when painful. Treatment relies on the recognition of pain followed by effective analgesia. As with any clinical situation where pain is suspected, analgesia should be provided and the patient reassessed at an appropriate time. Provision of good analgesia improves anaesthetic stability and, most importantly, patient comfort. Incorporation of local anaesthesia techniques, where appropriate, along with more traditional methods is likely to improve efficacy of analgesic treatment.

Clinical signs of ophthalmic pain include blepharospasm, excessive tearing, photophobia, and head shyness. Clinical signs may be dependent on the structures involved, such as the cornea, conjunctiva, adnexal or intraocular structures. For example, most ophthalmic conditions will lead to blepharospasm and head shyness, but pain associated with intraocular disease may result in an increase in intraocular pressure (IOP), which is more likely to result in photophobia. When treating ophthalmic pain, it is important to consider the type of surgery to be performed, as this is likely to allow the clinician to choose the most appropriate methods to provide analgesia.

The most commonly performed ophthalmic procedures involve enucleation and surgery to the cornea and eyelids. Although provision of analgesia for intraocular surgery is just as important, it is beyond the scope of this text. As well as treating pain associated with surgical conditions, it is important to consider presenting ophthalmic conditions that may require pain management prior to further medical or surgical intervention. Corneal ulceration, often secondary to corneal drying, entropion, distichiasis or ectopic cilia, is extremely painful and requires good analgesia.

Analgesics suitable for treatment of ocular pain include opioids, non-steroidal anti-inflammatory drugs (NSAIDs) and local anaesthetics. Additional analgesia may be provided using ketamine and the alpha-2 agonists, although the possibility of these drugs increasing IOP should be considered. Due to this, the use of ketamine or alpha-2 agonists is not advised with a fragile eye or during intraocular surgery.

BSAVA Guide to Pain Management in Small Animal Practice. Edited by Ian Self. ©BSAVA 2019

Eyelid pain

Intraoperative pain management for eyelid surgery can be particularly challenging and several analgesic options should be available to deal with treatment failure. Both systemic analgesia and topical local anaesthesia are useful in these cases. Local anaesthetic techniques will be discussed later in this chapter. Alongside opioid, topical local anaesthesia and NSAID analgesia, adjunct therapy with ketamine as a continuous infusion may be useful to provide intra-operative analgesia.

Corneal pain

The cornea contains a high density of nociceptors and a marked response is often noted with conditions such as corneal ulceration, along with any surgical intervention, due to exposure of nociceptors. Analgesia should be provided using a multimodal approach, with a combination of systemic and local analgesics. Topical local anaesthesia provides excellent, rapid onset analgesia and will facilitate further clinical examination. Tetracaine has a more rapid onset, but shorter duration, than proxymetacaine and results in less conjunctival irritation on application. Tetracaine followed by proxymetacaine may be used in the conscious patient. Repeated application of single drops of drug solution (Monclin et al., 2011) has been shown to provide improved analgesia of longer duration in horses compared with that provided by flooding the cornea. Good corneal lubrication is essential and the contralateral cornea should also be treated. Systemic analgesia may be provided with the use of opioids, such as methadone or buprenorphine, which provide excellent to good analgesia, respectively. It has been suggested that the cornea has opioid receptors within its structure, although evidence of the effectiveness of topical opioids is inconsistent (Thomson et al., 2013). NSAIDs also provide good analgesia and should be utilized unless any contraindication is evident.

Deep ocular pain

Intraocular diseases such as uveitis and glaucoma often result in a marked pain response due to an increase in intraocular pressure. Topical local anaesthesia is minimally effective in these cases and therefore analgesia should be provided with opioids, adjunct analgesics and, where appropriate, NSAIDs.

Enucleation

Analgesia for enucleation should be achieved with a multimodal approach utilizing opioid analgesia and, where appropriate, NSAIDs, alongside local anaesthesia. Retrobulbar or peribulbar anaesthesia can be administered prior to surgical incision or, when not possible, a splash block may be performed following globe removal. Local anaesthetic-soaked gelatin sponge material (Ploog et al., 2014) may also be used to aid haemostasis and provide postoperative analgesia. Where a preoperative local anaesthetic technique is not possible, alternative systemic intraoperative analgesia should be provided.

Local anaesthetic techniques

Where possible, a local anaesthetic technique should be incorporated into an analgesia plan. Calculation of a maximum dose of local anaesthetic should be performed, and aspiration is mandatory prior to injection.

Retrobulbar nerve block

Retrobulbar nerve block (RBA) is an effective technique to provide intra- and postoperative analgesia for enucleation and exenteration. The inferior temporal palpebral technique (Accola et al., 2006) has been documented to be a reliable method in the dog. A retrobulbar needle (Figure 7.12) or a 22 G spinal needle bent to a 20-degree angle is inserted midway between the lateral canthus and mid lower eyelid. It is directed along the ventral orbit and

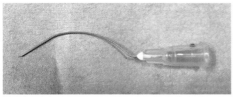

7.12 A curved retrobulbar needle suitable for use in the dog.

then redirected dorsomedially to reach the caudal aspect of the globe (Figure 7.13). Following aspiration, 1 to 4 ml of local anaesthetic solution is injected, depending on patient size. Although used in the cat, some controversy exists over whether this technique is appropriate in this species; care should be taken as brainstem anaesthesia has been reported in the cat following its use (Oliver and Bradbrook, 2013).

Peribulbar nerve block (PBA)

This technique has been shown by Shilo-Benhamini *et al.* (2014) to be superior to RBA in the cat and is used by the author. Local

anaesthetic is injected subconjunctivally around the globe to provide regional anaesthesia to the extraocular muscles. The injection site is 2 mm from the limbus and 0.1–0.2 ml/kg bupivacaine is administered using a 2.5 cm needle (Figure 7.14).

Subtenon nerve block

This technique provides anaesthesia, analgesia and akinesia for corneal and intraocular procedures (Ahn *et al.*, 2013). It is not used by the author for enucleation as it does not provide effective eyelid anaesthesia. Following induction of anaesthesia the patient is positioned in dorsal recumbency, topical local anaesthesia applied to the cornea and eyelid retractors placed. An incision is made 5 mm from the limbus in the dorsomedial aspect of the bulbar conjunctiva. The conjunctiva and tenon capsule are bluntly dissected from the underlying sclera. A curved spatulated cannula is directed dorsocaudally and 1–2 ml of lidocaine 2% solution is injected following aspiration (Figure 7.15).

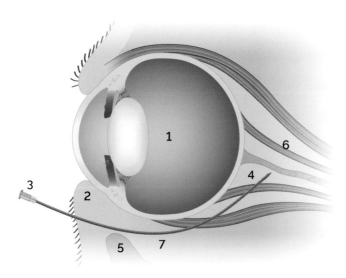

7.13 A cross-sectional diagram of the orbit, globe and associated structures: 1 = globe; 2 = eyelids; 3 = needle placement for a retrobulbar injection; 4 = intraconal space; 5 = orbit; 6 = extraocular muscles, nerves and blood vessels; 7 = injection site for peribulbar block.

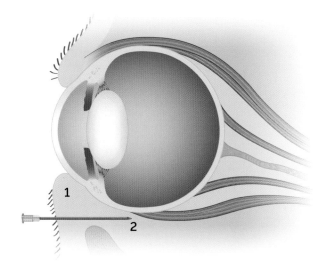

7.14 Injection site for a peribulbar block: 1 = eyelid; 2 = injection site in peribulbar tissue.

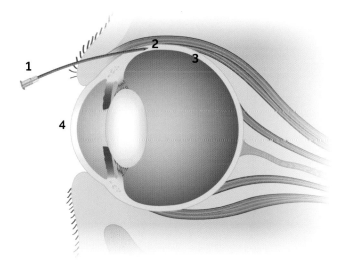

7.15 Injection site for a subtenon block: 1 = spatulated cannula used for injection; 2 = Tenon's capsule; 3 = sclera; 4 = cornea.

Eyelid blocks

Specific blocks for eyelid surgery are not well documented in small animals, and the author does not use them routinely. If appropriate, local anaesthetic may be infiltrated post-surgery, but care should be taken to monitor for and treat lid swelling. Cold packing of the lid region is a useful technique to employ in the postoperative period.

References and further reading

Accola PJ, Bentley E, Smith LJ *et al.* (2006) Development of a retrobulbar injection technique for ocular surgery and analgesia in dogs. *Journal of the American Veterinary Medical Association* **229**, 220–225

Ahn J, Jeong M, Lee E *et al.* (2013) Effects of peribulbar anesthesia (sub-Tenon injection of a local anesthetic) on akinesia of extraocular muscles, mydriasis, and intraoperative and postoperative analgesia in dogs undergoing phacoemulsification. *American Journal of Veterinary Research* **74**, 1126–1132

Giuliano EA and Walsh KP (2013) The eye. In: *Small Animal Regional Anesthesia and Analgesia*, ed. L Campoy and MR Read. Wiley-Blackwell, Oxford

Jolliffe C (2016) Ophthalmic surgery. In: *BSAVA Manual of Canine and Feline Anaesthesia and Analgesia, 3rd edn*, ed. T Duke-Novakovski, M de Vries and C Seymour. BSAVA Publications, Gloucester

Monclin SJ, Farnir F and Grauwels M (2011) Duration of corneal anaesthesia following multiple doses and two concentrations of tetracaine hydrochloride eyedrops on the normal equine cornea. *Equine Veterinary Journal* **43**, 69–73

Oliver JAC and Bradbrook CA (2013) Suspected brainstem anesthesia following retrobulbar block in a cat. *Veterinary Ophthalmology* **16**, 225–228

Ploog CL, Swinger RL, Spade J, Quandt KM and Mitchell MA (2014) Use of lidocaine-bupivacaine-infused gelatin hemostatic sponges *versus* lidocaine-bupivacaine retrobulbar injections for postoperative analgesia following eye enucleation in dogs. *Journal of the American Veterinary Medical Association* **244**, 57–62

Shilo-Benhamini Y, Pascoe PJ, Maggs DJ *et al.* (2014) Comparison of peribulbar and retrobulbar regional anesthesia with bupivacaine in cats. *American Journal of Veterinary Research* **75**, 1029–1039

Thomson S, Oliver JA, Gould DJ, Mendl M and Leece EA (2013) Preliminary investigations into the analgesic effects of topical ocular 1% morphine solution in dogs and cats. *Veterinary Anaesthesia and Analgesia* **40**, 632–640

Case example 1: Bilateral lower lid entropion correction

HISTORY AND PRESENTATION

A 2-year-old male Bulldog was presented for anaesthesia for correction of bilateral lower lid entropion. The dog had a history of chronic, intermittent conjunctivitis and moderate upper respiratory tract noise with stridor consistent with signs of brachycephalic obstructive airway syndrome (BOAS).

CLINICAL SIGNS

Ocular discharge, marked upper respiratory tract noise and poor exercise tolerance.

SIGNS OF PAIN

Blepharospasm, conjunctival hyperaemia, head shyness and excess tearing.

ANALGESIC PLAN

- Opioid: methadone 0.2 mg/kg i.m.
- Topical anaesthesia: proxymetacaine.
- NSAID: administered following blood pressure measurement (MAP >60 mmHg).
- Ketamine infusion: 10 µg/kg/min i.v. during surgical procedure.
- Infiltration of lidocaine (volume 0.2 ml per lid, maximum 2–4 mg/kg) into lids following surgical procedure, followed by cold packing of the area.

POSTOPERATIVE CARE

- Continue methadone 0.2 mg/kg i.m. every 4 hours.
- Sedation/anxiolysis should be considered to reduce stress during hospitalization.

Case example 2: Enucleation

HISTORY AND PRESENTATION

A 10-year-old female neutered Labrador Retriever was presented for enucleation due to chronic glaucoma. The dog had a 6-month history of medically managed glaucoma of the right eye, which was now intractable to medical treatment.

CLINICAL SIGNS

Exophthalmos, head shyness, conjunctival hyperaemia, uveitis and raised intraocular pressure.

SIGNS OF PAIN

Photophobia, reluctance to allow clinical examination and uncharacteristic aggression.

ANALGESIC PLAN

- Opioid: methadone 0.3 mg/kg i.m.
- NSAID: administered following assessment of minimal risk of further haemorrhage.
- Local anaesthesia technique: retrobulbar block; bupivacaine maximum dose 1 mg/kg (see Figure 7.13); volume required 2–3 ml.

POSTOPERATIVE CARE

Assess for pain taking into consideration bupivacaine duration of action (6–8 hours). Methadone 0.2 mg/kg i.m. every 4 hours starting at maximum of 6 hours post-retrobulbar block.

Chapter 7g

Orthopaedic pain

Kinley Smith

Whether acute or chronic, orthopaedic pain can be severe and debilitating. Treatment should be tailored to each individual patient and the use of non-pharmacological therapies encouraged.

Acute musculoskeletal injury

Opioids provide a rapid, powerful and relatively safe way to control pain in acute injury. Full mu agonists such as methadone are preferred, ensuring continuity of analgesia through possible anaesthesia and postoperative pain control. A continuous rate infusion (CRI) of opioids in combination with lidocaine and ketamine should be used in refractory cases. Non-steroidal anti-inflammatory drugs (NSAIDs) are valuable for the trauma patient but must not be used before the patient's condition has been stabilized. Hypothermia (cold packing) of acute orthopaedic injuries may reduce swelling as well as pain. While specialized equipment is available for delivery, typically a freezer ice pack wrapped in a thin towel is applied to the area for 10–20 minutes three times daily.

Chronic musculoskeletal disease

Osteoarthritis is an incurable condition that is painful, debilitating and progressive. Understanding chronic pain is essential in formulating a treatment plan for osteoarthritis. While osteoarthritis may be the most commonly diagnosed painful chronic orthopaedic disease, chronic pain from bone, muscle and tendons may exist in addition to joint pathology; accurate diagnosis is essential to pain management. Further details are provided in Chapter 4.

Treatment
Drug therapy
Figure 7.16 provides dose rates of selected oral drugs used in the management of orthopaedic pain.

NSAIDs: NSAIDs are usually the first choice in the management of osteoarthritis. They are effective, easy to administer and have a relatively low incidence of side effects. Long-term use may be associated with improved analgesia without increased side

Drug	Dogs	Cats	Notes
Amantadine	3–5 mg/kg q24h	1–4 mg/kg q24h	Start at lowest dose in cats
Amitriptyline	1–2 mg/kg q12–24h	0.5–1 mg/kg q24h	
Buprenorphine	–	0.02–0.03 mg/kg q24h	Oral transmucosal
Gabapentin	10–15 mg/kg q8–12h	2–5 mg/kg q12h	
Paracetamol	10 mg/kg q8–12h	DO NOT USE	Licensed dose is 33 mg/kg
Pregabalin	3–4 mg/kg q12h	–	Start at 2 mg/kg then increase

7.16 Dose rates of selected oral drugs used in the management of orthopaedic pain.

effects. Indeed, several human studies have suggested that continuous use was associated with fewer and less severe osteoarthritis flare ups. Tapering of NSAIDs to the minimum effective dose is commonly practiced but may result in inadequate pain control and there is no evidence for reduced side effects.

Amantadine: Amantadine has been shown to improve pain control in osteoarthritic dogs when combined with an NSAID. The author has had success using amantadine as a primary treatment for osteoarthritis in dogs.

Gabapentin: Gabapentin is a safe and effective drug for chronic pain in dogs and cats. It can be used in combination with NSAIDs and the author believes it is an effective primary treatment for chronic orthopaedic pain in dogs where NSAID use is not possible. Side effects are uncommon but may be more frequent at doses above 15 mg/kg.

Pregabalin: Pregabalin is similar to gabapentin but has a longer half-life and a higher bioavailability. It may provide improved analgesia where the response to gabapentin has been unsatisfactory.

Tramadol: Tramadol has unpredictable absorption and pharmacokinetics in dogs. This is reflected in clinical use where lack of efficacy and side effects are common and it is therefore becoming less popular as an analgesic agent. Tramadol should not be used with amitriptyline due to the serotonin reuptake effects.

Paracetamol: Licensed in combination with codeine, paracetamol is frequently used in dogs where NSAID use is not tolerated. At present, there is no published evidence to support its use as a sole treatment in osteoarthritis and its analgesic effect in dogs has recently been questioned. However, it is commonly used as part of multimodal analgesia regimes in the dog.

Amitriptyline: Amitriptyline, a tricyclic antidepressant, has proven efficacy in canine neuropathic pain and the author has used it in combination with NSAIDs in the management of osteoarthritis in dogs refractory to other drugs.

Structure-modifying drugs: Pentosan polysulphate and polysulphated glycosaminoglycan are considered to have the potential to retard cartilage degeneration. Clinical trials have reported mixed results but their use may provide a moderate level of comfort in canine osteoarthritis.

Nutraceuticals: Essential fatty acids of the n-3 group may have an anti-inflammatory effect and studies have shown dietary supplementation with eicosapentaenoic acid and docosahexaenoic acid improved mobility in dogs with osteoarthritis. Many laboratory studies showing potential benefits of glucosamine and chondroitin exist but data on efficacy in pain relief in both human and veterinary literature are lacking. Combinations of nutraceuticals in supplements and complete diets are increasingly available. Some clinical data showing efficacy are emerging and the author advises a 6-week trial of the client's preferred combination before assessment of clinical response.

Grapipant: This is a new non-COX inhibiting NSAID. It targets the EP4 prostaglandin receptor which is the primary mediator of canine osteoarthritis pain and inflammation. It potentially has fewer side efffects than traditional NSAIDs.

Cats: Osteoarthritis is extremely common in cats with one study showing 92% of cats having osteoarthritis. NSAID use in cats is limited with only meloxicam licensed for long-term use (14 days). However, continuous use may be tolerated and tapering the dose is recommended in cats. In longer term use, haematology, biochemistry, urinalysis and blood pressure monitoring are recommended (at least every 6 months). Gabapentin is an effective analgesic in cats with orthopaedic pain and amantadine has been used experimentally. Oral transmucosal delivery of buprenorphine can provide good analgesia.

Surgery
Joint replacement may provide a rapid and marked improvement in pain control and is readily available for the hip and stifle. Outcomes for elbow replacement are more variable. Hip replacement is also available and reliable for small dogs and cats. Early intervention may be preferable and such procedures should be discussed with the client early in the course of the disease. Arthrodesis offers an effective treatment for intractably painful joints and arthroplasty techniques offer improved limb use although the outcome is less predictable than joint replacement or arthrodesis. Extra-articular osteotomy techniques have been used to manage pain in the elbow and arthroscopy may offer clinical benefit in osteoarthritic joints.

Exercise
Exercise intolerance is a common finding in animals with osteoarthritis but little research is available. One study showed that trotting dogs for 1.2 km increased lameness in the short term. What the benefits of exercise are in the long term are unknown and it has been suggested that there may be an overall benefit of controlled exercise. A risk factor of ball and stick chasing in the development of elbow and hip dysplasia has been shown. Short periods of intense exercise (such as chasing balls, jumping and bursts of intense running) may be more likely to induce lameness in dogs with osteoarthritis than controlled lead exercise over longer periods. In the absence of research on this matter clients may be asked to identify exercise patterns associated with increased lameness and modify their pet's routine accordingly.

Physiotherapy
A review of the evidence for physiotherapy in companion animals is beyond the scope of this chapter. In humans, water- and land-based exercises are useful in the management of osteoarthritic joints and the author believes a combination of water- and land-based exercises is an important part of multimodal therapy for chronic orthopaedic pain (see Chapter 6b).

Weight loss management
Obesity is often identified in patients with osteoarthritis. While increased joint loading is undoubtedly a contributing factor to joint pain, the relationship between obesity and osteoarthritis is complex. Increased body fat has been associated with osteoarthritis in dogs and weight loss is likely to be beneficial in the treatment of canine osteoarthritis.

Cell-based therapies
Intra-articular injections of mesenchymal stem cells and of platelet-rich plasma have shown efficacy in clinical trials in patients with osteoarthritis. While there are no studies in dogs comparing efficacy with more conventional treatment, cell therapies may offer adjunctive treatment options in refractory cases.

Other therapies
Extracorporeal shockwave therapy (Figure 7.17) has been used successfully in a number of orthopaedic conditions and beneficial effects in hip osteoarthritis have been described. Transcutaneous electric nerve stimulation (TENS) has been shown to have a short-term

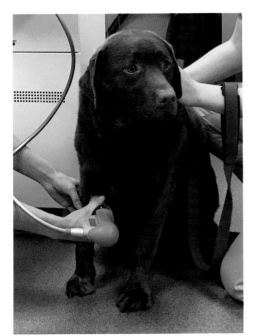

pain relieving effect (3–4 hours) in dogs, although its use in cats is not recommended. Acupuncture, massage, therapeutic laser and therapeutic ultrasound may have some benefit in companion animals.

References and further reading

Benitez ME, Roush JK, KuKanich B and McMurphy R (2015) Pharmacokinetics of hydrocodone and tramadol administered for control of postoperative pain in dogs following tibial plateau leveling osteotomy. *American Journal of Veterinary Research* **76**, 763–770

Beraud R, Moreau M and Lussier B (2010) Effect of exercise on kinetic gait analysis of dogs afflicted by osteoarthritis. *Veterinary and Comparative Orthopaedics and Traumatology* **23**, 87–92

Cashmore RG, Harcourt-Brown TR, Freeman PM, Jeffery ND and Granger N (2009) Clinical diagnosis and treatment of suspected neuropathic pain in three dogs. *Australian Veterinary Journal* **87**, 45–50

Hunt JR, Dean RS, Davis GN and Murrell JC (2015) An analysis of the relative frequencies of reported adverse events associated with NSAID administration in dogs and cats in the United Kingdom. *Veterinary Journal* **206**, 183–190

Innes JF, Clayton J and Lascelles BD (2010) Review of the safety and efficacy of long-term NSAID use in the treatment of canine osteoarthritis. *Veterinary Record* **166**, 226–230

Johnston SA, McLaughlin RM and Budsberg SC (2008) Nonsurgical management of osteoarthritis in dogs. *Veterinary Clinics of North America: Small Animal Practice* **38**, 1449–1470

7.17 Administration of extracorporeal shock wave therapy to treat flexor tendon enthesiopathy secondary to elbow dysplasia.

Author's perspective

- Review the diagnosis
    - Is the diagnosis correct?
    - Are there other co-morbidities?
    - Are these caused by or do they contribute to the clinical presentation?
    - Can these be resolved by other means (e.g. surgery, weight loss)?
- Review the medication(s)
    - Are they appropriate?
    - Is there a history of adverse reactions?
    - Consider multimodal pain therapy
        - Typical sequence of drug use (used in combination)
            - o NSAID
            - o + Gabapentin
            - o + Amantadine
            - o + Paracetamol (dogs only)
    - Consider nutraceuticals and structure-modifying drugs
- Start physiotherapy/hydrotherapy
- Discuss exercise control
- Discuss weight control
- Consider other treatments such as extracorporeal shockwave therapy or acupuncture

KuKanich B (2016) Pharmacokinetics and pharmacodynamics of oral acetaminophen in combination with codeine in healthy Greyhound dogs. *Journal of Veterinary Pharmacology and Therapeutics* **39**, 514–517

Lascelles BD, Gaynor JS, Smith ES *et al.* (2008) Amantadine in a multimodal analgesic regimen for alleviation of refractory osteoarthritis pain in dogs. *Journal of Veterinary Internal Medicine* **22**, 53–59

Lascelles BD, Henry JB III, Brown J *et al.* (2010) Cross-sectional study of the prevalence of radiographic degenerative joint disease in domesticated cats. *Veterinary Surgery* **39**, 535–544

Marshall W, Bockstahler B, Hulse D and Carmichael S (2009) A review of osteoarthritis and obesity: current understanding of the relationship and benefit of obesity treatment and prevention in the dog. *Veterinary and Comparative Orthopaedics and Traumatology* **22**, 339–345

Mehler SJ, May LR, King C, Harris WS and Shah Z (2016) A prospective, randomized, double blind, placebo-controlled evaluation of the effects of eicosapentaenoic acid and docosahexaenoic acid on the clinical signs and erythrocyte membrane polyunsaturated fatty acid concentrations in dogs with osteoarthritis. *Prostaglandins, Leukotrienes and Essential Fatty Acids* **109**, 1–7

Roush JK, Cross AR, Renberg WC *et al.* (2010a) Evaluation of the effects of dietary supplementation with fish oil omega-3 fatty acids on weight bearing in dogs with osteoarthritis. *Journal of the American Veterinary Medical Association* **236**, 67–73

Roush JK, Dodd CE, Fritsch DA *et al.* (2010b) Multicenter veterinary practice assessment of the effects of omega-3 fatty acids on osteoarthritis in dogs. *Journal of the American Veterinary Medical Association* **236**, 59–66

Sallander MH, Hedhammar A and Trogen ME (2006) Diet, exercise, and weight as risk factors in hip dysplasia and elbow arthrosis in Labrador Retrievers. *The Journal of Nutrition* **136**, 2050S–2052S

Sanderson RO, Beata C, Flipo RM *et al.* (2009) Systematic review of the management of canine osteoarthritis. *Veterinary Record* **164**, 418–424

Smith GK, Lawler DF, Biery DN *et al.* (2012) Chronology of hip dysplasia development in a cohort of 48 Labrador Retrievers followed for life. *Veterinary Surgery* **41**, 20–33

Souza AN, Ferreira MP, Hagen SC, Patricio GC and Matera JM (2016) Radial shock wave therapy in dogs with hip osteoarthritis. *Veterinary and Comparative Orthopaedics and Traumatology* **29**, 108–114

Sparkes AH, Heiene R, Lascelles BD *et al.* (2010) ISFM and AAFP consensus guidelines: long-term use of NSAIDs in cats. *Journal of Feline Medicine and Surgery* **12**, 521–538

Wernham BG, Trumpatori B, Hash J *et al.* (2011) Dose reduction of meloxicam in dogs with osteoarthritis-associated pain and impaired mobility. *Journal of Veterinary Internal Medicine* **25**, 1298–1305

Zhang W, Nuki G, Moskowitz RW *et al.* (2010) OARSI recommendations for the management of hip and knee osteoarthritis: part III: Changes in evidence following systematic cumulative update of research published through January 2009. *Osteoarthritis and Cartilage* **18**, 476–499

Chapter 7h

Cancer pain

Iain Grant and Jenny Helm

In 1998, The Morris Animal Health Foundation Survey stated that cancer was a leading cause of death in both dogs and cats. Although the figure for dogs was higher than for cats (47% *versus* 32%), companion animal cancer is clearly a major concern for veterinary surgeons (veterinarians) and pet owners.

Human studies indicate a high prevalence of cancer pain, particularly in patients with advanced tumours (Keefe *et al.*, 2005). As many veterinary patients present with advanced cancer (Mason *et al.*, 2013), a significant proportion may therefore have experienced pain before undergoing any medical evaluation or treatment; however, the precise prevalence of cancer pain is unknown.

In advanced cases, the majority of pain is associated directly with the infiltrative growth of the tumour or its metastases, with a smaller proportion due to the side effects of therapy (Christo and Mazloomdoost, 2008). To include both direct and treatment-related effects, the authors believe that the term 'cancer-associated pain' better describes this problem. Cancer-associated pain has significant implications in terms of patient welfare and is likely, therefore, to strongly influence the clinician's approach to therapy.

Quality of life and cancer-associated pain

Many owners and professionals agree to a protocol of cancer management if it is possible to maintain a pet's 'quality of life' (QoL) throughout. QoL is a multi-dimensional concept, which includes assessment of a patient's pain (Velikova *et al.*, 1999; see Chapter 2 and Appendix 1). For the majority of pet owners, the occurrence of cancer-associated pain and particularly the inability to control it effectively defines a diminishing QoL and is a common reason to elect for euthanasia. The importance of recognizing cancer-associated pain and trying to treat it effectively, therefore, cannot be understated.

Recognizing or predicting cancer-associated pain

Similar to infants, veterinary patients are unable to provide information first hand of their subjective pain experience, for example where pain is localized or its intensity or nature. This relies on assessment by the owner or the health care professional who are termed proxy-informants (Yazback and Fantoni, 2005). Cancer-associated pain may also be complex in nature and may be persistent or intermittent. Due to such challenges, it can be assumed that cancer-associated pain is potentially under-diagnosed and therefore under-treated (Yazback and Fantoni, 2005).

A number of factors can be assessed to help to predict the occurrence of pain in veterinary patients affected by cancer:

- Tumour type and location
- Presence of co-morbidities
- Occurrence of paraneoplastic effects
- Therapies and associated side effects
- Inference from human reporting.

Patient history and physical examination

The owner interacts with their pet every day and can describe changes in behaviour or personality that may indicate the presence of pain. It is important to recognize that the species, age, breed and personality of the individual animal may influence the expression of these behaviours. Furthermore, some behaviours may occur spontaneously and others may be evoked by physical examination; and some may occur frequently and others rarely (Hansen, 2003). See Chapter 2 and Appendix 1 for information on pain assessment tools.

Management of the veterinary cancer patient typically involves repeat visits and re-examinations. This positions the clinician ideally for two-way communication with the owner and for frequent pain reassessment. This highlights the value of one single clinician or a clinician and veterinary nurse within the practice being assigned to the management of an individual cancer patient throughout its care, if possible.

Tumour type and location

Tumours that exhibit invasive or destructive growth, or are associated with necrosis (Figure 7.18a), ulceration (Figure 7.18b) or inflammation are likely to be associated with significant pain. Assessment of the degree of tumour

invasiveness within sites including body cavities, soft tissues, bone and nervous tissues may require both physical examination and advanced imaging studies (Figure 7.19).

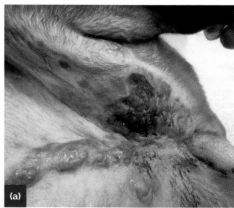

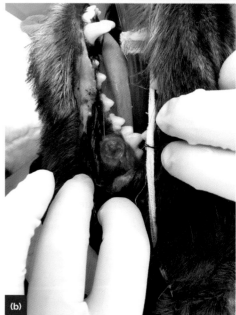

7.18 Tumours associated with ulceration, necrosis or inflammation are likely to be painful. **(a)** Tissue necrosis secondary to dermal lymphatic invasion of an inflammatory mammary carcinoma in a Hungarian Visla. **(b)** An ulcerated oral tumour in a crossbreed dog.

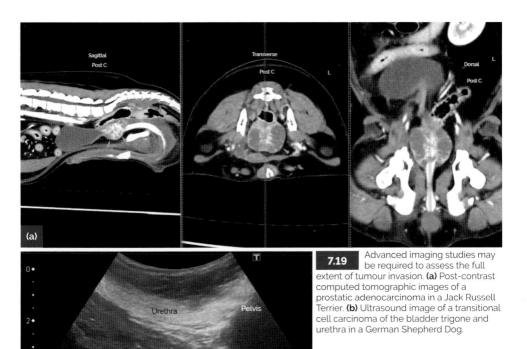

7.19 Advanced imaging studies may be required to assess the full extent of tumour invasion. **(a)** Post-contrast computed tomographic images of a prostatic adenocarcinoma in a Jack Russell Terrier. **(b)** Ultrasound image of a transitional cell carcinoma of the bladder trigone and urethra in a German Shepherd Dog.

Presence of co-morbidities

The prevalence of many tumours rises after middle age in canine patients (Dobson *et al.*, 2002). In this age group, and often in specific breeds, painful, chronic co-morbidities may also arise, adding to the overall impact on quality of life. These include degenerative joint disease, inflammatory skin disease, dental disease, chronic pancreatitis, cystitis or prostatitis. Co-morbidities (e.g. chronic renal or hepatic disease) may also complicate the choice of drug treatments used to manage cancer-associated pain and may necessitate ongoing assessment of therapy and any treatment side effects.

Occurrence of paraneoplastic effects

Paraneoplastic syndromes are systemic disorders that result from the presence of cancer but occur at sites distant from the primary tumour (Bergman, 2012). They occur secondary to the release of hormones, cytokines, growth factors or other peptides from the tumour or as a result of tumour-related autoimmunity. Paraneoplastic syndromes associated with significant pain may include:

- Polyneuropathies
- Polymyopathies
- Immune-mediated polyarthritis

- Vasculitis
- Hypertrophic osteopathy
- Necrolytic migratory erythema
- New tumour formation.

Therapies and associated side effects

Cancer therapy and specifically treatment-related side effects, can lead to pain. A clinician should provide multimodal pre-emptive analgesia whenever possible according to the clinical circumstances (Gaynor, 2008).

Surgery, performed with either therapeutic or diagnostic intent (e.g. tumour biopsy) causes pain. Typically, surgery is associated with acute pain, which follows bodily injury and tends to be self-limiting following appropriate healing.

Adjuvant therapies used in cancer management include radiotherapy and chemotherapy. Although advances in modern treatment planning systems allow for targeted radiation treatment and a clinician may choose appropriate dosing and fractionation, both acute and late side effects can occur, which can result in significant pain (Gaynor, 2008). Due to the advances in modern planning systems allowing for targeted radiation and also appropriate dosing or 'fractionation', side effects are controlled during treatment; however, both acute and late side effects are described.

Acute effects usually occur 2–5 weeks after starting definitive therapy, and resolve within 2–4 weeks. These may include, depending on the site of radiation treatment:

- Skin reaction, either moist or dry desquamation
- Oral mucositis following radiation therapy for nasal or oral tumours (Figure 7.20)
- Proctitis.

Late effects, which occur months to years after treatment is completed, are permanent, irreversible changes. These occur more commonly following hypofractionated or palliative radiation protocols and include:

- Ocular changes, such as keratoconjunctivitis sicca
- Bowel strictures
- Soft tissue fibrosis

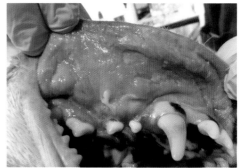

7.20 Acute radiation therapy side effect (mucositis) in the oral cavity of a Dalmatian following treatment for a soft tissue tumour.

- Bone necrosis
- Fistula formation.

Chemotherapy can be associated with pain through the drug infusion itself, if extravasation injury occurs with certain cytotoxics (Figure 7.21). Drug-induced neuropathies, although rarely significant clinically, are reported with cisplatin, vincristine, and vinblastine treatment (Cudden, 2002).

Inference from human reporting

The similar biological behaviour of neoplasia between species and treatment methods employed suggests that tumours or interventions associated with pain in humans are likely to be associated with pain in dogs and cats.

In Figure 7.22, examples of some types of cancers that occur in companion animals and which may be associated with significant pain are listed (Fan, 2014).

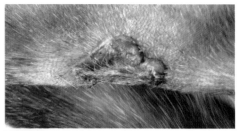

7.21 Full-thickness cutaneous necrosis at the site of extravasation of a chemotherapy drug in a Greyhound.

Musculoskeletal (commonly associated with pain)

- Primary bone and joint tumours (e.g. osteosarcoma, histiocytic sarcoma, synovial cell sarcoma)
- Digital tumours (e.g. melanoma, squamous cell carcinoma)
- Soft tissue tumours (sarcomas) depending on site and extent of infiltrative growth
- Round cell tumours with bone involvement (multiple myeloma, lymphoma)

Head and neck

- Oral tumours (tumours invading bone and soft tissues often traumatized during eating, e.g. malignant melanoma, squamous cell carcinoma, fibrosarcoma, epulides, epitheliotophic lymphoma mucosal lesions)
- Nasal tumours (tumours invading bone, soft tissues and neural tissues, e.g. adenocarcinoma, lymphoma)
- Calvarial tumours
- Ear canal tumours
- Ocular tumours (causing uveitis, e.g. primary or secondary intraocular lymphoma, melanoma, metastatic disease)

Skin and subcutaneous tissues and mucosal surfaces

- Cutaneous metastases (e.g. carcinomas, sarcomas, melanomas)
- Tumour-associated effusions with inflammation (e.g. mesothelioma, carcinomatosis)
- Infiltrative and ulcerated tumours (e.g. soft tissue sarcomas, squamous cell carcinoma, round cell tumours such as epitheliotrophic lymphoma)

Body cavities

- Tumours associated with inflammation (e.g. mast cell tumours – histamine release)
- Tumour-associated visceral bleeding (e.g. haemangiosarcoma, metastatic tumours)

Viscera (associated with capsular stretching or hollow organ obstruction)

- Hepatobiliary and splenic tumours
- Gastrointestinal tumours (e.g. lymphoma, adenocarcinoma, gastrointestinal stromal tumours)
- Urinary tract tumours (e.g. renal carcinoma, lymphoma, prostatic carcinoma, transitional cell carcinoma of the bladder or multiple sites in the upper and lower urinary tract)

Mammary gland

- Mammary tumours (e.g. inflammatory mammary carcinoma, anaplastic carcinoma, osteosarcoma)

Nervous tissue

- Central nervous system (e.g. meningioma, glioma – experience of type and intensity of pain is typically unknown in veterinary species)
- Peripheral nervous system (e.g. brachial plexus tumours)
- Spinal cord compressive lesions (e.g. vertebral body tumours, vertebral body fracture due to tumour infiltration (e.g. myeloma)
- Metastatic disease

7.22 Tumours in companion animals potentially associated with pain. This list is not intended to be exhaustive but provides some common examples.

Assessment of cancer-associated pain

Cancer-associated pain can be described based on its duration, type and localization.

Duration

Acute pain occurs in response to tissue damage and is self-limiting. Examples include surgical pain after tumour removal, acute subcapsular bleeding from a splenic haemangiosarcoma (Figure 7.23) or inflammation due to degranulation and histamine release from a mast cell tumour. Acute pain is often inflammatory in nature.

Chronic pain is pathological and non-protective. It persists beyond initial tissue damage and for a prolonged period of time, generally more than 3 months (International Association for the Study of Pain, 2012). Chronic

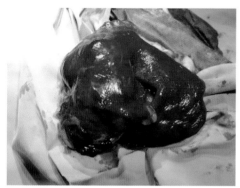

7.23 Splenic mass in a Labrador Retriever associated with an acute haemoabdomen.

pain may be associated with the presence of the tumour itself or may be a complication of cancer surgery (e.g. phantom pain after limb or digit amputation). It can also be associated with the use of adjuvant therapies or the presence of chronic co-morbidities (see above).

Cancer-associated pain may initially be acute but if a tumour is allowed to reach an advanced stage before pain is recognized and managed effectively, a chronic pain state of varying severity may develop (Gaynor, 2008). It is widely recognized that cancer pain therefore more often mimics a chronic rather than an acute pain model (Christo and Mazloomdoost, 2008).

A patient with chronic cancer-associated pain may also experience episodes of breakthrough pain. An example would be the occurrence of a pathological fracture at the site of a primary bone tumour (Figure 7.24). A period of weeks of chronic pain may precede an acute pain episode associated with collapse of the cortical bone.

Type and localization

Cancer-associated pain may be somatic, visceral or neuropathic in origin (Gaynor, 2008). Our understanding of the associated pain sensations is inferred from human reports and by examining an animal's behaviour.

- Somatic pain arises through tumour- or treatment-associated damage to bones, joints, muscle or skin; it is localized, constant and throbbing or aching in nature.

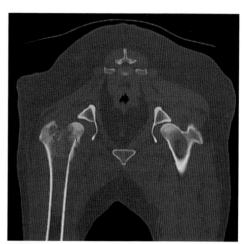

7.24 Pathological fracture in the femoral neck of a Leonberger at the site of a primary bone tumour (osteosarcoma).

- Visceral pain arises from stretching, distension or obstruction of viscera. This type of pain is poorly localized and is associated with a dull, deep, cramping and aching sensation (see Figure 7.22 for examples of tumours that can cause visceral pain).
- Neuropathic pain occurs due to a lesion or disease that affects the tissues of the somatosensory nervous system itself. This type of pain may occur through direct tumour compression or infiltration of nerves or nerve roots or may be associated with tumour treatment. It is associated with a burning, shooting or electric shock-like sensation.

Two other important concepts in the pathophysiology and management of cancer-associated pain are the processes of wind-up and sensitization. Wind-up occurs due to persistent nociceptive input to the spinal cord leading to potentiation of sensory pathways and contributes to sensitization. Sensitization is associated with a state of pain hypersensitivity (termed allodynia and hyperalgesia).

The complexity of managing cancer-associated pain therefore reflects the need to take into account its origin, intensity, duration and the occurrence of additional factors including wind-up and sensitization.

Cancer, inflammation and pain

It is now clear that virtually every tumour mass contains both neoplastic cells and immune cells present in varying densities. Rather than reflecting an attempt by the immune system to eradicate the tumour, there is increasing evidence that these cells and associated inflammation provide vital support to tumour development and progression. In fact, tumour-associated inflammation has recently been designated as a tumour enabling characteristic (Hanahan and Weinberg, 2011). This may explain why tumours may develop at sites of chronic inflammation.

The presence of immune cells in the tumour mass and microenvironment provides compelling evidence for the association of neoplastic growth and relevant inflammatory pain. This suggests widespread benefits of anti-inflammatory medications in both cancer pain management and potentially in the control of tumour progression.

Treatment of cancer-associated pain

The goal of pain management is to provide symptom relief and improve an individual's level of functioning in daily activities and therefore QoL. This is achieved in the following ways:

- Treatment of the tumour
- Provision of analgesia
- Use of complementary methods for palliative care.

It is beyond the scope of this chapter to describe treatment of specific tumour types and therefore we shall focus on provision of analgesia and complementary care.

In 1986, the World Health Organization introduced a three step analgesic 'ladder' that has been widely accepted in human cancer pain management (see Appendix 3). Broadly speaking, as the intensity of pain increases, patients are moved progressively higher on the ladder.

In human medicine, despite the popularity and proposed utility of the pain management ladder, few controlled clinical trials have been performed to support its effectiveness in managing cancer pain (Zech, 1995). In veterinary patients, it therefore forms part of a structured approach to the problem of cancer-associated pain; however, there are several important considerations and limitations:

- Difficulty in establishing the efficacy and safety of individual analgesic medications within and between species
- Difficulty in establishing effective dosing of human medications in veterinary species
- Specific toxicities of medications in veterinary species, e.g. paracetamol can never be given to cats
- Difficulties in drug dosing due to failure of owner or patient compliance; in particular, issues of drug palatability for oral dosing, which may be required long term
- Reformulation of medications or use of liquid preparations may be useful for smaller patients
- There are legal guidelines established by the drug Prescribing Cascade and the use of non-licensed medications is not encouraged
- Consideration of possible drug interactions or treatment-related side effects, especially if a patient is receiving chemotherapy. For example, certain tumours respond well to treatment with corticosteroids, ruling out concurrent use of non-steroidal anti-inflammatory drugs (NSAIDs)
- Consideration of the most appropriate analgesic for an individual's cancer type rather than always following a step-wise approach
- Many dogs and cats are presented with advanced cancer and therefore may be experiencing chronic pain at the time of initial presentation. Specific medications may be more suited to the management of chronic pain.

Throughout this book, specific descriptions of drugs are provided listed in various classes, including dose rates in dogs and cats, which may also be used in the management of cancer-associated pain.

In Figure 7.25, some important considerations are presented regarding the use of medications in this clinical setting. As certain medications are not licensed for use in veterinary species, despite their recognized efficacy, the owners must be informed of the off-label use of these products, their potential efficacy and side effects and provide signed consent following the rules dictated by the drug Prescribing Cascade.

Therapy	Considerations
Non-steroidal anti-inflammatory drugs (NSAIDs) (COX-1 and -2 inhibitors; level 1 analgesia) Examples: meloxicam, piroxicam (not licensed in the UK), carprofen, ketoprofen, tolfenamic acid, etodolac, firocoxib, deracoxib, robenacoxib, cimicoxib, mavacoxib	• Highly effective in managing acute and chronic cancer-associated inflammatory pain in veterinary patients. Range of drugs and formulations available • Check national product licence for species-specific use, dose and duration of therapy • Adverse effects (gastrointestinal, renal, coagulopathies, hepatotoxicity) must be monitored for in long-term use of these products and may be increased due to concurrent treatment with chemotherapy or co-morbidities in elderly patients. Many chemotherapy drugs are also associated with significant side effects of gastrointestinal toxicity • Care with hepatotoxic drugs including lomustine, renally excreted or potentially nephrotoxic drugs including platinum drugs in dogs and doxorubicin (and other anthracyclines) in cats and tyrosine kinase inhibitors (e.g. toceranib, masitinib) • Contraindicated in patients concurrently receiving corticosteroids for cancer management (e.g. lymphoma, mast cell tumour) • May be contraindicated in patients with uncontrolled hypercalcaemia of malignancy (e.g. lymphoma, anal sac adenocarcinoma, multiple myeloma) due to compromised renal blood flow and dehydration increasing renal toxicity • COX inhibition may however have antineoplastic as well as anti-inflammatory action in certain neoplasms such as transitional cell carcinoma of the bladder (Fulkerson and Knapp, 2015). NSAIDs may also be used in continuous low-dose oral (metronomic) chemotherapy protocols for the management of a range of tumours in combination with alkylating agents (Biller, 2014) • Piroxicam suppositories are useful in the management of colorectal adenomas and limit the extent of systemic adverse effects (Knottenbelt, Simpson and Tasker, 2000)
Endogenous cannabinoid-1 (CB-1) receptor and vanilloid subtype-1 (TRPV1) receptor activator and inhibitor of descending serotonergic pathways (level 1 analgesia) Examples: paracetamol	• Paracetamol should **NEVER** be administered to cats as they lack cytochrome P-450 dependent enzymes required for its metabolism (Booth, 1982) • Side effects in dogs are rare and much less frequent than with NSAIDs (above) but when extrapolated from the human literature can include similar toxicities including hepatotoxicity • The mechanism of action of paracetamol is complex; it has both analgesic and antipyretic effects but minimal anti-inflammatory activity • Synergistic effect reported with opioids and can be used cautiously with other NSAIDs or corticosteroids to manage breakthrough pain • Can be used for patients that do not tolerate NSAIDs or patients receiving glucocorticoids as chemotherapy • Cheap and readily available across the counter but only as unlicensed products. Available as a paediatric suspension for smaller patients and also as an injectable solution (Perfalgan). For oral suspensions containing sorbitol, this sweetening agent may have laxative effects in dogs. Suspensions containing xylitol should never be given to dogs • Can reduce fever in neutropenic patients after chemotherapy • May be useful for both acute and chronic cancer-associated pain

7.25 Important considerations regarding the use of medications in a clinical setting. (continues) ▶

Therapy	Considerations
Combination products (level 1/2 analgesia) Examples: predno-leucotropin (PLT, prednisolone + cinchophen), Pardale-V (paracetamol + codeine)	• PLT is a compound preparation containing cinchophen and prednisolone and may be a cheap and effective analgesic combination in cancer-associated pain including bone pain; it is generally well tolerated • Pardale-V is cheap and widely available and is a licensed product in dogs. **It should never be given to cats** • Long-term side effects are poorly documented • Recommended dose of Pardale-V contains a relatively high dose of paracetamol and therefore monitor for side effects including gastrointestinal. Licensed for 5 days of therapy • Codeine is an opiate with weak mu-receptor agonist activity
Corticosteroids Examples: prednisolone, dexamethasone, methylprednisolone	• Provide excellent anti-inflammatory effects and have additional antineoplastic action in certain neoplasms (e.g. lymphoma, mast cell tumours, leukaemias, and multiple myeloma) • Weak analgesics but reduction of inflammation can have significant beneficial effects • Adverse effects are common and include iatrogenic hyperadrenocorticism, muscle wasting and gastrointestinal adverse events • Effective in managing hypoglycaemia medically, a paraneoplastic effect associated with certain tumours, including insulinoma
Opioids (full and partial mu-opioid receptor agonists; level 2/3 analgesia) Examples: buprenorphine, codeine, methadone, fentanyl, tramadol	• Best used 'to effect' • Considered a stalwart of cancer pain relief. Deliver dose dependent, reliable and predictable analgesic effects when using full mu agonists • Particularly useful for acute pain management in hospitalized patients. Effective use in chronic pain and long-term pain management is thwarted by lack of availability of suitable medications and formulations for use at home • Oral transmucosal buprenorphine can be useful for management of feline pain at home; this route of administration is not thought to be as effective in dogs (Robertson et al., 2003) • Codeine is a weak analgesic with a risk of gastrointestinal upset – therefore it is not recommended for use alone • Fentanyl patches are useful to provide full opioid analgesia without the need for injectable drugs; however, transcutaneous absorption of the drug is very unreliable • Tramadol is not licensed in veterinary species and its effects may be unpredictable based on individual patient metabolism. It is metabolized to its active form and works through serotonin and noradrenalin reuptake inhibition and is a weak mu opioid receptor agonist. It is often used in combination with NSAIDs or corticosteroids and is useful in the management of chronic cancer-associated pain. • In cats, high concentrations of active metabolites mean lower doses and a longer dosing interval are recommended
Alpha-2 adrenergic agonists Examples: medetomidine, dexmedetomidine	• Require parenteral administration • May be administered as an infusion • When administered at low doses can provide effective analgesia with arousable sedation • These drugs may have significant cardiovascular effects
N-methyl-D-aspartate (NMDA) antagonists Examples: ketamine, amantadine	• Provides reasonable analgesia. Plays a role in reducing central sensitization and 'wind-up'. Particularly useful for pre-emptive cancer analgesia and can be effective at low doses as a constant rate infusion during and after surgery to reduce postoperative pain and opioid requirements, e.g. following limb amputation (Wagner et al., 2002) • Amantadine has the added advantage of being available as an oral medication. It can reduce chronic post-surgical pain in amputees (Pud et al., 1998) • Can be used in combination with NSAIDs for effective management particularly of chronic pain

7.25 (continued) Important considerations regarding the use of medications in a clinical setting. (continues) ▶

Therapy	Considerations
Anti-convulsants Examples: gabapentin, pregabalin	• Especially useful for chronic and neuropathic cancer pain • Can be effective in combination therapy, e.g. with concurrent NSAIDs and/or tramadol
Antihistamines Examples: chlorphenamine, loratidine	• Effective for specific tumour types, e.g. mast cell tumours where inflammation may be associated with histamine release • May reduce radiation-induced dermatitis • Available as injectable and oral formulations • May also have anti-nausea and appetite stimulatory effects; therefore useful in patients receiving chemotherapy
Sedatives and antidepressants Examples: amitriptyline, clomipramine	• May be useful for the management of chronic and neuropathic pain • Alter re-uptake of serotonin and noradrenaline in the central nervous system
Local analgesic techniques Examples: intercostal nerve blocks, intrapleural local anaesthetic, brachial plexus nerve block, opioid or local anaesthetics administered by epidural injection or infusion catheter, craniofacial (maxillary, mandibular, mental, infraorbital nerve blocks), 'wound soaker' local anaesthetic catheters	• Generally useful for the management of acute or surgical pain. Can be highly effective in the short term and are associated with minimal systemic side effects • Some techniques require specialist knowledge and expertise • Lidocaine 5% patches: may be suitable for local bruising, surgical wounds. No apparent systemic toxic effects have been noted. Must be stapled in place and hair clipped for contact (Weiland et al., 2006)
Radiotherapy	• Highly effective at 'palliative' doses for the management of osteolytic bone pain in human cancer patients (Fan, 2014). Mechanism of action is complex but may be by inducing apoptosis in malignant osteoblasts and activated osteoclasts and reduced secretion of prostaglandins by tumour-associated inflammatory cells. Also has direct anti-neoplastic activity (Milner et al., 2004) • Its use is well described for management of bone cancer pain in dogs with osteosarcoma, where amputation is declined. May be useful for primary tumours that invade bone, e.g. squamous cell carcinoma of the oral cavity in cats, or for management of secondary bone metastases, e.g. from prostatic carcinoma in dogs. Can be highly effective in the treatment of round cell tumours with bone involvement (lymphoma, myeloma) • Radiotherapy may be the chosen primary treatment modality for tumours associated with pain, e.g. brain tumours or nasal tumours • Requires referral for access to specialist equipment and treatment planning • Expensive • Most palliative protocols involve 2–4 individual treatments delivered 1 week apart. Five daily fraction protocols are also employed • Late side effects theoretically of greater concern although patients may not live long enough to develop these • May be used in combination with other analgesic drugs, bisphosphonates and chemotherapy agents. Radiotherapy can enhance analgesic drug effectiveness by reducing tumour bulk (e.g. in intracranial tumours or mediastinal tumours)

7.25 (continued) Important considerations regarding the use of medications in a clinical setting. (continues) ▶

Therapy	Considerations
Bisphosphonates Examples: pamidronate, clodronate, zoledronate, aledronate	• Reduce bone pain and the risk of pathological fractures in humans with malignant skeletal lesions (Fan, 2014) • Mechanism of action is principally through induction of osteoclast apoptosis, attenuating pathological bone resorption (Spugnini *et al.*, 2009). They also promote apoptosis, inhibit angiogenesis, cancer cell division and osteoclastogenesis • Used for relief of osteolytic bone pain in veterinary patients from primary and metastatic tumours and can help to control hypercalcaemia of malignancy, e.g. with round cell tumours (lymphoma, myeloma) and anal sac adenocarcinoma • Intravenous pamidronate, as a single agent or in combination with palliative radiotherapy or and chemotherapy, has been shown to successfully alleviate bone cancer pain and increase weight bearing in dogs (Fan, 2004). The use of oral bisphosphonates and injectable zoledronate has also been reported in canine osteosarcoma (Gaynor, 2000; Tomlin *et al.*, 2000) • Both oral and intravenous formulations are available. Amino-bisphosphonates are the most potent • There may be poor absorption of oral bisphosphonates from the gastrointestinal tract, especially in the presence of food (Spugnini *et al.*, 2009) • Oesophageal injury can occur if the oral medication is not swallowed quickly and completely, leading to prolonged contact with the mucosa • There is a theoretical risk of renal injury associated with use of these drugs in dogs but this has not been clearly demonstrated; however, monitoring renal function during use is recommended
Complementary therapies including traditional acupuncture and electroacupuncture	• Used for acute and chronic pain, lymphoedema and reduction of post-surgical swelling in human medicine. May reduce treatment-related nausea • Side effects are minimal • For further information see Chapter 6 and specialist texts (Sliwa and Marciniak, 1999)
Other physical therapies including massage, hot and cold therapy, laser therapy	• Physical supportive therapy is expanding in veterinary medicine, however the evidence base is still sparse. Despite this many of these therapies have been shown to be beneficial in the human field (Looney, 2010)
Nutrition and supplementary therapies Examples: omega 3 free fatty acids, omega 6 fatty acids	• Omega 3 free fatty acids have been shown to decrease joint inflammation in osteoarthritis. They have also been shown to be beneficial in *in vitro* and *in vivo* studies in humans and dogs with cancer (such as lymphoma, nasal tumours, haemangiosarcoma and osteosarcoma) • Omega 6 fatty acids may be beneficial in the management of epitheliotrophic lymphoma in dogs by reducing painful skin inflammation
Topical therapies Examples: steroids, antihistamines, aqueous agents, silver sulfadiazine, aloe, honey, colloidal oatmeal, capsaicin	• May be useful to aid healing and reduce inflammation in some oral, mucosal, mucocutaneous or cutaneous lesions (secondary to cancer or its treatment) • Seek specialist advice before applying any topical therapy to open surgical wounds or in the case of radiotherapy side effects
Surgical techniques Examples: neuroablative techniques	• Usually a last resort and infrequently used due to other quality of life issues. These techniques may be explored more over the next decade in both human and veterinary medicine

7.25 (continued) Important considerations regarding the use of medications in a clinical setting.

Monitoring pain in the cancer patient

Veterinary surgeons treating small animal patients with cancer are perfectly positioned to study and improve the management of cancer-associated pain. The practice of oncology requires detailed and open communication between veterinary surgeon and owner, a level of communication that is required to fully evaluate the changing pattern of a patient's pain experience. Frequent revisits are typical in cancer management and allow repeat pain assessments to be made in addition to assessment of response to analgesic therapy. Modifications should be made to therapy whenever required. Pain assessment should be carried out and the results accurately recorded for future comparison in 'every patient, every time' it visits the oncology clinic.

A number of studies have attempted to evaluate health-related QoL questionnaires as assessment tools for animals with cancer and more specifically cancer pain (Yazbek and Fantoni, 2005). The authors are currently exploring the use of a daily quality of life diary in their cancer clinics. Questions are answered and scores assigned in four broad categories, attempting to assess the following semi-objectively:

- Clinical signs of disease and side effects from therapy
- Physical activity
- Social interaction with the owner and other animals
- Psychological impact of the diagnosis and progress of treatment on the owner.

Early trials show good owner engagement and a possible benefit of continuous assessment over previous intermittent questionnaire-based evaluations.

References and further reading

Bergman PJ (2012) Paraneoplastic hypercalcaemia. *Topics in Companion Animal Medicine* **27**, 156–158

Biller B (2014) Metronomic chemotherapy in veterinary patients with cancer: Rethinking the targets and strategies of chemotherapy. *Veterinary Clinics of North America: Small Animal Practice* **44**, 817–829

Booth NH (1982) Non-narcotic analgesics. In: *Veterinary Pharmacology and Therapeutics, 5th edn*, ed. NH Booth and LE McDonald, pp. 297–320. Iowa State University Press, Ames

Christo PJ and Mazloomdoost D (2008) Cancer pain and analgesia. *Annals of The New York Academy of Science* **1138**, 278–298

Cudden PA (2002) Acquired canine peripheral neuropathies. *Veterinary Clinics of North America: Small Animal Practice* **32**, 207–249

Dobson JM, Samuel S, Milstein H *et al.* (2002) Canine neoplasia in the UK: estimates of incidence rates from a population of insured dogs. *Journal of Small Animal Practice* **43**, 240–246

Fan TM (2014) Pain management in veterinary patients with cancer. *Veterinary Clinics of North America: Small Animal Practice* **44**, 989–1001

Fulkerson CM and Knapp DW (2015) Management of transitional cell carcinoma of the urinary bladder in dogs: A review. *Veterinary Journal* **205**, 217–225

Gaynor JS (2000) Acupuncture for management of pain. *Veterinary Clinics of North America: Small Animal Practice* **30**, 875–884

Gaynor JS (2008) Control of cancer pain in veterinary patients. *Veterinary Clinics of North America: Small Animal Practice* **30**, 1429–1448

Goblirsch M, Mathews W, Lynch C *et al.* (2004) Radiation treatment decreases bone cancer pain, osteolysis and tumour size. *Radiation Research* **161**, 228–234

Hanahan D and Weinberg RA (2011) Hallmarks of cancer: the next generation. *Cell* **144**, 646–674

Hansen BD (2003) Assessment of pain in dogs: veterinary clinical studies. *Institute for Laboratory Animal Research* **44**, 197–205

Keefe FA, Abernethy AP and Campbell CL (2005) Psychological approaches to understanding and treating disease related pain. *Annual Review of Psychology* **56**, 1–22

Knottenbelt CM, Simpson JW, Tasker S *et al.* (2000) Preliminary clinical observations on the use of piroxicam in the management of rectal tubulopapillary polyp. *Journal of Small Animal Practice* **41**, 393–397

Looney A (2010) Oncology pain in veterinary patients. *Topics in Companion Animal Medicine* **25**, 32–44

Mason SL, Maddox TW, Lillis SM *et al.* (2013) Late presentation of canine nasal tumours in a UK referral hospital and treatment outcomes. *Journal of Small Animal Practice* **54**, 347–353

Milner RJ, Farese J, Henry CJ *et al.* (2004) Bisphosphonates and cancer. *Journal of Veterinary Internal Medicine* **18**, 597–604

Muir WW and Gaynor JS (2009) Pain behaviours. In: *Handbook of Veterinary Pain Management 2nd edn*, ed. WW Muir and JS Gaynor, pp. 62–77. Mosby Elsevier, St Louis

Pud D, Eisenberg E, Spitzer A *et al.* (1998) The NMDA receptor antagonist amantadine reduces surgical neuropathic pain in cancer patients: a double blind, randomised, placebo controlled trial. *Pain* **75**, 349–354

Robertson SA, Taylor PM and Sear JW (2003) Systemic uptake of buprenorphine by cats after oral mucosal administration. *Veterinary Record* **152**, 675–678

Schwab JM, Schluesener HJ and Laufer S (2003) Just another COX or the solitary elusive target of paracetamol? *Lancet* **361**, 981–982

Sliwa JA and Marciniak C (1999) Palliative care and rehabilitation of cancer patients. *Cancer Treatment and Research* **100**, 75–89

Spugnini EP, Vincenzi G, Caruso A *et al.* (2009) Zoledronic acid for the treatment of appendicular osteosarcoma in a dog. *Journal of Small Animal Practice* **50**, 44–46

Tomlin JL, Sturgeon C, Pead MJ *et al.* (2000) Use of the bisphosphonate drug alendronate for palliative management of osteosarcoma in two dogs. *Veterinary Record* **147**, 129–132

Velikova G, Stark D and Selby P (1999) Quality of life instruments in oncology. *European Journal of Cancer and Clinical Oncology* **35**, 1571–1580

Wagner AE, Walton JA, Hellyer PW *et al.* (2002) Use of low doses of ketamine administered by constant rate infusion as an adjunct for post-operative analgesia in dogs. *Journal of the American Veterinary Medical Association* **221**, 72–74

Weiland L, Croubels S, Baert K *et al.* (2006) Pharmacokinetics of a lidocaine patch 5% in dogs. *Journal of Veterinary Medicine Series* **A53**, 34–39

Yazbek KVB and Fantoni DT (2005) Validity of a health-related quality of life scale for dogs with signs of pain secondary to cancer. *Journal of the American Veterinary Medical Association* **8**, 1354–1358

Zech DF (1995) Validation of World Health Organization guidelines for cancer pain relief: a 10-year prospective study. *Pain* **63**, 65–76

Useful websites

International Association for the Study of Pain – IASP Taxonomy:
www.iasp-pain.org/Education/Contentaspx?ItemNumber=1698

Morris Animal Foundation:
www.morrisanimalfoundation.org

WHO's cancer pain ladder for adults:
www.who.int/cancer/palliative/painladder/en

Case examples

In the following case examples we try to demonstrate how a systematic approach to the assessment of cancer-associated pain in a veterinary patient provided a framework for planning an effective pain management protocol.

Through examining the local and systemic extent of a tumour and considering the tumour's growth rate and growth pattern, conclusions could be made regarding the possible nature of the tumour-associated pain. The characterization of the pain with respect to its type, localization, duration and intensity helped to guide therapy.

Case example 1: Transitional cell carcinoma

HISTORY AND PRESENTATION

A 7-year-old male neutered French Bulldog with transitional cell carcinoma of the prostate and bladder. Disease localized to the lower urinary tract based on ultrasound imaging, with no evidence of bone metastases.

CLINICAL SIGNS

Marked dysuria, stranguria, haematuria and faecal tenesmus.

TYPES OF PAIN

Moderate to severe, complex pain: inflammatory and visceral pain components; probable chronic pain associated with central sensitization with the potential for neuropathic pain.

CLINICAL EXAMINATION

Enlarged and painful prostate on rectal examination. Concurrent urinary tract infection was also diagnosed following clinical pathology.

→ CASE EXAMPLE 1 CONTINUED

ANALGESIC PLAN

Analgesic ladder level 2: initially, meloxicam (0.1 mg/kg orally q24h) and tramadol (2 mg/kg orally q12h), followed by amitriptyline (1 mg/kg orally q12h; **discontinuing tramadol** to prevent potential serotonin syndrome); antibiotic therapy (co-amoxiclav 15 mg/kg orally q12h); faecal softeners (lactulose, 5 ml/meal up to q8h); physical touch by the owner during particularly painful episodes of straining.

Tips from the authors

Transitional cell carcinoma is a highly invasive tumour; involvement of the prostate is commonly seen in male dogs. Metastatic sites can include lungs, liver and bone. Concurrent bacterial cystitis is common, especially in female dogs and contributes to inflammatory pain. The tumour causes muscle damage, nerve ending compression and infiltration and visceral outflow obstruction and distension as it occurs commonly in the trigone of the bladder and proximal urethra. The tumour has often been present for a period of time prior to diagnosis, with clinical signs frequently assumed to be associated with a urinary tract infection rather than neoplasia.

NSAIDs improve clinical signs rapidly in a high percentage of patients and through COX-2 inhibition may have anti-cancer benefits. The tumour may be managed with a range of systemic chemotherapy agents with a low to moderate response rate. Other medications that may be considered in the management of this condition include gabapentin (10 mg/kg orally q8–12h) for chronic pain and diazepam (2–5 mg dose orally q8–12h) to reduce acute urethral spasm. Urinary retention can be a side effect of amitriptyline in canine patients.

Case example 2: Soft tissue sarcoma with spinal cord involvement

PRESENTATION AND HISTORY

A 10-year-old, female neutered Labrador Retriever diagnosed with a poorly differentiated soft tissue sarcoma affecting the spinous process of T7 with spinal canal invasion and severe spinal cord compression (diagnosis made following MRI and surgical biopsy with histopathology). The disease was localized with no evidence of metastases.

CLINICAL SIGNS

Pelvic limb ataxia and vocalization, progressing to pelvic limb hemiparesis.

TYPES OF PAIN

Severe and complex pain; acute somatic inflammatory pain; chronic pain associated with central sensitization; neuropathic pain.

CLINICAL EXAMINATION

Based on the neurological examination the lesion was localized to the T3–L3 spinal cord segments although a multifocal localization was not excluded.

→ **CASE EXAMPLE 2 CONTINUED**

ANALGESIC PLAN

- Analgesic ladder level 3 initially: methadone (0.1–0.3 mg/kg i.v. q4h); radiotherapy (20 fractions of radiotherapy to a total dose of 50 Gy); prednisolone (0.5 mg/kg orally q12h); gabapentin (10–15 mg/kg orally q8h); fentanyl patch placement (changed every 72 hours); zoledronate (4 mg over 15 minutes with 0.9% NaCl i.v. infusion).

- Analgesic ladder level 2 for management at home: paracetamol/codeine (33 mg/kg Pardale-V orally q8–12h); tramadol (4 mg/kg orally q12h); gabapentin (10–15 mg/kg orally q8h); prednisolone (oral tapering dose).

Tips from the authors

In this case the invasive nature of the sarcoma was associated with severe pain and neurological dysfunction. Euthanasia was offered from the outset given the poor overall prognosis. However, the owners wanted to pursue treatment if her QoL could be improved and maintained.

Case example 3: Appendicular osteosarcoma

HISTORY AND PRESENTATION

A 2-year-old male neutered Labrador Retriever was diagnosed with appendicular osteosarcoma. There was local osteolytic bone disease at the time of presentation with no nodal or distant metastases. The right forelimb was amputated and a course of chemotherapy with carboplatin implemented. Thirty days after amputation, spontaneous pain episodes began and were subsequently documented in a pain diary kept by the owner.

TYPES OF PAIN

Severe, intense, short duration but multiple episodes daily. Possible inflammatory somatic pain at surgical site; clinical signs most compatible with neuropathic pain including central sensitization (leading to hyperalgesia).

ANALGESIA PLAN

Analgesic ladder level 2: meloxicam (0.1 mg/kg orally q24h); tramadol (2–4 mg/kg orally q8–12h); gabapentin (10 mg/kg orally q8h); verbal and physical comforting by the owner following pain episodes.

Tips from the authors

Phantom limb pain is under-reported in veterinary amputees but occurs in the majority of human amputees. It is part of a complex of symptoms that can also include stump pain (neuroma formation at the surgical site) and phantom sensations. It is chronic in nature, neuropathic in origin (although local neuroma formation may be concurrent with local inflammation) and appears to respond well, as in this case, to gabapentin therapy. Chronic pain prior to amputation may contribute to wind-up and central sensitization. Multimodal pre- and perioperative analgesia appears to reduce the incidence and severity of phantom pain in human amputees.

Case example 4: Cutaneous epitheliotrophic lymphoma

HISTORY AND PRESENTATION

A 10-year-old male neutered Jack Russell Terrier was diagnosed with cutaneous epitheliotrophic lymphoma; widespread local ulcerative lesions generalized to the skin and oral mucosa with nodal and hepatic involvement (Figure 7.26).

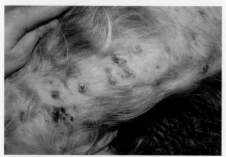

7.26 Papular, pustular and nodular skin lesions associated with epitheliotrophic lymphoma in a terrier dog.

CLINICAL SIGNS

Severe pruritus, pain on touching the skin, hypersensitivity to stimuli including subcutaneous injections, anorexia due to gingival pain on eating, facial oedema due to lymphadenopathy, secondary pyoderma.

TYPES OF PAIN

Severe and debilitating; inflammatory somatic pain, visceral pain (organ distension: lymph nodes, liver), chronic pain leading to central sensitization and allodynia on the skin surface.

ANALGESIC PLAN

Analgesic ladder level 3: methadone (0.4 mg/kg i.v. q4–8h) in hospital then specific anti-neoplastic therapy including systemic glucocorticoids (dexamethasone 0.2 mg/kg i.v. q24h) and L-asparaginase (400 IU/kg s.c. once). Reduced to level 2 for management at home with oral glucocorticoids (prednisolone 2 mg/kg orally q24h); paracetamol and codeine (paracetamol 10 mg/kg orally q8h); gabapentin (10 mg/kg orally q8h); antibiotics (cephalexin 15 mg/kg orally q12h); antihistamines (chlorphenamine 4 mg orally q8h) and topical local anaesthetic ointment on more painful skin lesions (EMLA cream (lidocaine 2.5% + prilocaine), topically q12h, avoiding ulcerated bleeding lesions and covered with a patch to prevent oral ingestion of cream).

Tips from the authors

Epitheliotrophic lymphoma is a slowly progressive form of cutaneous neoplasia that in advanced cases can involve nodal and distant sites of visceral progression. It is associated with significant chronic pain associated with the skin and mucous membranes. Advanced lesions are often widespread and ulcerated. This form of lymphoma is poorly responsive to chemotherapy and carries a very poor long-term prognosis. Palliation of pain requires consideration of the extent and severity of the lesions and can be managed with oral medications or in the most severe cases, localized palliative radiotherapy.

Chapter 7i

Pain in rabbits

Joanna Hedley

Despite a marked increase in the number of pet rabbits kept in the UK, our ability to interpret the behaviour of this prey species is still lacking. Signs of illness and of pain are generally hidden until disease is advanced. Careful and prolonged observation is required (ideally while the rabbit is unaware that it is being observed), as even subtle changes in behaviour may be significant.

It can, however, be difficult to distinguish between behavioural changes due to stress or underlying disease from those due to pain. An added challenge is that these changes may be non-specific, such as a reduction in the range of normal behaviours seen in the healthy pain-free animal, rather than the rabbit exhibiting specific pain-associated behaviours. The range of normal behaviours will vary for each individual, so thorough history-taking is required. Response to pain may also vary depending on whether the pain is acute or chronic and visceral or somatic, as shown by the case examples below. In laboratory situations, pain scoring systems such as the Rabbit Grimace Scale have been used to provide a more objective method of assessing pain, and these may also be useful to help evaluate rabbits in clinical practice (Keating *et al.*, 2012) (Figure 7.27).

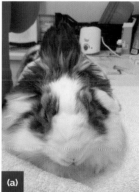
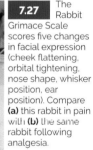
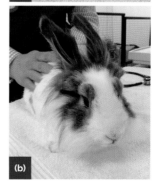

7.27 The Rabbit Grimace Scale scores five changes in facial expression (cheek flattening, orbital tightening, nose shape, whisker position, ear position). Compare **(a)** this rabbit in pain with **(b)** the same rabbit following analgesia.

Due to the difficulties in assessing pain in this species, analgesics should be used for any potentially painful procedure or disease condition, even if no obvious signs of pain are apparent. Doses may vary significantly from those used in other animals and so should be checked in each case. Suggested doses are listed in Figure 7.28. It is, however, important to appreciate that none of these drugs are licensed for rabbits and suggested doses are often anecdotal or based on studies in young healthy laboratory individuals. It is up to clinicians to use their own judgement to tailor these doses to the individual patient. In addition, appropriate hospitalization and good nursing care are always important considerations for a painful rabbit. Comfortable bedding, tempting food (within easy reach) and calm quiet surroundings should all be provided, preferably away from predator species. Behaviour should be regularly assessed, ideally by the same person for consistency, and analgesia adjusted as necessary.

References and further reading

Barter L (2011) Rabbit analgesia. *Veterinary Clinics of North America: Exotic Animal Practice* **14**, 93–104

Delk KW, Carpenter JW, KuKanich B, Nietfeld JC and Kohles M (2014) Pharmacokinetics of meloxicam administered orally to rabbits (*Oryctolagus cuniculus*) for 29 days. *American Journal of Veterinary Research* **75**, 195–199

Hawkins MG and Pascoe PJ (2012) Anesthesia, analgesia and sedation of small mammals. In: *Ferrets, Rabbits and Rodents: Clinical Medicine and Surgery, 3rd edn*, ed. K Quesenberry and J Carpenter, pp. 429–451. Saunders, Missouri

Johnson-Delaney C and Harcourt-Brown F (2013) Analgesia and postoperative care. In: *BSAVA Manual of Rabbit Surgery, Dentistry and Imaging*, ed. F Harcourt-Brown and J Chitty, pp. 26–38. BSAVA Publications, Gloucester

Keating SC, Thomas AA, Flecknell PA and Leach MC (2012) Evaluation of EMLA cream for preventing pain during tattooing of rabbits: changes in physiological, behavioural and facial expression responses. *PLoS One* **7**, e44437

Meredith A (2014) *BSAVA Small Animal Formulary, 9th edn – Part B: Exotic Pets*. BSAVA Publications, Gloucester

Shafford HL and Schadt JC (2008) Effect of buprenorphine on the cardiovascular and respiratory response to visceral pain in conscious rabbits. *Veterinary Anaesthesia and Analgesia* **35**, 333–340

Souza MJ, Greenacre CB and Cox SK (2008) Pharmacokinetics of orally administered tramadol in domestic rabbits (*Oryctolagus cuniculus*). *American Journal of Veterinary Research* **69**, 979–982

Weaver LA, Blaze CA, Linder DE, Andrutis KA and Karas AZ (2010) A model for clinical evaluation of perioperative analgesia in rabbits (*Oryctolagus cuniculus*). *Journal of the American Association for Laboratory Animal Science* **49**, 845–851

Wenger S (2012) Anaesthesia and analgesia in rabbits and rodents. *Journal of Exotic Pet Medicine* **21**, 7–16

Drug	Dose
Meloxicam	0.3–0.6 mg/kg s.c., orally q12–24h
Buprenorphine	0.03–0.05 mg/kg s.c., i.m., i.v. q6–12h
Morphine	0.5–5 mg/kg s.c., i.m. q2–4h – care is advised using high dosages in sick patients. The lower end of the dose range is recommended for most cases
Methadone	0.3–0.7 mg/kg slow i.v., i.m.
Tramadol	5–10 mg/kg orally q8–12h
Gabapentin	2–5 mg/kg orally q8h

7.28 Suggested drug doses for analgesia in rabbits. It is important to note that there are no drugs licensed for analgesia in rabbits in UK. All drugs should therefore be prescribed by the clinician according to the Cascade. The author normally recommends beginning at the top end of the dosing range except where indicated.

Case example 1: Reduced gastrointestinal motility (gut stasis)

Gut stasis is a common presentation seen in the pet rabbit, with many different causes. Pain may occur as a result of gastrointestinal distension or, alternatively, gastrointestinal motility may be reduced as a consequence of pain. Providing adequate analgesia is therefore vital to break the cycle in these patients.

HISTORY AND PRESENTATION

A rabbit with gut stasis may present as an acute emergency or, alternatively, the owner may have noticed subtle behavioural changes over the preceding few days.

CLINICAL SIGNS

Reduced or abnormal faecal output is usually the main sign, often in association with a reduced appetite.

SIGNS OF PAIN

Early subtle signs of pain seen in the rabbit with gut stasis may include slightly depressed behaviour, out of character aggressive behaviour, hiding away, sitting hunched up or bruxism. More severe signs of pain include a lack of interest in surroundings and stretching flat out with the abdomen pressed to the floor (Figure 7.29). Respiratory rate and heart rate may also increase, although not consistently in every case.

TREATMENT

No matter what the underlying cause, if the condition is left to progress untreated, pain will increase as the gastrointestinal system distends. Supportive treatment, including

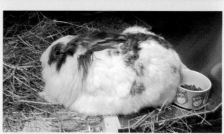

7.29 This rabbit shows signs of severe abdominal pain as shown by the hunched posture and abdomen pressed to the floor.

analgesia, fluid therapy, and supplementary feeding ± prokinetics, will be indicated and, if an obstruction is suspected, surgical intervention may be necessary.

For rabbits with mild signs of pain, non-steroidal anti-inflammatory drugs (NSAIDs) are a useful treatment choice. Meloxicam is the most commonly used NSAID in rabbits, either by the oral or parenteral route. Although relatively high doses may be better tolerated in rabbits than in many other species, the risks of renal toxicity or gastrointestinal ulceration should be considered, especially in the hypovolaemic patient, and doses tailored to the individual case.

For rabbits with moderate to severe signs of pain, a partial opioid agonist such as buprenorphine may be used, often in combination with an NSAID. There have been concerns about the effects of opioids reducing gastrointestinal motility but, in practice, the beneficial analgesic effects more than outweigh the potential negative effects on gastrointestinal motility for these patients. Doses should, however, be tailored to the individual to avoid excessive sedation.

Case example 2: Fractured limb

HISTORY AND PRESENTATION

Orthopaedic injuries are not uncommon in rabbits, especially giant breeds. There may be a known history of trauma, such as the rabbit having fallen or been dropped. Alternatively, as rabbits often spend large periods of the day unsupervised, the owner may have returned home to find the animal non-weight bearing on one limb.

CLINICAL SIGNS

The most obvious clinical sign is usually lameness and a reluctance to move around. The limb may be held up or at an abnormal angle. However, some animals will continue to weight bear despite severe fractures. On clinical examination, a fracture may be palpated.

SIGNS OF PAIN

Signs of pain are not always obvious and can be difficult to assess in a consulting room situation. The animal may appear depressed and reluctant to move, but many rabbits initially continue to eat, pass faeces and may not even react to palpation of the fracture site.

TREATMENT

If left untreated, the rabbit is likely to show reduced activity and this may progress to reduced appetite and reduced faecal output. Both NSAIDs and opioids are likely to be indicated for these patients. Full opioid agonists such as morphine and methadone may be used successfully for initial stabilization of these patients. The fracture will need to be immobilized if possible and the patient confined to a clean padded area to minimize further pain and injury.

Longer-term, if surgical repair is performed, multimodal analgesia should be considered including local anaesthetic blocks, epidural analgesia and ketamine constant rate infusions. Additional help with grooming and feeding is often required during this time.

Case example 3: Dental abscess

Dental abscesses may be seen in the pet rabbit as a consequence of chronic dental disease or following a traumatic injury or foreign body.

HISTORY AND PRESENTATION

The rabbit may be presented for obvious clinical signs, with the owner having detected a facial mass. Alternatively, abscesses may sometimes be detected incidentally on a routine health check.

CLINICAL SIGNS

Rabbits may have a reduced appetite or be favouring softer food types. Drooling may be noted and the animal may choose to chew preferentially on the unaffected side. However, many patients

→ CASE EXAMPLE 3 CONTINUED

continue to eat normally even with fairly large facial abscesses and appetite may only be reduced as a consequence of concurrent dental disease.

SIGNS OF PAIN

Signs of pain are not always apparent with dental abscesses. Some rabbits may react to palpation of the abscess site or strongly resist oral medication. Grooming behaviour may also be reduced leading to secondary skin problems.

TREATMENT

Abscesses can grow quickly into large space-occupying lesions often involving multiple teeth and underlying bone. Surgical treatment will usually be required, although in most cases ongoing medical management will also be necessary. Adequate analgesia is vital and initial treatment with a non-steroidal anti-inflammatory drug ± buprenorphine is recommended.

For long-term treatment of ongoing abscesses, tramadol or gabapentin may also be considered for use in rabbits. Effective doses have not yet been proven in this species, but clinician experience appears to indicate a reduction in signs of pain in many individuals.

Chapter 7j

Pain in birds

Steve Smith

Recognition and evaluation of pain in birds

Effective assessment, treatment and prevention of pain in birds remains challenging. Most birds are prey species and mask the signs of pain to reduce the chance of predation or to prevent movement down their hierarchy. Birds often fail to demonstrate outward signs that are typically associated with pain in other animals, for example birds exhibit minimal facial expression; a characteristic often used to aid pain assessment. There are also intra-species differences in pain sensitivity and even genetic variability. For example, response to pain has been demonstrated at the individual level in different strains of chickens (Hughes, 1990). Behavioural changes can be cryptic and subtle and do not manifest uniformly among different types of bird (Figure 7.30). Knowledge of normal species-specific behaviour, as well as individual behavioural characteristics, are important, hence, owners are often best at detecting early signs of pain and assessing response to analgesia.

Some behaviours that birds exhibit, which have evolved over thousands of years for

- Fluffed-up appearance
- Sleepy, partially closed eyes
- Separation from other flock members
- Reduced social/self-grooming
- Excessive preening/feather plucking
- Vocalization
- Increased/excessive movement
- Reduced activity/movement (such as beak clicking or climbing)
- Absence of vocalization
- Failure to engage with owner
- Guarding behaviour
- Aggression
- Any other abnormal behaviour

7.30 Observed signs of pain in birds. It should be noted that the signs of pain can be wide and varied (and sometimes conflicting).

survival, can hinder decision making; for example, immobility under observation may or may not be associated with pain. Feather grooming is another behaviour that can change variably in relation to pain: birds may stop grooming when in pain or, conversely, preen excessively when in pain as an intentional distraction.

Successful treatment of bird pain relies on accurate pain assessment. This remains highly subjective and the clinician is left to rely on

BSAVA Guide to Pain Management in Small Animal Practice. Edited by Ian Self. ©BSAVA 2019

vague, inconsistent signs/behaviours and often simply uses clinical judgement and experience to choose the type, level and duration of analgesia to provide. Pain scales and score sheets can improve the provision of analgesia as pain occurs on a gradient rather than 'all or nothing', but these are still in the development stage for avian medicine due to the difficulty in observing and appreciating signs of pain. Simple 1–10 scales and more detailed numerical scales have been trialled and show significant correlation (Hawkins and Paul-Murphy, 2011). Effective analgesia is expected to result in discernable changes in posture or behaviours that will translate to a change in the pain score. If no change in pain score occurs, drugs, dose, or frequency of administration need re-evaluation for that individual. In clinical practice, where pain scoring may not be commonplace, simply administering analgesia where appropriate and seeing if it helps is a good and reasonable way to determine if pain is present. Where there is doubt, it is advisable to assume pain is present and to treat it, rather than risk leaving the bird without analgesia and suffering the negative effects of pain.

Painful conditions in birds can be loosely grouped into the following areas:

- Orthopaedic trauma (fractures, luxations and sprains)
- Soft tissue injury (cuts, deep bruises, blunt trauma)
- Visceral pain (pancreatitis, bowel obstruction or distension, kidney injury, tumour-related)
- Osteoarthritic pain (age-related, degenerative joint disease, inflammatory or immune-mediated).

Common clinical presentations where pain relief is indicated include any form of trauma, age-related degenerative joint disease, soft tissue injuries such as broken nails and skin wounds, and abdominal distension caused by coelomitis or some other form of space-occupying disease such as an obstruction or tumour.

Evaluation of analgesics

Determining the likely efficacy of a chosen analgesic can be problematic in birds. To do this effectively it is important to know the pharmacokinetic (PK) and pharmacodynamic (PD) properties of the drugs in the target species. Extrapolation across species with respect to dose and dose frequency has been shown to be unreliable. However, due to the relatively small number of PK and PD studies in birds, the clinician often has no choice but to do this, or rely on anecdotal reports, to select analgesia for their avian patients. Doses from the literature, along with the recommended doses from this author, can be found in Figure 7.31.

The Veterinary Medicines Directorate Cascade must also be considered, as analgesics are invariably used 'off-licence' due to lack of licensed products for birds.

Opioids

Opioids vary in their receptor specificity and efficacy in mammals, resulting in a wide variety of clinical effects. In birds, there is a lack of published data on opioid receptor distribution, density and functionality. Mansour *et al.* (1988) showed that in pigeons, kappa and delta receptors were more prominent in the forebrain and midbrain than mu receptors and 76% of opioid receptors were kappa type. There is still much to be learned; some birds fail to respond well to mu agonists and others respond similarly to mammals to both mu and kappa agonists. It has been postulated that birds may not possess distinct mu and kappa receptors or that they have similar function (Concannon *et al.*, 1995).

Non-steroidal anti-inflammatory drugs

It is generally assumed that the chemistry and mechanism of action is similar in birds and mammals (Mathonnet *et al.*, 2001). There is little scientific support for a 'washout' period (Papich, 2008) and this could put the bird at risk of having untreated pain, although multiple non-steroidal anti-inflammatory drugs (NSAIDs)

Drug	Notes*	Dose range in literature*	Author recommendations and guidance
Opioids			
Morphine	• Relatively short-acting mu receptor agonist • Infrequently used due to conflicting early studies; even strain-dependent differences in the same species are reported • There are reductions in MAC with increasing doses (0.1, 1 and 3 mg/kg) and anecdotal reports of analgesia at 'normal' clinical doses but not well evaluated	0.1 mg to 200 mg/kg	0.1–0.5 mg/kg i.m. q2–4h could be used but other opioid options may be better
Fentanyl	• Very short-acting mu receptor agonist with a fast elimination making it more suitable as a CRI • 0.2 mg/kg s.c. was effective but caused hyperexcitability • CRI in red-tailed hawks reduced MAC without significant cardiovascular effects	10–30 µg/kg/min	Use at the doses in the literature should be accompanied by careful monitoring of cardio-vascular parameters
Butorphanol	• Mixed agonist/antagonist with low intrinsic activity at the mu receptor and strong agonist activity at the kappa receptor • One of the most commonly used opioids in birds despite the reported need for frequent dosing • Not associated with dysphoria that is seen in mammals • Dose ranges in literature from 0.5–6 mg/kg – more usually 1–4 mg/kg used clinically in psittacines • Minimal efficacy in American kestrels • Frequency is empirical but studies suggest q2–4h may be required	0.5–6 mg/kg	1–4 mg/kg i.m. q2–4h depending on pain assessment Use with care and at lower end of the dose range for birds of prey Can prolong recovery from anaesthesia
Bupre-norphine	• Slow-onset, long-acting; thought to act as a partial mu agonist but its kappa receptor activities are uncertain • Dissociation from binding sites is slow • No effect at 0.1 mg/kg in African grey parrots • Some effect at 0.25 mg/kg and more at 0.5 mg/kg in pigeons • Effective at 0.1–0.6 mg/kg in American kestrels for up to 6 hours with sedation at the top end of the dosing range • More data in other species needed	0.1–0.6 mg/kg	0.3–0.5 mg/kg i.m. q6h Use the lower end of dose range for birds of prey to avoid increased sedation without additional analgesia Some believe it has no effect and blocks other opioids
Nalbuphine	• Newer human kappa agonist and partial mu antagonist • Effective at 12.5 mg/kg i.m. for 3 hours in Hispaniolan parrots	12.5 mg/kg	Refer to literature dose

7.31 Analgesia drugs used in birds. *Information referenced from Hawkins *et al.*, 2016. CRI = continuous rate infusion; MAC = mean anaesthetic concentration; NSAID = non-steroidal anti-inflammatory drug; PD = pharmacodynamic; PK = pharmacokinetic. (continues)

▶

Drug	Notes*	Dose range in literature*	Author recommendations and guidance
Opioids continued			
Tramadol	• Provides analgesia by opioid (mu), serotonin and norepinephrine pathways with minimal adverse effects • It is a potent oral analgesic that is not currently under tight medication regulations • Effective doses reported include 5 mg/kg orally q12h in bald eagles, 5 mg/kg i.v. in Hispaniolan Amazon parrots, 11 mg/kg orally for 4h in red-tailed hawks and 30 mg/kg orally for 6h in Hispaniolan Amazon parrots (where 10 and 20 mg/kg were ineffective) • In American kestrels, 5 mg/kg orally was only effective for 1.5 hours	5–30 mg/kg orally q4–6h	5–10 mg/kg orally every 8–12h in birds of prey and every 6–8h in parrots The dose may need to be higher in parrots but this dose appears to have some effect anecdotally. More data required
Hydro-morphone	• Semi-synthetic mu receptor agonist • 3–4 times more potent than morphine • When evaluated at 0.1, 0.3 and 0.6 mg/kg, showed a dose-dependent response when given to American kestrels but only sedation when given to cockatiels	0.1–0.6 mg/kg q6h	Never been used by this author Refer to literature dose
NSAIDs			
Ketoprofen	• High bioavailability orally in mammals, but limited oral PK data in birds. Lack of convenient oral formulations mean it is used mainly parenterally • 2–5 mg/kg resulted in deaths of male eiders (may be related to behaviour leading to dehydration) • 5 mg/kg in mallards appeared effective for 12h • 2.5 mg/kg q24h for 7d caused renal tubular necrosis in budgies.	2–5 mg/kg	Not recommended due to potential renal effects
Meloxicam	• Most widely used NSAID in avian medicine • Convenient to use as injectable and oral formulations in two different strengths • Survey to determine NSAID toxicity in captive birds treated in zoos reported zero fatalities associated with meloxicam (700 birds from 60 species) • PK studies in multiple avian species • 1 mg/kg of meloxicam i.m. q12h in Hispaniolan Amazon parrots was necessary to achieve analgesia (lower bioavailability orally) • 1.6 mg/kg q12h orally for 15d in parrots and 2 mg/kg i.m. q24h for 14d in quail had no adverse effects • 1 mg/kg i.m. for 7d was effective in African grey parrots • In pigeons, 2 mg/kg orally q12h was effective but 0.5 mg/kg was not • Despite meloxicam's large therapeutic range and relative safety compared with other NSAIDs, adverse effects in different species should continue to be evaluated	0.1–2 mg/kg	0.5–1 mg/kg i.m. q24h (or q12h) and 1.5–2 mg/kg orally q24h (or q12h) Anecdotally, once daily dosing appears effective to this author but PK and PD data in the literature do not always support this. There is evidence that the anti-inflammatory and analgesic effects of NSAIDs continue longer than predicted by plasma half-lives Avoid if hypoperfusion is likely (dehydration or anaesthesia)

7.31 (continued) Analgesia drugs used in birds. *Information referenced from Hawkins *et al.*, 2016. CRI = continuous rate infusion; MAC = mean anaesthetic concentration; NSAID = non-steroidal anti-inflammatory drug; PD = pharmacodynamic; PK = pharmacokinetic. (continues) ▶

Drug	Notes*	Dose range in literature*	Author recommendations and guidance
NSAIDs continued			
Carprofen	• Much work is needed to determine appropriate doses, dosing routes, and dosing frequency of carprofen in birds • 1 mg/kg improved the speed and walking ability of lame chickens but another study showed 30 mg/kg i.m. was needed for analgesia • 3 mg/kg i.m. q12h was effective initially but the action was very short-lived	1–30 mg/kg	2–4 mg/kg q24h Use with caution as there are very limited data
Flunixin	• Used at a wide variety of doses in several avian species but reports in many species associated with glomerular lesions even at low doses	3–5.5 mg/kg i.m.	Not recommended due to potential renal effects
Local anaesthetics			
Lidocaine	• Use formulation 'without adrenaline' • Wide ranges used (up to 15 mg/kg) but not always shown to be effective • Empirical dosing generally accepted to be 2–3 mg/kg	2.5–15 mg/kg	2 mg/kg perineurally Use with caution to avoid overdose and toxicity
Bupi-vacaine	• Used with caution in birds due to its longer duration of action and potential for toxic effects to take longer to resolve • Potential for delayed toxicity at 6 and 12 hours	2–8 mg/kg	2 mg/kg perineurally Use with caution to avoid overdose and toxicity
Other			
Gabapentin	• Precise mechanism of action unknown • Considered synergistic with other drugs • Stepwise increases in dose thought to be required	10 mg/kg orally q12h	Never been used by this author Refer to literature dose
Dietary supplements	• No studies have been conducted in birds evaluating efficacy • Glucosamine, chondroitin and Boswelia extract may be beneficial in the treatment of osteoarthritis through their anti-inflammatory effects • Polysulfated glycosaminoglycans (PSGAGs) have been used anecdotally but fatal coagulopathies in different avian species have been reported	Unknown	Dose empirically based on other species Most joint supplements have a wide safety margin so safe to use, even if efficacy in birds is unproven Avoid PSGAGs in birds
Physical therapy	• Application of adjunctive therapy should be considered for acute and chronic pain, but there is no evidence of efficacy in birds to date • Thermotherapy and lasers may diminish pain/decrease indicators of neuropathic pain • Anecdotal reports of efficacy of acupuncture • Cold and/or heat therapy has been shown to be effective in other species • Photobiomodulation therapy (coid laser)	–	These methods are worth trying if available and the owner is able to carry them out without causing increased stress to the bird

7.31 (continued) Analgesia drugs used in birds. *Information referenced from Hawkins et al., 2016. CRI = continuous rate infusion; MAC = mean anaesthetic concentration; NSAID = non-steroidal anti-inflammatory drug; PD = pharmacodynamic; PK = pharmacokinetic.

should not be used concurrently. Selection is often determined by ease of administration (e.g. injection at the time of surgery followed by oral medication during the recovery period). PD and PK studies are also lacking across multiple species and allometric scaling is shown to be ineffective at predicting an accurate dose for different bird species. The most common problem with NSAIDs in birds is an adverse effect on renal tissue and function, as manifested by the deaths of vultures in Asia which led to the banning of diclofenac in hoof stock (Oaks *et al.*, 2004; Meteyer *et al.*, 2005; Naidoo and Swan, 2008).

Regional anaesthesia and analgesia

Where used, local line blocks or splash blocks are most common, although the thin subcutaneous space in most avian species makes accurate placement a challenge. Regional blocks (such as a brachial plexus block) have not been shown to be particularly effective (Brenner *et al.*, 2010). Systemic uptake of the local anaesthetics can be rapid in birds, and metabolism can be prolonged, leading to increased risk of toxicity. This risk, and lack of proven efficacy in some studies, makes local anaesthesia controversial and more research is required. Toxic effects reported in birds include fine tremors, ataxia, recumbency, seizures, cardiovascular effects and death. For smaller birds, dilution may be required to produce a useful volume for the block but it is unknown if dilution alters the action of the drug or reduces the tissue concentration below effective levels. Local anaesthetics in the form of transdermal patches and creams, epidural infusions, spinal blocks, and intravenous blocks have not been reported.

References and further reading

Brenner DJ, Larsen RS, Dickinson PJ *et al.* (2010) Development of an avian brachial plexus nerve block technique for perioperative analgesia in mallard ducks (*Anas platyrhynchos*). *Journal of Avian Medicine and Surgery* **24**, 24–34

Concannon KT, Dodam JR and Hellyer PW (1995) Influence of a mu- and kappa-opioid agonist on isoflurane minimal anesthetic concentration in chickens. *American Journal of Veterinary Research* **56**, 806–811

Hawkins MG and Paul-Murphy J (2011) Avian Analgesia. *Veterinary Clinics of North America: Exotic Animals* **14**, 61–80

Hawkins MG, Paul-Murphy J and Guzman DS (2016) Recognition, assessment, and management of pain in birds. In: *Current Therapy in Avian Medicine and Surgery*, ed. B Speer, pp. 616–630. Elsevier, Missouri

Hughes RA (1990) Strain-dependent morphine-induced analgesic and hyperalgesic effects on thermal nociception in domestic fowl (*Gallus gallus*). *Behavioral Neuroscience* **104**, 619–624

Mansour A, Khachaturian H, Lewis ME, Akil H and Watson SJ (1988) Anatomy of CNS opioid receptors. *Trends in Neuroscience* **11**, 308–314

Mathonnet M, Lalloue F, Danty E, Comte I and Lièvre CA (2001) Cyclo-oxygenase 2 tissue distribution and developmental pattern of expression in the chicken. *Clinical and Experimental Pharmacology and Physiology* **28**, 425–432

Meteyer CU, Rideout BA, Gilbert M, Shivaprasad HL and Oaks JL (2005) Pathology and proposed pathophysiology of diclofenac poisoning in free-living and experimentally exposed oriental white-backed vultures (*Gyps bengalensis*). *Journal of Wildlife Diseases* **41**, 707–716

Naidoo V and Swan GE (2008) Diclofenac toxicity in *Gyps* vulture is associated with decreased uri c acid excretion and not renal portal vasoconstriction. *Comparative Biochemistry and Physiology–Part C: Toxicology and Pharmacology* **149**, 269–274

Oaks JL, Gilbert M, Virani MZ *et al.* (2004) Diclofenac residues as the cause of vulture population decline in Pakistan. *Nature* **427**, 630–633

Papich MG (2008) An update on nonsteroidal anti-inflammatory drugs (NSAIDs) in small animals. *Veterinary Clinics of North America: Small Animal Practice* **38**, 1243–1266

Useful websites

The Veterinary Medicines Directorate Cascade
https://www.gov.uk/guidance/the-cascade-prescribing-unauthorised-medicines

Case example 1: Fracture repair

HISTORY AND PRESENTATION

An 8-year-old female (DNA sexed) pet African grey parrot was presented with sudden onset non-weight bearing on her left leg for the past 3–4 hours.

The bird had been owned for 7 years, fed a seed mix with a high percentage of sunflower seeds, plus various fruits, vegetables and human food treats. She was kept in cage at night but allowed free range of the house during the day. There are no other birds or pets in the house and no previous health problems. The owner heard squawking in the other room and found the bird on the floor, standing on one leg.

CLINICAL SIGNS

No previously reported health problems. The bird was overweight with a body condition score of 4/5. She had a small area of plucked feathers around the neck and a build-up of dry crusted deposits in the nares.

SIGNS OF PAIN

Holding the leg up, not using the foot, fluffed-up appearance, aggressive when approached.

TREATMENT

The general clinical signs are typical for a seed-fed bird that is kept indoors and likely reflect hypovitaminosis A and obesity from a high-fat, low-nutrient diet. Clinical examination revealed a mid-shaft fracture of her tibiotarsus bone, presumed to be from trauma sustained at home. She otherwise appeared stable so the main concern was control of pain.

Immediate pain relief is provided with opioids (e.g. butorphanol as it is relatively quick-acting). Non-steroidal anti-inflammatory drugs (NSAIDs) could also be considered but if the bird is likely to be anaesthetized or may be in early circulatory shock, there is a risk of hypoperfusion and renal problems when using NSAIDs. Once the bird is stable for surgery, pain relief can be continued with butorphanol, and additional analgesia with a continuous rate infusion or local anaesthesia may be attempted (although there is limited evidence of efficacy and safe dosing). The limb should be immobilized to stabilize the fractured bone ends to reduce further pain (and soft tissue damage); this may be with a splint prior to surgery.

Postoperatively, continue with butorphanol and NSAIDs (assuming good hydration) and then the parenteral opioids can be reduced in favour of tramadol if opioid pain relief is required in the days following surgery. Cold therapy may aid reduction of swelling and hot therapy may increase blood flow and healing. NSAIDs (meloxicam) can be continued at home until the bird exhibits fewer signs of pain.

Photobiomodulation therapy may also help to increase the speed of bone healing.

Case example 2: Degenerative joint disease

HISTORY AND PRESENTATION

A 17-year-old male working Snowy Owl was presented, not perching normally. The bird had been owned for 12 years and used for pest control and in the entertainment industry (e.g. displays). He was kept in a moderately-sized outdoor aviary and fed a variety of killed whole prey foods; his bodyweight was monitored daily.

CLINICAL SIGNS

The owl had no abnormal general clinical signs. His plumage was in good condition and weight a little above 'flying weight'. The bird was very bright and alert. The feet appeared slightly swollen and warm to the touch.

SIGNS OF PAIN

The owl was restless on his perches, shifting his weight from one foot to the other and sometimes knuckling and holding the feet in odd positions. He was less keen to work for food and more 'nippy' with the handler than normal.

TREATMENT

Further palpation of the feet revealed stiffness and crepitus; some form of age-related foot problem was suspected. Bloods were taken and were unremarkable. Radiographs showed moderate to marked soft tissue swelling and bony changes around many of the joints in the toes of both feet. This was consistent with moderate degenerative joint disease.

In this case, it is very important to teach the client how to assess the bird's pain level since treatment will vary depending on how uncomfortable the bird is on a day-to-day basis. Where the pain appears mild then keeping the bird lean, flying the bird more and using dietary supplements (glucosamine, chondroitin, Boswelia) may be adequate to control the pain signs. NSAIDs (meloxicam) can be used as needed but if the signs become more persistent then NSAIDs should be used daily, titrating down to the minimum effective dose for that individual. As pain becomes more severe, adding in other medications such as tramadol and gabapentin is indicated. Eventually, euthanasia is likely to be required on welfare grounds.

Chapter 7k

Pain in other exotic pets

Jenna Richardson and Kevin Eatwell

Alleviating pain in exotic species is often overlooked, or the extent of pain is underestimated. However, the level of veterinary care provided to species such as rodents and reptiles is increasing, led by both client expectations and increased veterinary awareness and training. In the same manner as with canine and feline patients, the level of analgesia provided to exotic pets should match the severity of the injury or disease process and the complexity of the procedures being undertaken.

Rodents and reptiles hide clinical signs of pain very well and so are often presented when chronic diseases have reached the point of displaying acute clinical signs (Figure 7.32).

The side effects of analgesics can be overestimated in exotic patients and this is often used as the clinical reasoning behind not providing adequate pain relief. Identifying appropriate dosing regimens can also be difficult and the dosages used in dogs and cats are generally insufficient for those species with high metabolic rates (such as rodents) or risk overdosing those species with low metabolic rates (such as reptiles). It is important to realize that the full range of analgesics that can be used in other species can generally be applied

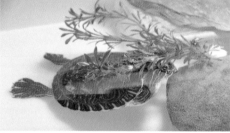

7.32 Rodent and reptile species often do not display overt signs of pain.
© Jenna Richardson

to exotic species. A good starting point when considering appropriate analgesia in exotic species is to identify the level of analgesia that would be provided to a canine patient with a similar disease process. Doses for the commonly used analgesics in exotic species can be found in the *BSAVA Small Animal Formulary – Part B: Exotic Pets*.

Owner and animal compliance, as well as method of administration, are important factors to consider when creating a therapeutic regime. Most agents are not licensed for use in exotic animal species and the client must give informed consent for their use. It is also important to ensure movement of painful

BSAVA Guide to Pain Management in Small Animal Practice. Edited by Ian Self. ©BSAVA 2019

areas is minimized, although, bandaging options can be limited in some species. The weight of the bandage can apply traction to painful tissues rather than stabilizing them. Preventing further trauma to a wound can be facilitated in rodent species with the application of custom-designed 'buster' collar. This will prevent the patient from self-traumatizing.

The distress associated with the disease process, pain, hospitalization and even administration of treatments can lead to anorexia. This is particularly concerning in species with a high metabolic rate and repeated assisted feeding may be required. Additional problems such as self-inflicted trauma can occur due to chewing, grooming or as a result of attempts to remove the dressings or escape from the hospital environment.

References and further reading

Baker BB, Sladky KK and Johnson SM (2011) Evaluation of the analgesic effects of oral and subcutaneous tramadol administration in red-eared slider turtles. *Journal of the American Veterinary Medical Association* **238**, 220–227

Cannon CZ, Kissling GE, Hoenerhoff MJ, King-Herbert AP and Blankenship-Paris T (2010) Evaluation of dosages and routes of administration of tramadol analgesia in rats using hot-plate and tail-flick tests. *Laboratory Animals* **39**, 342–351

Curtin LI, Grakowsky JA, Suarez M *et al.* (2009) Evaluation of buprenorphine in a postoperative pain model in rats. *Comparative Medicine* **59**, 60–71

Gades NM, Danneman PJ, Wixson SK and Tolley EA (2000) The magnitude and duration of the analgesic effect of morphine, butorphanol, and buprenorphine in rats and mice. *Contemporary Topics in Laboratory Animal Science* **39**, 8–13

Hernandez-Divers SJ, McBride M, Koch T *et al.* (2004) Single dose oral and intravenous pharmacokinetics of meloxicam in the green iguana (*Iguana iguana*). *Proceedings of the Association of Reptilian and Amphibian Veterinarians*, Naples, Florida, pp. 106–107

Martin LBE, Thompson AC, Martin T and Kristal MB (2001) Analgesic efficacy of orally administered buprenorphine in rats. *Comparative Medicine* **51**, 43–48

Meredith A (2015) *BSAVA Small Animal Formulary – Part B: Exotic Pets, 9th edn.* BSAVA Publications, Gloucester

Sladky KK, Miletic V, Paul-Murphy J *et al.* (2007) Analgesic efficacy and respiratory effects of butorphanol and morphine in turtles. *Journal of the American Veterinary Medical Association* **230**, 1356–1362

Souza MJ, Greenacre CB and Cox SK (2008) Pharmacokinetics of orally administered tramadol in domestic rabbits (*Oryctolagus cuniculus*). *American Journal of Veterinary Research* **69**, 979–982

Thompson AC, Kristal MB, Salaj A *et al.* (2004) Analgesic efficacy of oral buprenorphine in rats: methodological considerations. *Comparative Medicine* **54**, 293–300

Case example 1: Mammary mass removal in rats

Mammary mass removal is the most common surgical procedure performed in rats. These are often older patients and may be suffering from other underlying diseases such as *Mycoplasma* pneumonia or other systemic disease. Rats are naturally curious, tend to explore their environment, and spend long periods of time chewing and gnawing. Of all the small rodent pets commonly encountered in clinical practice, rats are the most likely to self-traumatize a surgical site (Figure 7.33).

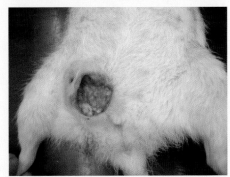

7.33 Rats are prone to self-traumatizing wounds.

© Jenna Richardson

→ CASE EXAMPLE 1 CONTINUED

HISTORY AND PRESENTATION

Both male and female rats possess a large amount of mammary tissue extending from the inguinal region to the shoulders. Mammary masses can develop ventrally, typically in the inguinal region or behind the front legs (Figure 7.34). Although usually benign (80–95% fibroadenomas), surgical removal may be necessary as the masses can grow very large and limit the mobility of the patient.

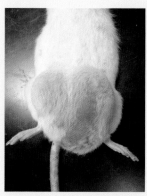

7.35
Inflammation, ulceration and infection of masses can increase the level of discomfort significantly.
© Jenna Richardson

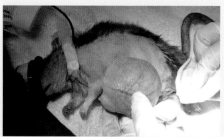

7.34 Fibroadenomas can grow very large and significantly affect mobility.
© Jenna Richardson

CLINICAL SIGNS AND SIGNS OF PAIN

Clinically overt signs of discomfort in the early stages can be limited. Reduced ambulation and feeding may be identified. Rats are social creatures so there may be increased bullying by companions. Large masses can become inflamed (Figure 7.35), ulcerated and infected, leading to significant pain, and the rat may persistently groom the site.

TREATMENT

Pre-emptive analgesia should be administered in these cases. The use of non-steroidal anti-inflammatory drugs (NSAIDs) such as meloxicam is encouraged and can be provided orally as a suspension. Opioids (e.g. tramadol provided orally in liquid form) are also commonly used. However, in many cases, the use of opioids is withheld until immediately prior to surgery. Parenteral NSAIDs and opioids can be given pre-emptively to the patient. Buprenorphine is often chosen as it has a 6–8 hour duration of action (Gades *et al.*, 2000) and is readily available in clinical practice in multi-dose bottles. A dose of 0.05 mg/kg administered subcutaneously has been shown to be most effective (Curtin *et al.*, 2009). For extensive procedures, consideration should be given to pure mu opioids such as methadone or morphine. These are shorter-acting drugs and will need repeated administration every 2–4 hours.

Typically, small rodents are induced for a general anaesthetic using inhalation anaesthesia of sevoflurane or isoflurane vaporized in oxygen in an induction chamber (Figure 7.36). They are then maintained via a

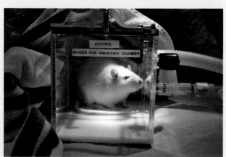

7.36 Inhalation anaesthetic offers no analgesic properties in rats.
© Jenna Richardson

→ CASE EXAMPLE 1 CONTINUED

mask with inhalation anaesthetic. This does not provide any analgesia. Some clinicians prefer to premedicate small rodents and typically an alpha-2 agonist (such as dexmedetomidine) and ketamine can be used alongside other analgesics. The advantage of this regimen is that both provide some additional analgesic effects but this has to be balanced alongside the cardiovascular side effects of the alpha-2 agonist in a higher risk patient.

Once anaesthetized, the use of local anaesthetics should not be overlooked. Lidocaine is short-acting (1–2 hours) but has a relatively fast onset of effect, whereas bupivacaine has a longer duration of action (4–8 hours) but takes longer for its initial effect (30 minutes). Generally, these two agents are provided together in the same syringe at a dose of 1 mg/kg lidocaine and 1 mg/kg bupivacaine. This increases the duration of the sensory blockade with reduced motor blockade. The top doses recommended are 4 mg/kg lidocaine and 2 mg/kg bupivacaine. Infiltration can be performed both under the mammary mass and subcutaneously under the incision site. The drugs can be diluted with saline to allow distribution over a greater area, therefore increasing the effectiveness of tissue infiltration. Gentle tissue handling and the use of moistened gauze swabs/sterile cotton tips will reduce tissue inflammation during the surgery. Selection of a monofilament suture material such as poliglecaprone 25 is important to minimize tissue reactions. Reactions can occur; multifilament material can lead to significant wound reactions. Immediately postoperatively the wound should be gently cleaned using moist gauze swabs. Postoperatively, the rat should be transferred to an incubator providing a quiet and warm environment (Figure 7.37). A suitable hiding place full of shredded paper or a towel can be provided for further insulation. Once mobile, spoon or syringe

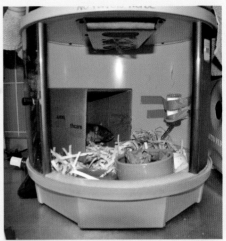

7.37 A warm, quiet area should be provided postoperatively.
© Jenna Richardson

feeding can be provided with a warm critical care liquid diet (e.g. Emeraid Omnivore). Parenteral opioid therapy should continue while the rat is hospitalized; typically, buprenorphine is the drug of choice.

When the rat is recovered and sent home it is important to continue to provide analgesia. An NSAID such as meloxicam should be continued for 3–5 days and can be provided orally. Tramadol can be used to replace the buprenorphine given in a clinical setting; alternatively, buprenorphine can be given orally or mixed with jelly. The typical recommended dose is 0.5 mg/kg orally but it has been shown not to be as effective as parenteral dosing (Thompson *et al.*, 2004). It is important to increase the dose to 5–10 mg/kg to ensure effectiveness, but palatability may be poor at this concentration (Martin *et al.*, 2001). The effectiveness of oral tramadol is uncertain, even at doses as high as 50 mg/kg (Cannon *et al.*, 2010). Dose ranges are often extrapolated from the rabbit dose of 11 mg/kg by mouth once daily (Souza *et al.*, 2008); however, the effectiveness of the drug in this species is also uncertain.

Case example 2: Shell trauma in tortoises

HISTORY AND PRESENTATION

Shell trauma is a common presentation in terrestrial chelonians. This is often due to trauma from dog bites, lawnmowers or simply being dropped by the owner. Tortoises rarely show evidence of pain despite having severe injuries. It can be difficult for owners and veterinary surgeons (veterinarians) to appreciate the urgency of these cases and the need for analgesia.

CLINICAL SIGNS AND SIGNS OF PAIN

Large deficits can be present exposing areas of pectoral or pelvic musculature in highly mobile areas that can be difficult to stabilize (Figure 7.38). Clinically overt signs of discomfort at this stage can be limited although some individuals may retreat into their shell, have reduced mobility or attempt to bite. This can make a detailed assessment of injuries problematic. With severe injuries, anaesthesia and surgical debridement or repair is indicated.

TREATMENT

The tortoise needs to be warmed to its optimal temperature in order to effectively absorb fluid therapy and metabolize therapeutic agents. It should be allowed to warm to 28°C; if facilities such as a vivarium are not available, then an incubator will suffice in the first instance while emergency care is undertaken. Depending on the severity of the injuries, the tortoise may benefit from stabilization with supportive care, and fluid therapy should be considered. Antibiotics including anaerobic cover should be provided as organisms from the mouth of a dog or soil can contaminate wounds. Once the tortoise is warmed attention should be paid to analgesia. Parenteral meloxicam at 0.2 mg/kg every 48 hours by injection (Hernandez-Divers *et al.*, 2004) should be used as standard. Opioids should always be used in situations where there has been extensive skeletal trauma. Pure mu opioids such as morphine are indicated. These can take up to 2 hours for an analgesic effect. Up to 6.5 mg/kg every 24 hours has been suggested (Sladky *et al.*, 2007).

The wounds can be managed in a similar fashion to open wounds of any species. Gentle flushing with sterile saline is required and physical debris can be removed. In severely contaminated wounds, surgical debridement is often required (Figure 7.39). This should be thorough with any remaining debris or bone fragments removed. Pre-medication with morphine prior to surgical debridement is indicated. The use of other premedicants is often overlooked but may

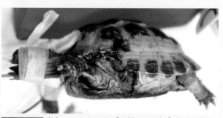

7.38 It is common to find large deficits in the plastron and carapace following a dog attack.
© Jenna Richardson

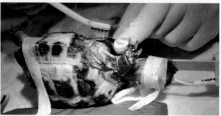

7.39 A sterile toothbrush can be useful for wound debridement.
© Jenna Richardson

➡

→ CASE EXAMPLE 2 CONTINUED

provide some additional analgesia. Ketamine at 10–30 mg/kg intramuscularly can be used alongside, although it should be remembered that higher doses can elongate anaesthetic recovery times.

Once cleaned, open wounds should be dressed and stabilized where possible (Figure 7.40). Topical hydrocolloid gels can be used and covered with foam style dressings designed to stimulate granulation and facilitate debridement of the wound. These can be held in place using conforming bandage (Figure 7.41).

Postoperatively, the tortoise should be kept warm under an even temperature until ambulatory. Analgesia should be continued during hospitalization.

Treatment at home can be problematic for owners as providing medication orally is very difficult and they may lack the confidence to provide parenteral medication. In these cases, placement of an

oesophagostomy tube to facilitate ongoing medication at home will be required (Figure 7.42). If such a tube is in place then oral therapy with both meloxicam (0.2 mg/kg once daily for 5 days) and tramadol (10 mg/kg once every 4 days) are possible, with oral tramadol being more effective than parenteral use (Baker *et al.*, 2011).

The wounds are likely to require a large amount of postoperative management and many clinicians will consider the tortoise returning for frequent consultations to facilitate wound care and parenteral antibiotics and analgesia. Shell damage takes time to heal fully and, until a granulation bed is formed (Figure 7.43) (typically 12–16 weeks after the original insult), infection is still possible. Hibernation will also reduce wound healing and tortoises that usually hibernate should be prevented from doing so until the wound has completely healed.

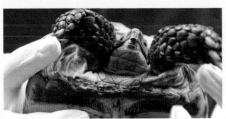

7.40 Skin deficits may require suturing as in other species.
© Jenna Richardson

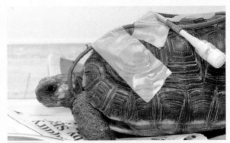

7.42 Placement of an oesophagostomy feeding tube will facilitate long-term administration of medication at home.
© Jenna Richardson

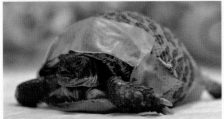

7.41 Wounds often need to be dressed and stabilized post-surgery.
© Jenna Richardson

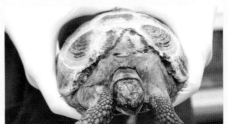

7.43 It can take 12–16 weeks for a wound to heal completely.
© Jenna Richardson

Appendix 1

Pain scales

Introduction

For all pain scales, training will improve the probability and consistency of pain identification. All team members involved in patient care should understand the importance of pain scoring and all patients that have undergone painful procedures should be assessed for pain. The scales are designed to decrease subjectivity in pain scores and, to best support that goal, the pain assessment protocols must be followed. It is best if the same person scores the patient at each assessment time, but this is not always possible.

The assessments should be repeated at scheduled times, and extra assessments added at 'important' times, such as after treatment. The interval between assessments should not automatically be set at a predetermined interval for all patients, but should be based on the nature of the pain (i.e. acute or chronic), the intensity of the pain, and the patient's response to analgesic therapy. (See Chapter 2 for more information.)

Commonly used pain scales for cats and dogs are included in this Appendix:

- Colorado Acute Canine Pain Scale
- Colorado Acute Feline Pain Scale
- UNESP-Botucatu Multidimensional Composite Pain Scale (Short Form)
- Glasgow Composite Measure Pain Scale (Canine – Short Form)
- Glasgow Composite Measure Pain Scale (Feline).

Using pain scales and scoring systems

A patient's pain score is a composite of multidimensional factors such as behaviour, body postures, facial grimaces and (for some scales) physiological parameters that might indicate pain.

- Change in behaviour between pre- and post-painful stimulus is the most consistent indicator of the presence of pain.
- When in doubt as to whether or not a patient is in pain, the default is to administer analgesia and reassess their comfort level.

BSAVA Guide to Pain Management in Small Animal Practice. Edited by Ian Self. ©BSAVA 2019

Colorado Canine Acute Pain Scale

Your Clinic
Name Here

Date _____

Time _____

Canine Acute Pain Scale

	Rescore when awake	☐ Animal is sleeping, but can be aroused - Not evaluated for pain ☐ Animal can't be aroused, check vital signs, assess therapy		
Pain Score	Example	Psychological & Behavioral	Response to Palpation	Body Tension
0		☐ **Comfortable** when resting ☐ **Happy, content** ☐ Not bothering wound or surgery site ☐ Interested in or curious about surroundings	☐ **Nontender** to palpation of wound or surgery site, or to palpation elsewhere	Minimal
1		☐ **Content to slightly unsettled** or restless ☐ **Distracted easily** by surroundings	☐ **Reacts to palpation** of wound, surgery site, or other body part by **looking around, flinching,** or **whimpering**	Mild
2		☐ Looks **uncomfortable** when resting ☐ May **whimper** or cry and may **lick or rub wound** or surgery site when unattended ☐ Droopy ears, **worried facial expression** (arched eye brows, darting eyes) ☐ **Reluctant to respond** when beckoned ☐ **Not eager to interact** with people or surroundings but will look around to see what is going on	☐ Flinches, whimpers cries, or guards/pulls away	Mild to Moderate **Reassess analgesic plan**
3		☐ **Unsettled, crying, groaning, biting or chewing** wound when unattended ☐ **Guards or protects** wound or surgery site by altering weight distribution (i.e., limping, shifting body position) ☐ **May be unwilling to move** all or part of body	☐ May be **subtle** (shifting eyes or increased respiratory rate) if dog is too painful to move or is stoic ☐ May be **dramatic**, such as a sharp cry, growl, bite or bite threat, and/or pulling away	Moderate **Reassess analgesic plan**
4		☐ **Constantly groaning or screaming** when unattended ☐ May bite or chew at wound, but unlikely to move ☐ **Potentially unresponsive** to surroundings ☐ **Difficult to distract** from pain	☐ **Cries at non-painful palpation** (may be experiencing allodynia, wind-up, or fearful that pain could be made worse) ☐ May react aggressively to palpation	Moderate to Severe **May be rigid to avoid painful movement** **Reassess analgesic plan**

○ Tender to palpation
✕ Warm
■ Tense

RIGHT   LEFT

Comments _____

© 2006/PW Hellyer, SR Uhrig, NG Robinson Colorado State University
Veterinary Teaching Hospital

(Reproduced with permission from Peter W Hellyer, Colorado State University, Veterinary Medical Center, USA)

Colorado Feline Acute Pain Scale

Your Clinic Name Here

Date _____

Time _____

Feline Acute Pain Scale

	Rescore when awake	☐ Animal is sleeping, but can be aroused - Not evaluated for pain ☐ Animal can't be aroused, check vital signs, assess therapy		
Pain Score	Example	Psychological & Behavioral	Response to Palpation	Body Tension
0		☐ **Content and quiet** when unattended ☐ **Comfortable** when resting ☐ Interested in or **curious** about surroundings	☐ **Not bothered** by palpation of wound or surgery site, or to palpation elsewhere	Minimal
1		☐ **Signs are often subtle and not easily detected in the hospital setting**; more likely to be detected by the owner(s) at home ☐ Earliest signs at home may be <u>**withdrawal from surroundings or change in normal routine**</u> ☐ In the hospital, may be content or slightly unsettled ☐ **Less interested** in surroundings but will look around to see what is going on	☐ May or may not react to palpation of wound or surgery site	Mild
2		☐ Decreased responsiveness, **seeks solitude** ☐ **Quiet**, loss of brightness in eyes ☐ **Lays curled up or sits tucked up** (all four feet under body, shoulders hunched, head held slightly lower than shoulders, tail curled tightly around body) with eyes partially or mostly closed ☐ **Hair coat appears rough** or fluffed up ☐ May intensively groom an area that is painful or irritating ☐ Decreased appetite, **not interested in food**	☐ **Responds aggressively or tries to escape** if painful area is palpated or approached ☐ Tolerates attention, may even perk up when petted as long as painful area is avoided	Mild to Moderate **Reassess analgesic plan**
3		☐ Constantly **yowling, growling, or hissing** when unattended ☐ May bite or chew at wound, but **unlikely to move** if left alone	☐ **Growls or hisses at non-painful palpation** (may be experiencing allodynia, wind-up, or fearful that pain could be made worse) ☐ **Reacts aggressively** to palpation, **adamantly pulls away** to avoid any contact	Moderate **Reassess analgesic plan**
4		☐ Prostrate ☐ Potentially **unresponsive** to or unaware of surroundings, difficult to distract from pain ☐ Receptive to care (even aggressive or feral cats will be more tolerant of contact)	☐ May not respond to palpation ☐ May be rigid to avoid painful movement	Moderate to Severe May be rigid to avoid painful movement **Reassess analgesic plan**

RIGHT   LEFT

○ Tender to palpation
✕ Warm
■ Tense

Comments _____

© 2006/PW Hellyer, SR Uhrig, NG Robinson   Colorado State University
Veterinary Teaching Hospital

(Reproduced with permission from Peter W Hellyer, Colorado State University, Veterinary Medical Center, USA)

UNESP-Botucatu Multidimensional Composite Pain Scale (Short Form)

Item	Description	Score (Circle)
Evaluate the cat's posture in the cage for 2 minutes.		
1	Natural, relaxed and/or moves normally	0
	Natural but tense, does not move or moves little or is reluctant to move	1
	Hunched position and/or dorsolateral recumbency	2
	Frequently changes position or restless	3
2	• The cat contracts and extends its pelvic limbs and/or contracts its abdominal muscles (flank) • The cat's eyes are partially closed (do not consider this item if present until 1h after the end of anaesthesia) • The cat licks and/or bites the surgical wound • The cat moves its tail strongly	
	All above behaviours are absent	0
	Presence of one of the above behaviours	1
	Presence of two of the above behaviours	2
	Presence of three or all of the above behaviours	3
Evaluation of comfort, activity and attitude after the cage is open and how attentive the cat is to the observer and/or surroundings		
3	Comfortable and attentive	0
	Quiet and slightly attentive	1
	Quiet and not attentive. The cat may face the back of the cage	2
	Uncomfortable, restless and slightly attentive or not attentive. The cat may face the back of the cage	3
Evaluation of the cat's reaction when touching, followed by pressuring around the painful site		
4	Does not react	0
	Does not react when the painful site is touched, but does react when it is gently pressed	1
	Reacts when the painful site is touched and when pressed	2
	Does not allow touch or palpation	3
	Total score	
Analgesia should be given when total score is ≥ 4		

(Reproduced with permission from Stelio P Luna, School of Veterinary Medicine and Animal Science, UNESP, Brazil)

Glasgow Composite Measure Pain Scale (Canine – Short Form)

Short form of the Glasgow Composite Measure Pain Scale

Dog's name.. Date.................. Time.............. Hospital number................

Procedure or condition..

In the sections below please circle the appropriate score in each list and sum these to give the total score

A. Look at dog in kennel

Is the dog?

(i)		(ii)	
Quiet	0	Ignoring any wound or painful area	0
Crying or whimpering	1	Looking at wound or painful area	1
Groaning	2	Licking wound or painful area	2
Screaming	3	Rubbing wound or painful area	3
		Chewing wound or painful area	4

In the case of spinal, pelvic or multiple limb fractures, or where assistance is required to aid locomotion, do not carry out section B and proceed to C. Please tick if this is the case then proceed to C

B. Put lead on dog and lead out of the kennel

(iii)	
Normal	0
Lame	1
Slow or reluctant	2
Stiff	3
It refuses to move	4

C. If it has a wound or painful area including abdomen, apply gently pressure 2 inches round the site

Does it?

(iv)	
Do nothing	0
Look round	1
Flinch	2
Growl or guard area	3
Snap	4
Cry	5

D. Overall

Is the dog?

(v)	
Happy and content or happy and bouncy	0
Quiet	1
Indifferent or non-responsive to surroundings	2
Nervous or anxious or fearful	3
Depressed or non-responsive to stimulation	4

Is the dog?

(vi)	
Comfortable	0
Unsettled	1
Restless	2
Hunched or tense	3
Rigid	4

Total score (i+ii+iii+iv+v+vi) = ...

(Reproduced with permission from Jacqueline Reid, University of Glasgow, School of Veterinary Medicine, UK)

Glasgow Composite Measure Pain Scale (Feline)

Glasgow feline composite measure pain scale: CMPS – Feline

Choose the most appropriate expression from each section and total the scores to calculate the pain score for the cat. If more than one expression applies choose the higher score.

Look at the cat in its cage:

Is it?

Question 1

Silent/purring/meowing	0
Crying/growling/groaning	1

Question 2

Relaxed	0
Licking lips	1
Restless/cowering at back of cage	2
Tense/crouched	3
Rigid/hunched	4

Question 3

Ignoring any wound or painful area	0
Attention to wound	1

Question 4

(a) Look at the following caricatures. Circle the drawing which best depicts the cat's ear position?

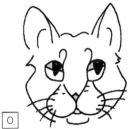 0

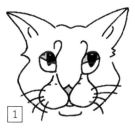 1

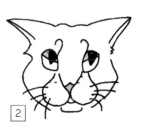 2

(b) Look at the shape of the muzzle in the following caricatures. Circle the drawing which appears most like that of the cat?

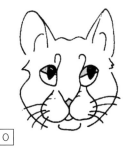 0

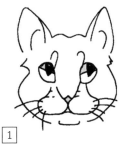 1

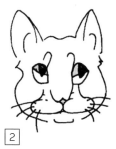 2

Glasgow feline composite measure pain scale: CMPS – Feline *continued*

Approach the cage, call the cat by name and stroke along its back from head to tail

Question 5

Does it?

Respond to stroking	0

Is it?

Unresponsive	1
Aggressive	2

If it has a wound or painful area, apply gentle pressure 5 cm around the site. In the absence of any painful area, apply similar pressure around in the hind leg above the knee

Question 6

Does it?

Do nothing	0
Swish tail/flatten ears	1
Cry/hiss	2
Growl	3
Bite/lash out	4

Question 7

General impression

Is the cat?

Happy and content	0
Disinterested/quiet	1
Anxious/fearful	2
Dull	3
Depressed/grumpy	4

Pain score .... /20

© Universities of Glasgow & Edinburgh Napier 2015. Licensed to NewMetrica Ltd. Permission granted to reproduce for personal and educational use only. To request any other permissions please contact jacky.reid@newmetrica.com.

(Reproduced with permission from Jacqueline Reid, University of Glasgow, School of Veterinary Medicine, UK)

Guidance for use of the Glasgow Composite Measure Pain Scales

Canine – Short Form

The short form composite measure pain score (CMPS-SF) can be applied quickly and reliably in a clinical setting and has been designed as a clinical decision making tool which was developed for dogs in acute pain. It includes 30 descriptor options within six behavioural categories, including mobility. Within each category, the descriptors are ranked numerically according to their associated pain severity and the person carrying out the assessment chooses the descriptor within each category which best fits the dog's behaviour/condition. It is important to carry out the assessment procedure as described on the questionnaire, following the protocol closely. The pain score is the sum of the rank scores. The maximum score for the six categories is 24, or 20 if mobility is impossible to assess. The total CMPS-SF score has been shown to be a useful indicator of analgesic requirement and the recommended analgesic intervention level is 6/24 or 5/20.

Feline

The Glasgow Feline Composite Measure Pain Scale (CMPS-Feline), which can be applied quickly and reliably in a clinical setting, has been designed as a clinical decision making tool for use in cats in acute pain. It includes 28 descriptor options within seven behavioural categories. Within each category, the descriptors are ranked numerically according to their associated pain severity and the person carrying out the assessment chooses the descriptor within each category which best fits the cat's behaviour/condition. It is important to carry out the assessment procedure as described on the questionnaire, following the protocol closely. The pain score is the sum of the rank scores. The maximum score for the seven categories is 20. The total CMPS-Feline score has been shown to be a useful indicator of analgesic requirement and the recommended analgesic intervention level is 5/20.

Major local anaesthetic blocks

With all blocks, the maximum dose of lidocaine in cats is 4 mg/kg and in dogs is 10 mg/kg. For bupivacaine and ropivacaine the dose is approximately 1 mg/kg in both dogs and cats. It may be necessary to dilute the agent in sterile saline if several sites are being blocked. It is not recommended to mix two agents together. In all cases, the skin should be aseptically prepared wherever possible, and always aspirate prior to injection to avoid intravascular administration.

For detailed instructions please refer to the *BSAVA Manual of Canine and Feline Anaesthesia and Analgesia*.

Dental blocks

Mental (A) and mandibular (B) nerve blocks

- Blocking the mental branch of the mandibular nerve as it exits the largest mental foraminae anaesthetizes the lower incisors and skin and tissues rostral to the foramen.
    - Insert the needle intraorally or percutaneously, parallel to the teeth, just rostral to the mental foramen.
    - The mental foramen is caudal and ventral to the canine tooth.
    - Inject between 0.25 and 1 ml depending on the patient's size and breed.
- Blocking the inferior alveolar branch of the mandibular nerve at its point of entry into the mandibular canal at the mandibular foramen anaesthetizes the entire hemi mandible and more reliably anaesthetizes the teeth of the lower jaw.
    - The foramen is located on the medial side of the mandibular ramus, just rostral to the angular process and can easily be palpated in most dogs and cats from the inside of the mouth.
    - The aim is to block the mandibular nerve before it enters the foramen.
    - Inject between 0.25 and 1 ml depending on the patient's size and breed.

Infraorbital (C) and maxillary (D) nerve blocks

- Local anaesthetic administration at the infraorbital foramen will provide anaesthesia rostral to the foramen. Local anaesthetic administration where the maxillary nerve courses perpendicular to the palatine bone, between the maxillary foramen and the foramen rotundum, will provide anaesthesia to the entire upper jaw, including the teeth, on the same side.

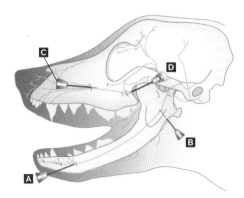

Anatomical landmarks for performing mental (A), mandibular (B), infraorbital (C) and maxillary (D) nerve blocks in dogs.

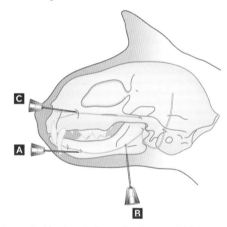

Anatomical landmarks for performing mental (A), mandibular (B) and infraorbital (C) nerve blocks in cats.

- To block the infraorbital nerve:
  - Insert a needle through the buccal mucosa over the foramen, which is usually found dorsal to the third premolar, and deposit local anaesthetic.
  - Inject between 0.25 and 1.5 ml depending on the patient's size and breed.
- To anaesthetize the entire upper jaw, including all of the teeth:
  - Block the maxillary nerve either via the use of a flexible cannula inserted into the infraorbital foramen, or insert a needle through the skin at a 90-degree

angle, in a medial direction, ventral to the border of the zygomatic arch and about 0.5 cm caudal to the lateral canthus, and then advance it toward the pterygopalatine fossa.
  - Slowly inject the local anaesthetic after test aspiration. Inject between 0.5 and 2 ml depending on the patient's size and breed.
  - This technique is more difficult to perform in cats.
- These blocks should be administered cautiously in brachycephalic dogs and cats because of the proximity of the orbit to the foramen and the potential for penetrating the globe.

Auriculotemporal (A) and great auricular (B) nerve block (dog)

- This block provides analgesia to the external ear canal and the auricular cartilage and is a useful technique for dogs undergoing total ear canal ablation and bulla osteotomy.
  - The auriculotemporal nerve is located by slowly advancing a needle between the rostral aspect of the vertical ear canal and the caudal aspect of the zygomatic arch perpendicular to the

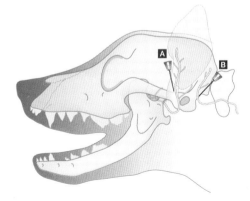

Anatomical landmarks for performing auriculotemporal (A) and great auricular (B) nerve block in dogs.

skin until bone is encountered, at which point the needle is withdrawn half the distance inserted and local anaesthetic (0.25–2 ml) injected.
- To block the greater auricular nerve, a needle is inserted superficially between the caudal aspect of the vertical ear canal and just cranioventral to the wing of the atlas, keeping the needle parallel to the vertical ear canal. Inject 0.25 to 2 ml of local anaesthetic.

Axillary brachial plexus block

- Brachial plexus block provides analgesia to the forelimb distal to, and possibly including, the elbow. The technique should be performed in the anaesthetized patient.

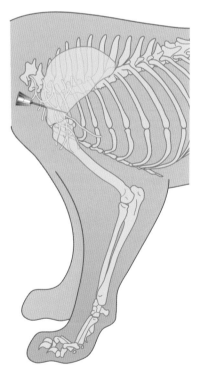

Anatomical landmarks for performing axillary blockade of the brachial plexus in cats.

- With the patient in lateral recumbency, aseptically prepare the skin and insert a spinal needle 5–20 cm into the axillary region, medial to and at the level of the shoulder joint caudally and parallel to the vertebral column. The needle's distal end should lie just caudal to the spine of the scapula.
- Always aspirate the syringe to avoid intravascular administration, and then inject the calculated dose as you slowly withdraw the needle.
- Maximum suggested doses of lidocaine are 8 mg/kg in dogs and 4 mg/kg in cats, and for bupivacaine and ropivacaine are 1–2 mg/kg in dogs and 1 mg/kg in cats. It may be necessary to dilute the local anaesthetic in normal saline to increase the volume available for injection.

Radial, ulnar, median and musculocutaneous nerve blocks

- For procedures of the elbow and distal forelimb, the radial, median, ulnar, and musculocutaneous nerves may be blocked proximal to the humeral epicondyles. These nerves can often be palpated, making this technique relatively straightforward.
  - After sterile preparation, approach the radial nerve on the lateral aspect of the distal humerus.
  - Palpable just proximal to the lateral epicondyle, the radial nerve is located between the brachialis muscle and the lateral head of the triceps.
  - The median, ulnar, and musculocutaneous nerves are located close to one another on the medial aspect of the forelimb, proximal to the medial epicondyle.
  - The brachial artery is situated among these nerves. The musculocutaneous nerve is cranial to the artery while the median and ulnar nerves are located caudally.

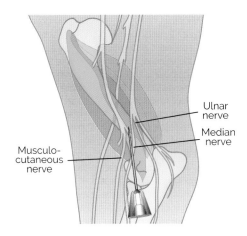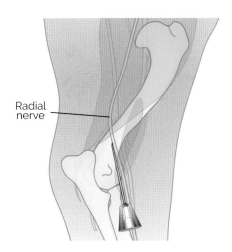

Musculo-cutaneous nerve

Ulnar nerve

Median nerve

Radial nerve

Anatomical landmarks for performing radial, ulnar, median and musculocutaneous nerve blocks in dogs.

- Identify the artery with palpation, and aspirate the syringe before depositing local anaesthetic avoiding intra-arterial, intravenous, and intraneural injection.

Femoral/sciatic nerve blocks

- Anaesthesia of the hindlimb can be achieved by blocking the lumbosacral plexus (L4–S2), which gives rise to the femoral and sciatic nerves plus the lateral femoral cutaneous nerve, obturator and the caudal cutaneous femoral nerves.
- Perhaps the most useful blockade (suitable for stifle surgery) is the femoral/sciatic block.
  - The proximal sciatic block is approached approximately two-thirds of the distance between the greater trochanter and the ischiatic tuberosity with the needle advanced perpendicular to the skin following surgical preparation. Electrolocation techniques are commonly utilized to ensure correct depth of needle insertion.

- The femoral nerve can be blocked inguinally, following sterile skin preparation, at the femoral triangle and electrolocation may be utilized to ensure proximity to the nerve.
- It is increasingly common to use ultrasound guidance ± electrolocation to ensure adequate proximity to the target nerve.

Epidural anaesthesia and analgesia

- The injection site is usually at the lumbosacral space in dogs, cats and rabbits with the animal positioned in sternal recumbency with the limbs drawn forwards. It is possible to palpate the space as a depression immediately caudal to the dorsal spinous process of L7 and immediately cranial to the fused dorsal spinous processes of the sacrum.
  - The area should be aseptically prepared, the operator gloved and the site draped.
  - Using a sterile disposable 2.5–7.5 cm, 20–22 G spinal needle position the spinal needle over the midline.

199

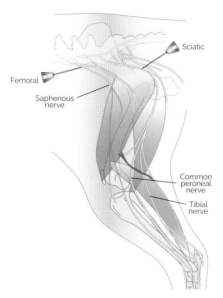

Anatomical landmarks for saphenous, common peroneal and tibial nerve blocks in dogs.

- Direct the needle bevel cranially, and advance the needle, with stylet in place, perpendicular to the skin. If the needle encounters bone, withdraw it slightly, redirect it caudally or cranially, and advance it again.
- Advance the needle perpendicular to the skin until a popping sensation is felt (ligamentum flavum), then remove the stylet, attach a 2 ml syringe and check for inadvertent intrathecal or intravenous injection (aspirate and ensure there is no cerebrospinal fluid (CSF) or blood). If blood is seen, a venous sinus has been penetrated and the needle should be withdrawn and repositioned. If CSF is noted, the subarachnoid space has been entered: withdraw or reposition the needle or, alternatively, inject

one-half of the calculated volume of the drug.

- Inject 2 ml of saline to confirm correct placement and follow with the solution to be injected ensuring there is a small air bubble in the syringe; minimal compression of the air bubble indicates lack of resistance to injection and correct placement in the epidural space. Administer slowly over 2 minutes. The needle is then withdrawn.

■ Typically, a mixture of bupivacaine (1 mg/kg) plus preservative-free morphine (0.1 mg/kg) will be injected.

■ Contraindications include coagulopathies, sepsis, infection at injection site and hypovolaemia or hypotension (use of local anaesthetics can cause hypotension due to sympathetic blockade).

■ Remember that successful epidural anaesthesia reduces the requirement for inhaled anaesthetic agents.

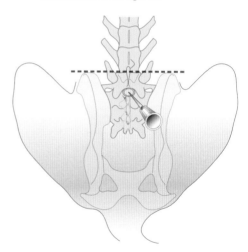

Anatomical landmarks for performing lumbosacral epidural anaesthesia and analgesia in dogs. The lumbosacral space can be found caudal to a line drawn between the cranial borders of the ilia (marked with a dotted line).

Appendix 3

WHO pain relief ladder

In 1986, the World Health Organization (WHO) introduced a three-step analgesic ladder that is widely used in adult human cancer pain relief.

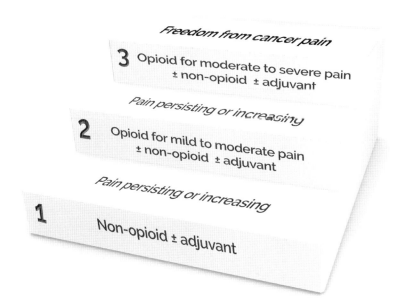

Freedom from cancer pain

3 Opioid for moderate to severe pain
± non-opioid ± adjuvant

Pain persisting or increasing

2 Opioid for mild to moderate pain
± non-opioid ± adjuvant

Pain persisting or increasing

1 Non-opioid ± adjuvant

Redrawn after the WHO,
http://www.who.int/cancer/palliative/painladder/en/

Index

BSAVA Guide to Pain Management in Small Animal Practice. Edited by Ian Self. ©BSAVA 2019